W0018365

Controversies
and
Dilemmas
in
Contemporary
Psychiatry

Controversies
and
Dilemmas
in
Contemporary
Psychiatry

Dusan Kecmanovic

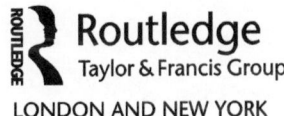

Routledge
Taylor & Francis Group

LONDON AND NEW YORK

First published 2011 by Transaction Publishers

2 Park Square, Milton Park, Abingdon, Oxfordshire OX14 4RN
711 Third Avenue, New York, NY 10017

*Routledge is an imprint of the Taylor & Francis Group, an informa
business*

First issued in paperback 2017

Copyright © 2011 Taylor & Francis

All rights reserved. No part of this book may be reprinted or
reproduced or utilised in any form or by any electronic, mechanical,
or other means, now known or hereafter invented, including
photocopying and recording, or in any information storage or retrieval
system, without permission in writing from the publishers.

Notice:
Product or corporate names may be trademarks or registered
trademarks, and are used only for identification and explanation
without intent to infringe.

Library of Congress Catalog Number: 2010031367

Library of Congress Cataloging-in-Publication Data

Kecmanovic, Dusan.
    Controversies and dilemmas in contemporary psychiatry /
Dusan Kecmanovic.
        p. ; cm.
    Includes bibliographical references and indexes.
    ISBN 978-1-4128-1460-7 (alk. paper)
    1. Psychiatry--Philosophy. 2. Psychiatry--Terminology. I. Title.
[DNLM: 1. Mental Disorders. 2. Models, Psychological. 3. Psy-
chiatry--methods. WM 140]

RC437.5.K43 2010
616.89--dc22

                                                    2010031367

ISBN 13: 978-1-4128-1460-7 (hbk)
ISBN 13: 978-1-138-50860-6 (pbk)

In loving memory of my parents, Milica and Ilija

Most psychiatric diagnoses can never be confirmed or refuted, for there is no external criterion to appeal to.

Robert E. Kendell
Companion to Psychiatric Studies
(1988: 208)

The hardest cause of all to imagine is the one that you don't know and you will probably never know. And that is what I have to think about all day to be an honest psychiatrist. That is why psychiatry is the hardest discipline.

Rachael E. Dew
"Why psychiatry is the hardest specialty"
(2009)

Contents

Contents

Preface

This monograph is timely in reminding psychiatrists and those who have an interest in the field that the discipline rests on a shaky set of assumptions. For very good reason, Professor Kecmanovic draws on the recent history of the evolving classification system of mental disorders as the starting point for his exegesis. The inception of the Diagnostic and Statistical Manual edition III of the American Psychiatric Association aimed to put psychiatry on a scientific footing: henceforth, mental health professionals would be able to apply accurate diagnoses to patients based on readily observable behavioural phenomena. This "operationalization" of diagnosis was seen as the passport that psychiatry needed to achieve final acceptance as a legitimate branch of medicine. To be doctors, we needed objective assessment methods to allow us to offer specific, evidence-based interventions. Hence, there was no longer any reason why the approach to diagnosing and managing depression should be different, in principle, to that for identifying and treating pneumonia. We have had 30 years of experience with this new model—and it has to be said that the report card is mixed in relation to the benefits and disadvantages of this experiment to medicalize Psychiatry.

What this revolution in diagnosis has achieved is greater reliability, that is, higher levels of agreement or consistency amongst diagnosticians, but only if they use structured instruments based on the specified diagnostic system. This does not mean, however, that there is greater validity, that is, that what we are measuring reflects the reality of mental illness in the real world; or that practicing psychiatrists actually use the DSM system in a rigorous manner in practice. There are several reasons for this disjuncture between the formal systems of modern Psychiatry and the exigencies of actual practice: psychiatrists may be ignorant of new developments or they may have a tendency to practice by habit based on what worked in the past; cases they encounter may not fit neatly into the diagnostic system; and the rank and file practitioners may have a deep distrust of the way the diagnostic system has been established and the motivations of those who control the process or who influence its content. This disjunction between diagnostic systems and practice may occur in other branches of medicine but not to the same extent or for the same reasons. For example, as Kecmanovic indicates, psychiatrists constantly face the problem of the mind-brain dichotomy and the related distinction between the subjective world of the patient (and, let us not forget, of the psychiatrist) and the objectification that occurs when we try to make a diagnosis based on verbal reports and observable behaviour. Diagnosing pneumonia generally can occur without entering the inner, subjective life of the patient.

An additional issue relates to the fact that psychiatrists diverge in the models of behaviour that they subscribe to; for example, some may regard brain mechanisms as the key determinant of pathological behaviour, the model that dominates at present, whereas others may believe that learning is the major factor, implicit in cognitive behavioural theories. Although lip service is paid to a comprehensive bio-psycho-social model, in reality, the discourses that take place in psychiatry clearly indicate that different professionals start from fundamentally different positions, some assuming psychological, others biological, and yet others social determinants of behaviour. There is much divergence in thinking and assumptions even within these three domains.

In addition, we cannot avoid the fact that psychiatric patients are regarded implicitly or explicitly as deviant, a central point made by Kecmanovic. Compared to the 1960s, the height of the anti-psychiatry movement, the debate about the challenges psychiatrists face in being part of wider social structures that enforce conformity has become somewhat of a marginal issue. Admittedly, few psychiatrists would continue to question, even in private, whether schizophrenia is an illness or not or that the illness drives certain behaviours that may be injurious to the self or others, requiring a protective response at times from Psychiatry. Nevertheless, given our uncertainties about diagnosis, there are still many issues that are not sufficiently challenged. For example, schizophrenia occurs in a personal and social context: how can we be sure that deviant behaviour manifested by persons with schizophrenia is being driven by the person, the context or the illness? Further, what do we do about conditions that have an adverse impact on others, for example antisocial personality disorder, sexual deviancy or impulse control disorders (gambling, aggression and the like), disorders located at the crossroads of Psychiatry and the criminal-justice system? As yet, no society appears to have resolved the many dilemmas that this fault line causes: whether a person should be excused criminal acts because of their putative psychiatric disorder; whether the responsibility for managing the person, and ensuring that adverse social outcomes are averted, rests with Psychiatry; or whether the criminal-justice system should remain the key agency enforcing social control and sanction in these cases. Although the media periodically sensationalizes these issues, there is an uncanny silence concerning these controversies within the psychiatric community itself, a self-imposed taboo presumably motivated to ensure that undue levels of controversy do not threaten our status as members of the medical establishment. Funding issues are not irrelevant to this issue—psychiatrists are largely supported by the same public or private funding arrangements that apply to other doctors, and controversy about diagnosis or treatment does little to guarantee this privilege.

In summary, Professor Dusan Kecmanovic confronts and explains these fundamental controversies in Psychiatry in a manner that is engaging and compelling for professionals and lay readers alike. Unlike other critics of Psychiatry, he does not stop at generalities but undertakes a close analysis of the key issues at stake in order to reveal the areas that are amenable to resolution—and those that are not. His approach is therefore honest, realistic and constructive; he does not claim to be able to provide answers for all dilemmas but he points out where we can make progress by applying critical thinking to the key problems we face. Remarkably, Professor Kecmanovic is able to stand back from the baggage of theoretical dogma and vested interest, the obstacles to clear thinking within the discipline. As a world renowned academic and someone who has worked at the clinical coal-face across very different environments and societies, Dusan Kecmanovic has the wisdom, breadth of experience and depth of knowledge to address this momentous task. He offers the reader a voyage of discovery in which the core controversies of psychiatry are revealed in a refreshingly direct and accessible manner. Unlike others who have questioned the fundamentals of psychiatry in the past, Professor Kecmanovic offers potential solutions that do not reject the value of psychiatric practice per se, but which aim to strengthen the foundations on which the discipline rests. Clearly, his ultimate aim, driven by the humanitarian instinct for which he is well known, is to improve the lives of patients and their families.

Derrick Silove, M.D.
Professor of Psychiatry
University of New South Wales, Sydney

Introduction

The controversies and dilemmas in psychiatry are so numerous and serious that, to a great extent, they define psychiatry.

Yet most psychiatrists pay little or no attention to the controversies in psychiatry. They maintain that talking about them tarnishes psychiatry's reputation and them along with it. That is why they act as though these controversies do not exist. They seem to expect that the controversies and dilemmas will disappear if they do not become topical. On the other hand, critics of psychiatry use the controversies and dilemmas and psychiatrists' unwillingness to discuss them in order to undermine psychiatry, questioning the very existence of mental disorder, the purpose of psychiatric therapy, and thereby psychiatry's *raison d'être*.

I have set out several basic controversies and dilemmas in contemporary psychiatry with no pretensions on enumerating them all. I have chosen to focus on those controversies and dilemmas which are the most important insofar as they first, might be instrumental for making controversial psychiatry itself, and second, because they include many other controversies and dilemmas or give rise to them.

A mentally ill person lives in two worlds.

A mentally ill person lives in the biological world and in a world of values and meanings. These two worlds are different.

The fact that no organic basis has been found for most of mental disorders underpins a great many hard to resolve questions related to the diagnosis and treatment of the mentally ill. Even if an organic basis of most or all mental disorders is one day established, the phenomenology of mental disorders will not change; not substantially, at least. The meaning of those sides of mental disorders that are not determined by brain pathology will not change, either.

Psychiatrists do not share the same view of the mind-body relationship.

Psychiatrists have a hard time conceptualizing the relationship between mind and body; this is the work of philosophers. As there are different philosophical answers to the question of the relationship between mind and body different schools of philosophy sow the seeds of conceptual discord in psychiatry.

Even when psychiatrists give no thought to the mind-body relationship, their attitude towards this relationship determines their approach to dealing with the mentally ill, their understanding of the origin and nature of the mental disorder, and the therapy they think has priority. Sometimes they cite a particular school of philosophy in order to find conceptual support for the theoretical approach and practice. The fact that psychiatrists do not speak the same language is the result of such circumstances. There can be no dialogue without the use of a common language, just as opposing views cannot converge without dialogue.

The proponents of each psychiatric model practice psychiatry as though only the model they advocate is legitimate.

There are several models in psychiatry (e.g., biomedical, psychological, sociocultural) that are distinguished by their epistemological, conceptual and practical, diagnostic-therapeutic aspects. No scientific or other evidence exists to show that any one of the models is more valid, useful or better than any other. Hence no unitary psychiatry exists in the general-theoretical and practical sense. This is not the case with any other medical discipline.

Psychiatrists are reluctant to acknowledge that they are inter alia the guardians of social peace and order.

A mentally ill person is a social deviant. Psychiatrists implicitly take into account this characteristic. A very small number of psychiatrists explicitly speak of the importance of the deviant nature of the mentally ill with regard to their social and psychiatric treatment.

The behavior of the mentally ill is socially dissonant. Such are their ideas, their feelings and how they express them, their attitude toward themselves and others. It is one of the main reasons why they are considered to be a menace. They threaten the prevailing manner of communicating, expressing one's thoughts and feelings, and the existing meaning of symbols in a given environment. Deviancy of a person with a mental disorder is specific. It is socially perceived as incomprehensible, irrational, and unpredictable. What is common to all reactions to the socially disruptive nature of a mental disorder is the desire to be protected from those with mental illness; in other words, to put them under control and supervision. Psychiatrists are professionally trained and socially authorized to mitigate the socially dissonant nature of mental illness. Whether they like it or not, they thus become the guardians of social peace and order. Psychiatrists today persistently refuse to acknowledge that they (also) carry out this function, because it is contrary to the image they have of themselves as medically educated experts dealing with organic functions and structures, facts with a neutral value.

Psychiatrists diagnose mental disorders every day, although there is no generally agreed upon definition of mental disorder.

Yet when someone seeks help, the psychiatrist is first expected to say whether this person has a mental disorder and if so, to diagnose it. When asked for a definition of mental disorder, the majority of psychiatrists are unable to answer this question. The definitions of mental disorder by those who are able to give one differ considerably one from the other. Mental disorder continues to elude a definition that would be of great assistance in clearly distinguishing mental disorder from non-disorder.

Psychiatrists reduce mental health to the absence of mental disorder.

Psychiatrists deal primarily, or even exclusively, with mental disorders and do not pay much attention to mental health, its definition, or how to achieve it. Such a lack of psychiatrists' interest for mental health does not match the role mental health plays in psychiatric research, diagnosing, and treatment.

In tune with their ignorance of numerous mental health related issues, most psychiatrists use a clinically-pragmatic definition for mental health whereby mental health is the absence of mental disorder and complying with the prevailing behavior and belief standard. Mental health is, however, much more than the mere absence of mental disorder and respecting the existing social norms.

Although the official classifications of mental disorders state that there is no difference between somatic disease and mental disorder, the dissimilarities of these pathological phenomena largely outweigh their similarities.

According to the official classifications of mental disorders there is no difference between physical disease and mental disorder. Nevertheless, physical diseases and mental disorders differ considerably in their etiological, diagnostic, and clinical aspects and particularly in their meaning for society.

Making a distinction between physical disease and mental disorder does not mean adhering to Cartesian dualism. But regarding mental disorder the same as any other disease means reifying mental disorder, i.e., neglecting the numerous and important specific attributes of mental disorders that make them transcend their organic foundation. The differences between physical disease and mental disorder cannot be removed by failing to discuss them.

Attempts to increase the reliability of mental disorder diagnoses have been made at the cost of the desubjectification and dexontectualization of mental disorders.

A higher degree of reliability of mental disorder diagnosis is necessary in order to establish the validity of mental disorders, achieve better understanding among psychiatrists, study the causes of individual mental disorders and determine the effectiveness of different types of therapy. The operational definitions of mental disorders set out in the *Diagnostic and Statistical Manuals* (from DSM-III) have tried to increase the reliability of mental disorder diagnosis but at the price of disregarding specific individual experience, and the context in which a particular mental disorder appears. Yet subjective experience and context are extremely important for the onset and experience of a mental disorder and thereby for its diagnosis. The question is how far formalizing diagnostic procedure can go without jeopardizing certain essential aspects of mental disorders, such as the patient's subjective experience, which unless it is translated in words or behavior cannot be perceived.

Thus, in diagnosing mental disorders psychiatrists are torn between the diagnostic rules defined in official classifications and paying attention to a patient's narrative. The first route is easier, it is like a shortcut, yet it does not provide insight into the richness of personal experience. The second one is longer and winding. In return, it helps psychiatrists to acknowledge the variety of experiential dimensions of those who suffer from one and the same kind of mental disorder, not to mention of those suffering from various types of mental disorders. Negligence of psychopathology and clinical phenomenology is the price paid for focusing on the symptoms rather than on the patient's story.

The categorical and dimensional concepts of mental disorders are difficult to reconcile.

In current classifications, mental disorders are conceived as categories, i.e., entities that are set apart from other entities (mental disorders). Numerous studies have shown, however, that a distinct border cannot be drawn between individual types of mental disorder. It seems that the dimensional concept of mental disorder is better suited to the nature of a great many mental disorders. According to this concept, a non-disorder state gradually transforms into a disorder. The problem is that it is difficult to reach an agreement on the number of dimensions that would be used to define a specific type of mental disorder. In addition, using the concept of "mental disorder" in some contexts, for example in epidemiological studies, requires that a clear distinction be made between mental disorder and non-disorder. This means that a cut-off point between mental disorder and non-disorder must be arbitrarily determined on disorder-non-disorder dimensions. Dimensional determination thereby becomes categorical. Eventually, the dimensional conceptualization of individual psychopathological phenomena such as for example delusion or psychosis can be (ab)used so as to negate their distinctiveness.

The methods of causal explanation and meaningful understanding, without which psychiatry cannot do, are two essentially different methods.

The specific characteristics of mental disorder are reflected by the fact that only the method of meaningful understanding, i.e., the intuitive understanding of what a specific event or state means for a specific individual, is suitable for some disorders as well as for particular symptoms of some disorders. The issue is unresolved as to which method, causal explanation or meaningful understanding, is more suitable for which mental disorders and/or their particular symptoms. There is also no undivided opinion as to whether understanding is an equal, inferior or superior method of knowledge compared to explanation. Finally, sometimes meaningful connections are wrongly interpreted as causal connections, as is done by psychoanalytically oriented psychotherapists.

Frequent changes in diagnostic classifications are not accompanied by a change in the diagnostic work of a large number of psychiatrists throughout the world.

As shown inter alia by the publication of several versions of mental disorder classifications in a relatively short time—in particular the *Diagnostic and Statistical Manual of Mental Disorders* (American Psychiatric Association) and the *International Classification of Diseases* (World Health Organization)—psychiatrists and particularly psychiatrist-researchers have focused their attention on diagnosing and classifying mental disorders in the last three dozen years. At the same time, psychiatrists who are not involved in research and do not work in the public sector, and in many environments they make up the majority, diagnose their clients' disorders without respecting the definitions of mental disorders set out in official classifications. The divide is thereby widened between psychiatric research and psychiatric practice, between academic and non-academic psychiatry.

Mental healthcare market reduces psychiatrist to a psychopharmacologist or pharmacopsychiatrist.

The opinion that several therapists should take part in the treatment of a patient has both financial and professional justification. With regard to the first, it is claimed that a psychiatrist, whose services are comparatively speaking the most expensive, should see the client once in every two or three months, or even less frequently. On he other hand, clinical psychologists, psychiatric nurses and/or psychiatric social workers, whose services are less expensive than those of a psychiatrist, according to the same line of reasoning, should see the client more frequently. With regard to the second justification, the best services are provided by those who are most experienced and knowledgeable in a specific field. Since no therapist can be equally well versed in every form of treatment, different experts should provide therapeutic treatment. Within the financial and professional justification of several therapists treating the same patient, the psychiatrist has been reduced to a pharmacotherapist. Furthermore, this treatment model does not provide conditions for the establishment of a therapeutic alliance between the client and the therapist. And the therapeutic alliance is said to play in many cases a more important role in the treatment of people with mental disorder than many other treatment modalities.

What psychiatrists should do to solve the controversies and dilemmas in psychiatry? What is the use of pointing out the problems and analyzing them if there is no solution proposed here to explore?

There are actually two questions: what *should* be done and what *can* be done. As the reader will see, the solution of a number of controversies and dilemmas in contemporary psychiatry is beyond the reach of psychiatrists. They can do little or nothing to clear them up. Also, there are controversies and dilemmas which psychiatrists cannot solve, but can take the edges off them. Finally, there are controversies and dilemmas which are more apparent than real. It suffices to expose their real nature to remove them.

Below I will set out why some controversies cannot be resolved, and what psychiatrists should do to alleviate or unravel others.

As to a mentally ill person living in two worlds psychiatrists cannot change anything in this. In the way in which they conceptualize a mentally ill person, psychiatrists can, as they often do, force them in just one world. If they do so they falsify the nature of mentally ill people, and open the gate to further misinterpretations of those with mental illness. It is noteworthy that many controversies and dilemmas in psychiatry originate from the fact that a mentally ill person lives in two worlds.

Kenneth S. Kendler writes that "more than other professionals on earth, psychiatrists 'live' the mind-body problems in their day-to-day work" (2008: 9). As there is not a widely agreed-upon view of this relationship it would be inappropriate to expect psychiatrists to share the same view of the mind-body relationship. Psychiatrists can provide data which might help philosophers in their endeavors to answer the question of how the mind and body relate to one another. So long as there is not one but different philosophical answers to the mentioned question, psychiatrists are entitled to nurture various views of the mind-body relationship.

Psychiatry cannot do without medicine. However necessary medicine (its principles, its way of reasoning) is, it is not sufficient if we want to get a comprehensive view and a true picture of people with mental illness. Psychiatrists cannot and should not change anything in this, either.

Psychiatrists should acknowledge that physical diseases and mental disorders are not the same. If this difference is the source of controversies and dilemmas—and it is quite often—psychiatrists have to live with them.

Mental disorder evades a definition. There are two main reasons for that. First, the definition of mental disorder should assign equal weight to both the biological part of mental disorder and that part of mental disorder that has to do with values and meanings. Second, the definition of mental disorder should comprise what is objective ("firm ground") in any mental disorder (be it low fertility, higher mortality, failure to perform evolutionary designed functions, impaired mental functions), and what is locally perceived as a mental disorder. However well articulated a definition of mental disorder has been, it has failed to equally respect each side of the two cited pairs of opposites. Finally, the unresolved mind-body puzzle cannot help but make the possibility of a universal and global definition of mental disorder even more uncertain. It is senseless, and it might be even counterproductive to make a particular definition of mental disorder mandatory for all psychiatrists and clinical psychologists. It seems more sensible to conceptually articulate the way in which most psychiatrists distinguish mental disorder from non-disorder. This is what I have done in chapter 1.

Psychiatrists should oppose any attempt at removing the boundary between mental disorder and non-disorder, between psychiatric populations and non-psychiatric populations. It might sound paradoxical: on one hand, psychiatrists cannot define mental disorder and on the other they are expected to resist the blurring of the boundary between disorder and non-disorder. That is one of the paradoxes which psychiatrists have to live with without being able to resolve them. They should stand against deleting the difference between people with mental illness and those who are mentally sound because no matter how fuzzy such difference is in many cases psychiatrists should not disregard it. Besides, those who endeavor to proclaim the cited difference non-existent or just a matter of degree often covertly target psychiatry. They are intended on dismissing psychiatry.

Psychiatrists should stop being entrenched in a particular concept of the origin and nature of mental disorders. Indeed, they cannot reconcile their conceptual positions because different epistemologies underlie them. Nevertheless, they are due to show interest in what is going on the other side of the fence of the concept they adhere to. In order to do that they have to refrain from dismissing approaches other than their own. If they do not do that psychiatry will become ever more fragmented. Moreover, psychiatrists cannot clear up psychiatric conceptual cacophony, nor can they form a conceptual framework in which different approaches would be reconciled unless the mind-body puzzle is resolved in a convincing way.

Psychiatrists have to pay due attention to mental health and the role that the notion of mental health plays in psychiatry. They should have a say in efforts to reach a definition of mental health, which at this stage seems as remote as ever. Psychiatrists' view of mental health as the absence of disorder is unacceptable.

Issues related to diagnosis and classification in general and the reliability and validity of mental disorders in particular are of utmost importance to psychiatry. Even though there are no hints that the validity of most psychiatric disorders has been established, not to mention increased, psychiatrists should invest more energy and knowledge in answering a great many questions related to the diagnosis and classification of mental disorders. At this stage, there are no hints that psychiatrists will be able to significantly increase the reliability of mental disorders' diagnoses, or to establish their validity in the near future; first, because in the diagnostic assessment, the subjective of the patient and psychiatrist alike cannot be excluded, and second, because organic foundation of most psychiatric illnesses is unknown.

If psychiatry is conceived of as an objective, value-free, (purely) scientific discipline, there is a controversy between such a concept of psychiatry and its function of preserving the existing social norms and system. However, if we accept that by being deviant the mentally ill are in a symbolic and realistic way opposed to the dominant values in the given society, in particular when they ignore them, the role of psychiatrists in defending and preserving the existent social system becomes evident. Psychiatrists make mentally ill people less deviant or non-deviant. One of the controversies and/or dilemmas in psychiatry has been created by psychiatrists' reluctance to acknowledge the kind of social role they are tacitly expected to perform.

The book comprises four chapters. Each chapter covers a specific topic: mental disorder, mental health, differences between physical disease and mental disorder, and psychiatric conceptual cacophony. These topics have been chosen because they offer the best opportunity to shed light on a large number of psychiatric dilemmas and controversies. What is common to these topics is that they are key issues for psychiatry. They simply cannot be dodged in any deliberation about psychiatry and its particularities.

Chapter 1 ("Toward a Definition of Mental Disorder") presents numerous dilemmas surrounding the definition of mental disorder. A critical analysis is given of previous attempts to define mental disorder and particularly of efforts to make definitions more instrumental in differentiating between mental disorder and non-disorder. There have also been attempts to make it harder to distinguish between mental disorder and non-disorder, and show that psychiatrists do not know how to distinguish between these two states. These have been critically analyzed as well.

To formulate my definition of mental health I started from the assumption that mental disorder should be defined so that it allows the best distinction possible between mental disorder and states that have similarities with mental disorder ("closest neighbors"). A detailed explanation is given of my definition of mental disorder that comprises four elements: (1) a mentally ill person deviates from the prevailing behavior and belief standard in a given environment; (2) one or more mental functions are impaired in such a person, and that is preceded or followed by a psychological dysfunction; (3) their deviation and the impairment of one or more mental functions happen against their will, and (4) cause mental suffering of the respective person.

Chapter 2 ("From Normality to Mental Health") is devoted to mental health. Psychiatrists primarily deal with mental disorder. Possible reasons are presented as to why psychiatrists pay little attention to issues related to the definition of mental health. An explanation is given as to why they should do this much more often and to a much greater extent. I distinguished three ways of defining mental disorder (clinical pragmatic,

positive psychology view of mental disorder, and humanistic-philosophical approach to mental disorder) and pointed out their perfections and
imperfections. Also, the reasons for developing a classification of mental
health states have been expounded.

Chapter 3 ("Physical Diseases and Mental Disorders: Should They be
Differentiated?") is concerned with differences between physical disease
and mental disorder. Mental disorder is the same as any other disease has
been stated in DSM-III and DSM-IV. In other words, physical disease
should be equated with mental disorder. A number of reasons underpin
this view (for example, the belief that progress in neurochemical research
and improvements in imaging techniques will lead to the discovery of
organic correlates to mental disorders; the need to reinforce the status of
psychiatry as a medical discipline; the desire to decrease or eliminate the
stigma of mental disorder; the need to maintain psychiatry as a medical
discipline). I have identified numerous substantial differences between
physical disease and mental disorder. They by far outweigh similarities
between these two pathological phenomena.

Finally, in chapter 4 ("Conceptual Cacophony in Psychiatry") the
origins and consequences of the existence of different models in psychiatry, each one as legitimate as any other, have been analyzed. There
are attempts to tone down the conceptual heterogeneity of psychiatry (for
example, eclecticism, the biopsychosocial model, methodical pluralism,
pragmatic psychiatry). None of these attempts has provided such a solution of conceptual cacophony that would result in widely accepting it as
the sole or dominant theoretical-practical model. It is hard to imagine
a conceptual homogeneity in psychiatry until philosophers agree on
a concept of the mind-body relationship. Moreover, particular social
and financial interests that will always favor the dominance of one of
the psychiatric models will remain a significant obstacle on the path to
creating psychiatry's conceptual unity.

Learning about the origin, nature and effects of at least a number
of psychiatric controversies and dilemmas is beneficial for several
reasons.

First, it is beneficial to psychiatrists since, as stated, a great many of
them are unaware of the importance that controversies and dilemmas
have for psychiatry or else, fearing that they will undermine psychiatry's
reputation, they minimize them in defense.

Second, it is beneficial to those who are interested in psychiatry for
whatever reason, enabling them to gain insight into important aspects

of psychiatric theory and practice about which they have no information or little information.

Third, it shows that the contradictions and dilemmas in contemporary psychiatry are not the dark side of psychiatry. They are both the dark and the bright sides of psychiatry, just the same as other less contentious issues related to psychiatry.

I would like to thank my eldest daughter, Jelena Kecmanovic, who provided valuable comments on drafts of the second chapter. Also, my thanks go to Alice Copple-Tosic who translated the first chapter from Serbo-Croatian, and to my younger daughter, Milica Kecmanovic, for her help in proofreading the manuscript.

1

Towards a Definition of Mental Disorder

Physicians, including psychiatrists, give a lot of
thoughts in their everyday work to answer the
question of whether or not a particular patient has
a disorder; they rarely give much thought to the
broader issue of what constitutes a disorder.
Robert L. Spitzer, 1999

Attempts to define *mental disorder* are as old as the very concept of *mental disorder*.

If I say that there is no satisfactory definition of mental disorder even today, the reader will know how difficult it is to define. Otherwise, the many psychiatrists, psychologists, sociologists and anthropologists who have been trying for decades to find the *real* answer would have come at least close to the *right* answer to the question: what is mental disorder? And it seems they have not.[1] Assuming, of course, that there is a right answer.

Why is it Important to Define Mental Disorder?

The question of the nature and borders of mental disorder is not as academic as it might seem. The answer is particularly important for a person whose psychological state is evaluated as disordered or non-disordered. Being diagnosed as mentally ill has serious consequences for such a person and the members of their family, and to a somewhat lesser extent for the people from their work or their neighbors. In addition, it is important to public health in distinguishing mental disorder and non-disorder accurately. The incidence rate and prevalence of mental disorder in a specific community depends on the definition of mental disorder. The frequency of mental disorders in a specific community

1

determines, or at least should determine, the amount of money that will be earmarked to treat and care for the mentally ill.

The definition of generic mental disorder is also essential when classifying mental disorders. In order to demonstrate the importance of the definition of mental disorder for diagnostics and classification, Allan V. Horwitz and Jerome C. Wakefield (2007: 8) used a figure. Imagine an inverted pyramid, a pyramid standing on its top. The construction of the pyramid is as strong as the top on which the pyramid is standing. The top of the pyramid is the definition of mental disorder and the different types of mental disorder constitute the rest of the pyramid.

Finally, defining mental disorder is also important for those who want to know more about a specific society. The definition of mental disorder has universal elements that apply to every mental disorder, in every society, in every historical era, and elements that refer to a specific sociocultural environment in which a specific behavior is diagnosed as a mental disorder. Anthropologists and sociologists are interested in that aspect of the definition of mental disorder that is linked to a specific sociocultural environment. They can use it to learn quite a bit about the prevailing value system in a given community, about its inhabitants' likes and dislikes.

General Issues Linked to the Definition of Mental Disorder

Many issues have stood in the way to a generally accepted definition of mental disorder. The reader will learn about them in the text that follows; at least most of the relevant issues. Let me mention right away one of the general dilemmas about mental disorder. Some people consider that mental disorder exists and others maintain that mental disorder does not exist, that it is a mental construct with a certain explanatory value.

Those who represent the first viewpoint, the *essentialists*, stress that mental disorder is in the nature of the thing (*in rerum natura*). Essentialists believe that mental disorder exists as *ens*, as an entity, and there is something like an articulation or demarcation line in nature between mental disorder and non-disorder. It is scientists' job to establish where this "articulation" or demarcation line exists. Representative of the other viewpoint, the *nominalists*, believe that concepts such as "mental disorder" are simply mental constructs that do not correspond to reality. According to nominalism, abstract concepts, general notions or universal ideas do not exist independently as doctrines, but only as names. There is nothing in reality that corresponds to the concept "mental disorder." People have simply come up with the idea of "mental disorder" in order to explain certain phenomena (to themselves and other people).

Whoever takes up the thankless job of defining mental disorder will have to say what it is about mental disorder that distinguishes it from other phenomena, particularly phenomena that have some common characteristics with mental disorder, that are, in other words, similar to it in some respects. They will also have to say whether there is a difference between mental disorder and physical disease and if there is, in what respects.

Here are a few more general remarks regarding the definition of mental disorder.

Those who claim that mental disorder is a social construct actually deny the existence of mental disorder so their views of mental disorder—the argument goes—should not be taken into account when discussing the definition of mental disorder.

I do not agree with this opinion. I feel that those authors, primarily sociologists from the field of symbolic interactionism, who claim that mental disorder is a social construct define it in their own way. For them, mental disorder exists as a social construct. Such a definition of mental disorder should be accepted as legitimate.

A number of authors (for example, Kendell, 1975b, 1993, 2001; Wakefield, 1992, 1999a) who deal with the definition of mental disorder first define a so-called physical (organic, somatic) disease and then apply that definition to mental disorder, thereby tacitly or openly equating somatic disease and mental disorder. Other authors (for example, Klein, 1978; Henriques, 2002; Margolis, 1976), who also apply the definition of physical disease to mental disorder, are careful to point out certain specific features of mental disorder. A small amount of authors (for example, Sedgwick, 1982; Maslow and Mittlemann, 1951) define mental disorder without referring to the definition of physical disease.

Owing to the considerable differences between the nature of physical disease and mental disorder, which the reader will learn in the chapter "Physical Diseases and Mental Disorders: Should They Be Differentiated?" it is very difficult to include both types of pathological events in the same definition. This is why it is better to restrict the definition to only physical disease or only mental disorder. This text will deal solely with the definition of mental disorder. Where necessary, the definition of physical disease will also be considered.

It is difficult to look for the definition of mental disorder on *only one* of the following three levels: the cause(s) of mental disorder, its clinical picture, and its consequences. It is therefore no wonder that the authors of past definitions of mental disorder sought its specific features simultaneously on two or even all three of the above levels.

Attempts to establish what is distinctive to mental disorder on for example only the level of its etiology show how erroneous it is to keep to just one level of events when defining mental disorder. Every such attempt quickly leads to the realization that the task cannot be completed, since the cause of most mental disorders is unknown.

In addition, since different models or general concepts about mental disorder provide different explanations as to why it appears, when attempting to define mental disorder on the level of its etiology alone, we must opt for one of the concepts about the onset and nature of mental disorder. If we do this, our definition of mental disorder will be valid only within the definition of such a general concept or approach to mental disorder. All those with the ambition of defining mental disorder prefer to avoid such a restriction.

Also mental disorder is hard to define using *only one* of its characteristics. If they exist, monothetic definitions of mental disorder are lacking. Polythetic definitions provide a fuller definition of mental disorder and include several characteristics which, in the opinion of the authors of these definitions, are specific to mental disorder.

Further on in the text, I will present my own definition of mental disorder. My understanding is that psychiatrists use this definition of mental disorder when deciding whether a person is mentally disordered. As noted in the motto of this text, almost as a rule, psychiatrists neither try to define mental disorder nor think about which definition of mental disorder they use in their daily professional work. Yet, when one analyzes criteria most psychiatrists use in differentiating mental disorder and non-disorder it is not difficult to grasp what sorts of gauges they make use of.

As I present my own definition of mental disorder, which is in tune with how psychiatrists diagnose mental disorder, I will critically analyze the definitions of disorder, or disease, put forward by authors who have dealt with the matter of defining mental disorder.

After presenting my own definition of mental disorder, I will analyze two of the most important definitions of mental disorder that came out in the past thirty years: the definition set out in the third and fourth editions of the Diagnostic and Statistical Manual of Mental Disorders of the American Psychiatric Association (here and henceforth DSM-III, 1980, and DSM-IV, 1994, are named DSMs) and the definition of mental disorder formed by Jerome C. Wakefield. Both of these definitions are attempts to create the clearest possible distinction between mental disorder and non-disorder.

I also feel it necessary to discuss attempts to blur the border between mental disorder and non-disorder. I have found such an attempt not in increasing indications of auditory hallucinations and delusions in non-psychiatric populations, but rather in the conclusions drawn on the basis of such findings.

Problems with the definition of mental disorder came up in psychiatric-epidemiological studies as well. I indicate that results of the psychiatric-epidemiological research of the rate of prevalence and incidence of mental disorders in the United States of America carried out in the past twenty years have revealed that the defects of this type of research has been caused mostly by an insufficiently clear distinction between mental disorder and non-disorder.

Several researchers (e.g., Rosenhan, Slater) using an unusual method (deceit), tried to show that psychiatrists do not know what mental disorder is and therefore cannot clearly distinguish the mentally ill from those who are not mentally ill. I have given a critical review of this research.

Also I have shown that sociological definitions of mental disorder do not provide a clear distinction between mental disorder and non-disorder.

Finally, the last section of this chapter presents the factors and circumstances that make it difficult to define mental disorder.

In the text that follows I will set out my definition of mental disorder, i. e., its defining characteristics.

Mental Disorder:
Deviating from the Individual and Social Standard

The very word mental *disorder* suggests that there was order and it has been disturbed, resulting in disorder.

When it is said that order has been disturbed, resulting in disorder, this means that there has been a deviation, a departure from something that is considered standard or at least from some previous state that is not considered disturbed.

It is therefore no wonder that the concept of *deviation* is found in most definitions of mental disorder. Regardless of their differences and similarities, they all feature deviation as an important characteristic of mental disorder.

Thus, David P. Ausubel, an American psychologist, writes that "disease is generally regarded as including any marked *deviations*, physical, mental, or behavioral, from normally desirable standards of structural and functional integrity" (1961, my emphasis). Peter Sedgwick, Lecturer of Political Science and Psychiatry at the University of Leeds, notes in the same spirit that *"all sickness is essentially deviancy"* (1982: 32, emphasis in original) and adds that denoting some state as a disease is always preceded by calculating the size of the difference between the present behavior and some social norm. "If we could all function according to approved social requirements within any range of body temperature, thermometers would disappear from the household medical kit," writes Sedgwick (1982: 34-5). Lester King, who was the editor of the reputable *Journal of the American Medical Association* (JAMA), in his essay "What is Disease" states that disease is "the aggregate of those conditions which, judged by the prevailing culture, are deemed painful, or disabling, and which, at the same time, *deviate* from either the statistical norm or from some idealized status" (King, 1954, my emphasis).

Ruth Macklin, author of numerous works on ethical questions in medicine, joins these views about deviation as an essential characteristic of mental disorder. She writes: "In actual practice psychiatrists use a composite approach. They diagnose behavior as clearly abnormal when it is seriously disabling, frustrating, and *deviates* from established cultural norms" (1972, emphasis in original). Henry Cohen, Professor at the School of Medicine in Liverpool, also maintains that "disease indicates *deviations* from the normal" (Cohen, 1955, my emphasis).

Emil Kraepelin, the father of clinical psychiatry, in his famous textbook, defined mental disorder as deviating from the normal or the average. Kraepelin writes that "the standard we use in recognizing the morbid features of a man's mental life is *the departure from the average* in the direction of inefficiency" (1917: 295, my emphasis).

The mentally ill deviate from what is considered in a given community to be the normal, standard form of behaving, thinking and feeling, and relating to oneself and others. This happens when with no apparent reason someone says that a certain group of people is poisoning their food, when they cannot recognize their near and dear, when in an extremely heightened mood they squander property acquired with hard work, when they say that their internal organs are rotten and it is amazing that they are still alive, and when periodically, without any apparent reasons, they are seized by paralyzing fear accompanied by sweating, pounding of the heart and suffocation. I have given only some of the symptoms of different mental disorders to show that, regardless of the type of disorder, every mentally ill person deviates from the behavior and belief standard in a given community.

Highlighting decreased functional efficiency as a component part of the definition of disorder, Kraepelin indicated one more important characteristic of the mentally ill: they are less functional in one or several areas. They *deviate* in the functional sense as well: when disordered, they are less functionally capable in one or more areas than when they were mentally non-disordered.

Mental disorders appear in different periods of life. Very few are in evidence from the youngest age. When the disorder appears, the individual starts gradually or suddenly carrying out their social roles and tasks less successfully than they did before they were disordered, or cannot carry out new roles and tasks as successfully as most of their peers with the same physical condition and level of education.

There are two types of deviations: deviation from the *individual* and deviation from the *social*. From the *individual* since the person deviates from their (own) previous level of social functioning. Since their previous level of social functioning most often does not differentiate greatly from the level of social functioning of their peers with the same physical condition and education level, this is deviation from the *social* as well. When a person is less socially functional than their peers from an early age, this too is deviation from the *social*.

Five Groups that Contravene the Prevailing Behavior and Belief Pattern

Roughly speaking, those who contravene the established behavior and belief standard can be divided into five large groups. The first group consists of artists, great scientists and creators, in a word all those whose work changes the world: current ideas, current views of the world and people in it, the current social-cultural pattern. They are all at the helm of their work. They create it; they alone decide to persevere in their creative efforts, regardless of the frequent lack of understanding and even disapproval and open resistance from their surroundings.

The second group consists of another kind of offenders: criminals, thieves, swindlers, thugs. They decide for themselves whether they will be offenders. A dozen reasons and motives might be cited—ranging from biological to personal and social—why someone has become a criminal or outlaw. Most often several factors are at play. But regardless of which and how large the combination of factors that results in someone coming into conflict with the law, those who break the law and are not mentally disordered, in the great majority of cases, decide for themselves to go against the current social-cultural behavior and belief standard. Regardless of the different circumstances that pressure them into choosing the path of the criminal, they always have enough freedom to take another path.

Revolutionaries make the third group. They are not happy with the existing social practice and underpinning ideas or ideology. They are most unhappy with the regime which they hold accountable for, mildly said, imperfections of the social reality. That is why they contravene the prevailing behavior and belief model, and strive to change it by revolutionary means. Depending on the side one takes they are sometimes renamed as terrorists.

The fourth group consists of interventionists. There are governments which, for whatever reason, believe that the prevailing ideas and corresponding social practice in a country other than their own should be changed. They usually say that such a job should be done for the sake of people of that particular country. Hence they enforce, or at least try to enforce, a new behavior and belief model in the country that is the target of their intervention.

The fifth group of offenders consists of the mentally ill. They do not deviate willingly from either the *individual* or the *social*. They do so under the pressure of changed, disordered, damaged mental functions. And the damage to mental functions, as the reader will see below, is also outside the control of the mentally ill.

The concepts of *incapacity* and *dysfunction* that are frequently used by those who try to define mental disorder refer to this social-functional damage in the mentally ill.

Deviating from the Individual and Social Standard is Undesirable

Within the context of analyzing deviation as one of the characteristics of mental disorder, it should be noted that mental disorder is viewed in all environments as undesirable (negative) because the mentally ill behave, think and feel, and relate toward themselves and others in a way that deviates from what is considered normal in a given community, and also because they are functionally less efficient since they are disordered.[2]

From the individual and particularly from the social viewpoint, it is desirable (positive) to be normal and socially functional (which is actually one and the same thing).

In a word, mental disorder and non-disorder are value concepts. "Our claim is that the traditional medical model, and the claim to value-free diagnosis on which it rests, is unsupportable; and that, to the contrary, diagnosis, although properly grounded on facts, is also, and essentially grounded on values" (Fulford, Thornton, Graham, 2006: 565).

The prevailing behavior and belief model is considered desirable until the majority of the members of a specific community decides, for whatever reason, that it is (no longer) good and should therefore be changed, either violently and quickly, or nonviolently and gradually. Until the majority of the members of a specific community adopt a new behavior and belief pattern, the old pattern is the example to follow, it is the gauge and criterion of what is good and desirable.

I do not claim that a specific behavior and belief model is desirable for someone outside that society. I also do not pass judgment on whether the behavior and belief pattern recognized by the majority of a community is good (desirable) according to some universal criteria. (This topic is considered in more detail in Chapter 2).

The dominant behavior and belief model is important for those involved in defining mental disorder because *the mentally ill always deviate from the prevailing behavior and belief pattern*, and because when evaluating whether someone is mentally ill, psychiatrists do not go outside the framework of the prevailing behavior and belief model in a given society as being good, desirable and even mentally non-disordered. (Hereinafter, the concept of "behavior" as the first part of the syntagma "behavior and belief" shall be used to denote not only behavioral but also cognitive and emotional aspects of conduct.)

Psychiatrists do not judge whether someone deviates from the prevailing behavior and belief model on the basis of some universal or extramundane criteria, and even less based on the opinions of any of the minorities in a given community. Psychiatrists do not ask themselves whether a specific individual's ideas and behavior, and how they relate to themselves and the environment, are consistent with the views, let's say, of humanistic or some other concept and ideology of the desirable model of how a person should behave, think, relate to themselves and others. They ask themselves whether and to what extent the ideas, behavior and perceptions of a specific individual clash with the ideas, behavior and perceptions found among the great majority of people in a given society, and whether, how much and why a specific individual functionally fails in one or several areas of their personal and social life. This is how it was long ago when people first suspected that someone might be mentally disordered based on their deviant behavior, their reasoning and feelings. And this is still true today.

Paul Hirst and Penny Woolley along the same lines write: "Psychiatry cannot be other than a practice adjusted to what subjects need to be in their conducts and relations to others" (1982: 105).

There is an exception here. Minorities, primarily most of the world's ethnic groups, try to preserve their identity by fostering traditions and languages that are different from the language spoken by the majority in a given society. In countries where multiculturalism is not only an official policy but a principle respected in daily life, and in countries where multiculturalism is not part of the official policy, a considerable number of people belonging to ethnic groups (ethnics) foster their customs, their system of values, their beliefs.

It sometimes happens that when an ethnic is outside their ethnic group and they publicly behave according to the behavior and belief model specific to their ethnic group, the majority population perceives them as being deviant and expresses doubts that "something is psychologically wrong with them." In order to avoid diagnosing people as disordered if they strictly hold to the behavior and belief model of their ethnic group, psychiatrists must bear in mind the specific customs and beliefs of different ethnic groups.

In some countries conflicts between the behavior and belief patterns of the minority and majority are rare; in others quite frequent. In either case they do not challenge the accuracy of the claim that breaching the prevailing norms is one of the characteristics of those with mental disorder.

Someone's deviation from the prevailing behavior and belief pattern does not have to be caused by mental disorder and not everyone who deviates because of mental disorder will reach a psychiatrist, but every person diagnosed by a psychiatrist as mentally ill deviates from the behavior of the majority in a given community.

Let me cite the example of homosexuals in different revisions of the Diagnostic and Statistical Handbook of Mental Disorders (DSM) of the American Psychiatric Association in support of the above assertion that the less unusual a person's behavior, in the broadest sense, is considered in a specific community, the smaller are the prospects that it will raise doubts that it is or could be an expression of mental disorder. In the first (1952) and second (1968) versions of this classification, homosexuality appears as a pathological entity, which means a mental disorder. In the final phases of preparing the third revision that was published in 1980, political activists of the increasingly well organized homosexuals put pressure for months on the authors of the third revision, particularly on Robert L. Spitzer, its executive editor, to take homosexuality off the list of mental disorders. And they succeeded. Not only because they fiercely fought to remove the label of mental disorder from homosexuality but also because the authors of DSM-III were aware that public opinion towards homosexuality was changing in the United States. And even though many religious groups (Catholics and evangelists, for example) condemn homosexuality at the top of their lungs today, the general social climate has changed and is still changing in the direction of viewing homosexuality as a form of sexual orientation that is as legitimate and legal as heterosexuality.

Finally, the very fact that no one creating a new revision of the American or any other classification of mental disorder in one of the highly industrialized countries of the part of the world called the West would think of reclassifying homosexuality among the mentally disordered, says that homosexuality has been substantially accepted as one of the standard forms of sexual orientation and, more broadly, behavior.

Now is the time to answer the question: is every deviation from the current behavior and belief standard negative, or at least something undesirable from the individual and social viewpoint? No. For example if someone has an extremely high intelligence quotient (IQ), they deviate from the intelligence level of most people in a given community. Neither psychiatrists nor lay people will consider them mentally disordered because of their high intelligence. I can also say that there is *abnormally* high intelligence, but this does not mean it is a mental disorder.[3] Furthermore, someone might have a special type of talent for artistic expression or acting, for example, that deviates from the average of this type of talent among the majority in a specific community. Here again, there are little prospects that this will be denoted as a mental disorder.

When evaluating whether a person is mentally disordered, individual deviations are considered negative if they are undesirable, and they are undesirable because they disturb the existing peace and order, challenge the meanings of different aspects of social life and because they handicap the person in the functional sense, making them less capable or incapable of normally functioning in one or more areas of individual or social life. In a considerable number of cases, a mentally disordered person continues to carry out their social roles and tasks, but less successfully compared to how they carried them out in the previous period of their life, or less successfully compared to people of the same age and level of education. (It is very rare for a mentally disordered person to stop carrying out all their social roles and tasks.)

It is not just about less successfully carrying out numerous social roles—ranging from conjugal, parental, familial, to professional, sociopolitical and so on—but about carrying out only one or at most two social roles instead of the dozen and even more social roles that people play in daily life. For example, if an artist seriously neglects all or most of their social roles and obligations, except for the role of artist, they run the risk of people considering them daft in the milder form and mentally disordered in a less mild form. And the more they neglect all their social roles except that as an artist (because the role of an artist is also a social role), the closer the artist draws to those known as eccentrics, and the greater the chances of their becoming the focus of psychiatrists' interest.

Average and Ideal on Equal Footing

In defining what is mentally (non) disordered, in addition to the criterion of social standard, which is actually a *statistical criterion*, one other criterion is usually mentioned, the *criterion of the ideal*. According to this latter criterion, mentally non-disordered is when a person's behavior and ideas are closest to a specific behavior and belief *ideal*, or *ideal* behavior and belief model, and mentally disordered is a person who deviates from the ideal behavior.

Who defines this ideal behavior and belief model? Do psychiatrists? Never. The ideal behavior and belief model is defined by the spirit of the era, *Zeitgeist*, society, regime, the economic, social, political environment, those that hold sway in society.

When psychiatrists assess whether someone might be mentally disordered, they cannot do it without bearing in mind the existing behavior and belief model. What is important for psychiatrists is the behavior and belief model that is the most widespread in the here and now. For them it is ideal, since they consider people to be mentally non-disordered if their behavior, thinking and how they relate toward themselves and others, reflects this very model. And being mentally non-disordered is an ideal category for every psychiatrist. (And not only psychiatrists, of course.) In this sense, psychiatrists equate the average and the ideal in people's behavior, in what they say and how they say it, how they act, how they perceive themselves and the world around them, what they want, what they fear, what they hope for.

In order to remove any possible misunderstanding regarding the first component in the definition of mental disorder—deviating from the current behavior and belief model—I would like to stress that someone's deviating from the current behavior and belief model is used by psychiatrists (and not only them) as only one of the indicators that a particular person (might) have "some psychological problems." Individual deviating from the behavior and belief model is a *necessary* but not *sufficient* indicator that this person is mentally disordered.

I repeat: *individual* and *not group* deviating. The deviating of a large number of people whose identical behavior, ideas, manner of dress, faith and so on comprises a separate group within a community or society, should not raise suspicions that "something is psychologically wrong" with the members of such a group. I am thinking of those groups that people join voluntarily and not out of external or internal pressure. Psychiatrists should not shed doubt that "something is psychologically wrong" with the members of such groups or subcultures based solely on the fact that they do not belong to the prevailing social, cultural, political, religious and ethno-national standard. By the same token, psychiatrists would not be justified in shedding doubt about the mental health of an individual who starts to deviate from the behavior and belief standard of one of these groups (subcultures). For example, members of alternative groups (e. g., hippies) are not less mentally healthy or "probably psychologically disturbed" because they belong to alternative groups. Neither is there any reason to suspect that someone who leaves the society (subculture) of an alternative group is "probably daft."[4]

Only an individual's and not a group's deviation from the prevailing behavior and belief, an individual's deviation that appears for no apparent reason, and does not arise under the pressure of specific larger or smaller groups, should raise (reasonable) doubt such a deviation might express a mental disorder (Kecmanovic, 1998).

It is noteworthy that there is no psychiatry of smaller or larger groups or subcultures within a community or society (dominant culture). In a word, there are not several types of psychiatry, particularly not within the same society.[5] There is one psychiatry and psychiatrists always use the dominant behavior and belief model in a given environment as a reference point when evaluating whether someone is mentally disordered, i.e., whether someone might be mentally disordered because, there are also other components to the definition of mental disorder, which will be discussed on the following pages.

Impairment of Mental Functions
That is Preceded or Followed by Psychological Dysfunction

When I say *mental functions*, I am thinking of mental functions such as feeling (emotion, affect, mood), volition, thinking, memory, perception, orientation in space, time and toward others, strength and control of impulses, concentration, motivation, intelligence, reasoning, self-perception, experiencing oneself and people around us. Damaged mental functions are an integral part of mental disorder.

Back in 1953 Aubrey Lewis considered impaired mental function(s) a *differentia specifica* of a mentally disordered deviant compared to a deviant who is not mentally disordered. "In mental disorder it is shown by the occurrence of say, disturbed thinking, as in delusions, or disturbed perceptions, as in hallucinations, or disturbed emotional states, as in anxiety neurosis or melancholia. Deviant, maladapted, nonconformist behaviour is pathological if it is accompanied by a manifest disturbance of some such functions."[6]

And what do I mean by *psychological dysfunction*? By this notion I mean a *disruption of coordination and harmony of individual mental functions.*

I will give some examples so as to show what I mean by the coordination (and harmony) of mental functions and its disruption, respectively.

In normal mental states, affect is in synchrony with speech content. For example, when you talk about the loss of a friend, you are expected to be crestfallen with a concomitant facial expression of sadness. That is not the case in some people with schizophrenia. Their affect is not in synchrony with their speech content. The coordination between them has been disrupted. As Emil Kraepelin put it, there is "a loss of inner unity of intellect, emotion and volition, in themselves and among one another" (1919: 34-35) in people suffering from schizophrenia. (Kraepelin used the term *dementia praecox* for schizophrenia). Erwin Stransky (1904), on his part, writes that "disturbances of the smooth interplay" between ideation and emotion of the psyche is the key characteristic of those diagnosed with schizophrenia. This psychiatrist also used the term *instrapsychic ataxia* to describe the state of mind of schizophrenic patients.

Here is another example. If you feel uncomfortable when, crossing squares due to an unpleasant event that you experienced while crossing a particular square, or you are afraid of crossing squares for no apparent reason, your memory tells you that you had crossed various squares or may be that particular square uneventfully dozens of times prior to the unfortunate event. Also, you have witnessed thousands of people crossing this or that square with not a bit of anxiety. Therefore, you have no reason whatsoever to be afraid of crossing squares. Memory, reasoning, and affect are in harmony; they are mutually coordinated and regulated; they correct one another. This is not the case with people with agoraphobia.

Here is still another example. A person with personality disorder repeatedly comes into conflict with the law because, among other reasons, they are not able to learn from experience in the way mentally sound people do. They are, sometimes severely, punished for their misbehavior, but they still keep on breaching the law. There is a disruption of coordination between experience and behavior in people with personality disorder. Experience does not exercise a corrective influence on people's desires, tendencies, and impulses; at least not to such a degree that it would keep experience, ideas, needs, and behavior in harmony. Nor do so poorly internalized social norms. In psychoanalytical terms, the individual instances of the personality (Id, Ego, Super-Ego) are not well coordinated; they are not harmonized.

Here is an example of the harmony and coordination of memory functions, experience, and affect, and of the disruption of such a harmony. If you are head over hills in love, you sometimes tend to be more or less jealous. And jealousy goes with suspiciousness. Yet whenever you start toying with the idea that your partner is cheating on you, you somehow manage to keep your suspicions under check due to your memory and experience. You know from experience that you partner is the last person who would be unfaithful. That is what your memories of your partner's behavior and the history of your relationship with them teach you. The disruption of the internal regulation, i.e., of the coordination and the harmonious relation between memory, experience, and affect, characterizes a pathological state—Pathological Jealousy (Delusional Disorder).

There is a "distortion," "disturbance," "loss of synchrony," "loss of coordination," "loss of inner unity," "loss of the smooth interplay;" there is, briefly, inner psychological dysfunction in all cited cases of mental pathology.

I said that the impairment of individual mental functions precedes or follows psychological dysfunction.

There are cases where a particular mental function is first affected, or more affected than other mental functions. For example, processes underlying Alzheimer's disease or senile dementia cause the impairment of primarily memory functions, at least in the first phase of these diseases. Then the impairment of memory functions effectuates psychological dysfunction, that is, the disruption of internal regulation and coordination of other individual mental functions.

In some other cases, psychological dysfunction can cause the impairment in individual mental functions.

In most cases, it is difficult to assess whether the impairment of individual mental functions precedes or follows the psychological dysfunction.

It is important to note that both the impairment of individual mental functions and (internal) psychological dysfunction can have various causes (biological, psychological, and sociocultural); most often all of them take part in the causative process.

Apart from dominant defense mechanisms, and other personal and sociocultural circumstances, symptoms of particular forms of mental disorder are determined by (a) the extent and kind of impairment of one or more individual mental functions, and (b) the extent and kind of (internal) psychological dysfunction.

The diversity of clinical pictures of individual types of mental disorder and the diversity of the manifestations of one and the same disorder stem *inter alia* from different forms of impairment of individual mental functions and different types of individual dysfunctions that result from it.

Deviating from the Individual and Social Pattern, and Impairment of Mental Functions are Beyond the Individual's Control

Mentally disordered people have *no willing impact* on their deviating from the prevailing behavior and belief standard or on the impairment of their mental functions. Both are outside their control. They do not decide, because they cannot decide, whether they will deviate from the social milieu's behavior and belief standard, whether they will have damaged one or more mental functions, and whether they will mentally suffer as a result of the above. Both deviating from the behavior and belief model that is characteristic of a given environment and impairment of one or more mental functions are essential elements of mental disorder that, figuratively speaking, have their hold on the mentally ill, and not the other way around.

It is mostly clear in psychotic patients that the psychotic event is outside their control. Also, when talking to people with impaired cognitive abilities, it is not difficult to conclude that the cognitive damage is beyond the reach of their will. Although the reader might think that a pathological mental event is less outside the individual control of neurotic patients (to use the concept of "neurosis," which has fallen out of use, although it might come back again) than with psychotic patients and patients with damaged cognitive abilities, I would remind them of the element of compelling, or more exactly, automatic repetition that is expressed in every neurosis. Without opening a Pandora's Box of different concepts on the origin and mechanism of the onset of neurosis, there are reasonable grounds to maintain that the symptoms of all forms of neurotic disorder automatically repeat. When I say *automatically repeat*, this is the same as saying they repeat despite or against or independent of a person's will and desire. Thus Laurence S. Kubie rightly notes, in the paper "The fundamental nature of the distinction between normality and neurosis," that mental illness is "unusually persistent pattern of behavior over which the individual has little or no voluntary control" (1954).

The mentally ill cannot think, feel or behave differently from the way they behave, how and what they think, how and what they feel, and how they relate to themselves and others. They are in the power of their disorder.[7]

Writing about Georges Canguilhem's concept of "mentally pathological," Victoria Margree (2002) states that the opposite of pathological is not normal but *normative*, understood as a person's ability to constantly reconsider and transcend themselves. A mentally disordered person is lacking this ability of self-revision and self-transcendence. Since mental disorder is outside the individual's will, they cannot revise *themselves as mentally disordered*, and willingly transcend their own mental disorder. That actually occurs very rarely, so rarely that this cannot be taken as a characteristic of mental disorder, i.e., of a mentally disordered person.

It seems that the incapacity for self-transcendence or self-correction as indicated by Margree, as a characteristic of mentally disordered people, partially results from the fact that the pathological develops *independently* of the individual's will. Just as a person has no influence on the development of the pathological, they cannot overcome it or correct it by themselves without someone's help.

An individual cannot willingly cause impairment of their mental functions. (This excludes very rare disorders where a person pretends to be crazy for the sake of some form of personal gain.) They cannot wish for, e. g., hallucinations or delusions or psychotic depression and have them. In this regard, someone might say that when defining mental disorder, it is enough to say that a mentally disordered person has impaired mental functions and psychological dysfunction. The fact that impairment of their mental functions happens independent of their will goes without saying and should not be given special emphasis, particularly not as the third important characteristic (of the definition) of mental disorder.

The reader making such a remark is right for the most part. Nevertheless, I feel it necessary to include in the definition of mental disorder the fact that a mentally disordered person deviates from the *individual* and from the *social* independent of their will and that they have impaired mental functions also independent of their will. I do this for several reasons.

When we say that someone's mental functions are impaired independent of their will, that there is nothing they can do to make them unimpaired, this—it seems to me—stresses the *pathological* nature of the impairment of mental functions. In the same vein, when we say that deviation from the *individual* and *social* happens against individual will, this suggests that mental disorder has most likely caused the deviation.

Emphasizing a mentally disordered person's powerlessness to willingly influence whether and how much they deviate from the prevailing behavior and belief standard, and whether and how much their mental functions are impaired, is useful when drawing the clearest possible distinction between mentally disordered people and those who, like the mentally disordered, deviate from the current behavior and belief standard, but are not mentally disordered.

What about artists like Charles Baudelaire and Aldous Huxley who willingly took various narcotics that caused damage to their mental functions, doing so in order to expand their sensitivity, experience other worlds and, as they believed, spur their creative potential? I would answer this question as follows. These artists are not mentally disordered for having willingly, consciously taken substances that cause temporary damage to their mental functions. If they became addicted to the substances they took, then they were mentally disordered, because then they would have to take them, and probably in increasingly larger quantities, *against their will*, following the dictate of the addiction. Then the damage to mental functions is usually not the slightest bit transitory or temporary but of long duration and even permanent.

I will use several examples to illustrate the assertion that there is reasonable doubt that a person is mentally disordered only when their behavior (in the broadest sense) has all three characteristics: they deviate from the prevailing behavior and belief pattern, one or more mental functions is impaired followed or preceded by psychological dysfunction, and all of this happens against their will.

If, for example, someone has ideas that are not shared by the great majority of people in a given community, ideas that the great majority consider to be a distortion and falsification of the reality that is seen and experienced by practically everyone in that community, and if, because of such ideas, they cannot carry out some or most of their social functions and tasks, and if, regardless of being shown proof that they are wrong, they cannot willingly change such ideas, such a person will be considered to have delusions, which most often means that they are mentally disordered.

The reader who has carefully read the above lines might wonder: was Copernicus insane when he claimed that the earth rotates around the sun and not the sun around the earth, at a time when no one else believed it? I would answer this question, first, that no one was able to offer Copernicus proof that he was wrong, and second, which is much more important for assessing whether Copernicus was crazy or not, is the fact that Copernicus willingly stated his opinion that the earth rotates around the sun, that is, he did it not against his will. He was quite able to control his "heretical" thoughts. They were not contrary to his knowledge, will and desire.

Here is another example. When someone is supposed to cross a square, if they are overcome by paralyzing fear accompanied by sweating and shaking hands and legs, they will be considered to have "something psychically wrong." It is a well-known fact that great majority of people are not afraid of open spaces and are not afraid of crossing squares. A person who is seized by paralyzing fear when they are supposed to cross a square or even at the thought of crossing a square, deviates from the behavior and belief standard of the given community. In addition, their emotions (as well as some other mental functions) are disordered and this all happens against their will.

A few more examples will be of help. If someone needs twenty or more seconds to remember the name of their near and dear; if they do not dare go a hundred meters from their house because they are not sure of finding their way back; if they cannot explain the point of the simplest folk saying, and if in spite of greatly wanting to remember a name, and be better oriented in space and time, they are unable to do so, then by their mental functions, specifically their memory functions, they deviate so much from people of the same age that almost everyone who knows them will be convinced that their "mind has strayed" or they have "turned senile." (Extreme cases are excluded, of course. For example, people who are over ninety years old are not expected to have memory functions in best shape.) In addition, in spite of the greatest desire to remember a name and to be better oriented in space and time, the specific individual is unable to do so.

All the above cases involve, first, deviating from the *individual* and the *social*. From the *individual* because, before they were mentally disordered, they did not have delusional ideas, were not afraid to cross a square, were not so forgetful. From the *social*, because the great majority of people do not have delusions, phobic fears, are not overly ("excessively") forgetful, do not show a lack of orientation in space, and so on. Second, in all these cases the "actors" have one or more impaired mental functions. Finally, deviating from the prevailing behavior and belief standard, and the impaired mental functions of all of them takes place against their will.

Can Mental Disorder be Prevented?

Robert M. Veatch, Professor of Medical Ethics at Georgetown University in Washington DC, has two critical remarks about the view that disease is beyond a person's control, something that happens to (and with) a person without their credit or blame (1973).

The first remark deals with diseases that an individual can prevent with conscious action, so onset is *not* something beyond their control. Is this assertion valid for mental disorder as well? Could it be applied to mental disorder as well?

Let us first see how much physical disease can be prevented by an individual's actions. Indeed, more and more is known about risk factors for the onset of many physical diseases. Many of the risk factors are linked to lifestyle. If someone smokes, for example, or is obese, or leads a sedentary lifestyle, if they have high "bad" cholesterol values in their blood and refuse to change their lifestyle and/or take pills to lower the "bad cholesterol," their risk of contracting cardiovascular disease is considerably higher than someone who does not have the above risk factors. These risk factors are not beyond a person's control and are not factors that cannot be removed or lowered with conscious, willful action.

Here are a few more examples where individual action can prevent certain diseases. During an epidemic of hepatitis B, if someone does not regularly wash their hands or uses unwashed cutlery used by someone who already has hepatitis, they risk coming down with it. If someone does not use a condom with a new, unknown partner, they risk contracting a sexually transmittable disease. If someone travels to regions where certain contagious diseases are endemic and they refuse to be vaccinated against those diseases before their trip, they also have great prospects of becoming infected. There are many examples of how an individual's conscious action can considerably decrease the risk of contracting certain diseases. In all these cases, it cannot be said that contracting this or that disease is beyond the individual's control, that they can do nothing to avoid getting sick. This is what the situation is like with physical diseases.

Veatch's fitting remark that the onset of a number of physical diseases is not (completely) beyond the individual's control, however, has no place where mental disorders are concerned.

I would recall, first of all, that physical disease is a deviation from the structural-functional norms or standards of individual organs or organic systems, while mental disorder is a dysfunctional deviation from the prevailing behavior and belief, sociocultural standard. So much for the character of deviation of those suffering from a particular physical disease and of those who suffer from a particular mental disorder.

It is an open question as to how a person should live and what they should do to decrease the risk of mental disorder. Primary psychiatric prevention includes general (nonspecific) and specific measures. The first includes the prevention of all those somatic diseases that directly or indirectly impair brain tissue, from the prenatal period to almost the last days of life. Nonspecific preventive measures also imply planning and carrying out measures to ensure the harmonious psychophysical development and growth of children and young people, creating healthy work and living environments, promoting a healthy lifestyle, comprehensive care for the elderly, and so forth. So-called mental-hygienic measures such as fostering harmonious relations in the family and work environment, establishing a balance between work and relaxation, fostering positive views, and duly resolving living and development crises, are also part of general primary preventive measures.

The number of *specific* primary preventive measures is comparatively limited. They include giving eugenic advice, avoiding the physical and chemical-toxic impairment of the brain, measures that decrease the risk of (early) development of arteriosclerosis, adding iodine to salt (food) and specific measures to prevent alcoholism and other forms of dependence. Except for these, no other specific measures exist whose application could prevent mental disorder with a high degree of certainty.

What, for example, should a person do (except bear hereditary factors in mind) not to contract schizophrenia, delusional disorder, bipolar disorder, obsessive-compulsive disorder, generalized anxiety disorder, panic disorder, personality disorder? Clinical psychology and psychiatry do not have the slightest reliable answer to these questions.[8]

Indeed, efforts have recently been made to identify so-called premorbid disorders (for example, prepsychotic syndromes). The idea is that early-case finding and early treatment will either prevent the development of fully-blown clinical picture or will prevent disorder from developing. However, as noted by Allen J. Frances, "there has been little attention given to the insoluble problem inherent in any current attempt to identify those at risk for developing more severe disorders. It is simply impossible given available knowledge, to create criteria sets that will be specific enough to avoid also identifying a large pool of false positives" (2009a).[9]

The reader may ask: what about dependence illnesses? Aren't dependence illnesses proof that deviating from the current sociocultural standard is not beyond the reach of one's will? Can't the wide variety of addicts decide for themselves about their dependence? Here is the answer to such a remark. It might be restated that future addicts usually take an addictive substance intentionally the first time or first several times. But as soon as they become dependent, their will ("resolute decision") has limited power to free them of the dependence, should they so decide, and ultimately be cured.

I would add that more and more findings indicate that people who easily become dependent on addictive substances have a special type of metabolism that favors the development of their dependence, which says that willpower has little or no say in whether or not they become addicts.

Individual (Lack of) Responsibility for the Onset of Mental Disorder and Individual Freedom

Veatch's second remark refers to the open question of the expediency of releasing people from blame when they are unable to willfully control their actions and behavior. Questions have been raised about the justification of releasing people from blame for their disease or disorder, which is one of the functions of the medical model.

I would note with regard to Veatch's second remark that we should first ask: who in most cases identifies the value of the blame that people should allegedly feel because they are sick or disordered? The value of the blame for disease and disorder is primarily identified by advocates of alternative lifestyles. They say that releasing people from responsibility for their somatic disease or mental disorder deprives them of dignity, autonomy, their right to be different and their freedom.

The answer to such radical views and demands might be that even though releasing a person with pneumonia or schizophrenia from responsibility for their disease or disorder might be interpreted as removing their autonomy and individual freedom—it is more *inhumane* (and harmful) to blame these sick people for their disease than to consider that they are not responsible for their disease (disorder). Finally, it is very questionable whether those suffering from pneumonia or schizophrenia, with all the health problems and accompanying personal and social difficulties, care more about autonomy and individual freedom which goes with their being responsible for their disease (disorder), or they prefer not to be responsible for their disease (disorder) in their own eyes and the eyes of those around them, regardless of how much this decreases their freedom and autonomy.

Based on several decades of psychiatric experience, I feel that those with physical diseases and mental disorders do not long for the freedom that goes with making them responsible for their disease (disorder).

Table 1.1
The Definition of Mental Disorder

Individual behavioral-functional deviation from the behavior and belief standard of the given society
Impairment of mental functions that either precedes or follows psychological dysfunction
Deviation from the behavior and belief standard of the given society, impairment of mental functions, and psychological dysfunction are beyond an individual's control
Mental suffering

Mental Suffering (Distress)

There is no mental disorder without mental suffering. Famous *la belle indifférence* of people suffering from Hysteria or Conversion Disorder is not a feature of other forms of mental disorder. (By the way, *la belle indifférence* is not adduced among DSM-IV diagnostic criteria for Conversion Disorder either.)[10]

Mental suffering of mentally ill people has multiple origins. It is one of the initial symptoms of mental disorder. It is a component part of an individual's reaction to the impairment of one or more of their mental functions and to psychological dysfunction, respectively. Also, it is a component part of an individual's reaction to (a) their reduced capacity to perform various tasks in numerous domains of private and social life; (b) their learning that they suffer from a mental disorder, or their fear of going mad, and (c) their experiencing of people's negative attitude towards them as mentally ill.

The often cited example of manic and hypo manic patients does not challenge the assertion that mental disorder goes with mental suffering. In those cases of Bipolar Disorder where depressive phases are distinct, depression is an integral part of that particular disorder. Needless to say that depression causes mental suffering. Yet in cases of Manic Episode, no matter how highly elevated their mood is, patients suffer from the consequences of their buying sprees, promiscuous behavior, reckless driving, and of being now and then physically threatening to others and assaultive. Moreover, irritability and enormous and exhaustive energy waste of manic patients does not always produce much enjoyment. At times, the case is quite opposite.

From what I have said so far about the four essential characteristics of mental disorder—deviation from the *individual* and the *social*, impairment in mental functions and psychological dysfunction, events happening against an individual's will, and mental suffering—it is clear that, first, all four elements participate in defining mental disorder, and second, they are interdependent. When someone becomes mentally disordered, they deviate from the *individual* and the *social* because their mental functions are impaired, and one and the other take place against their will.

How My Definition of Mental Disorder Helps Make the Distinction between Mental Disorder and States that May Look Like Mental Disorder

In introductory parts of the text I wrote that those who endeavor to define mental disorder have to provide a definition of it that helps make the distinction between mental disorder and "similar" states ("closest neighbors"). Let us see whether my definition of mental disorder is useful in differentiating mental disorder from (a) deviancy that is not caused by mental disorder; (b) normal psychic reaction, and (c) those mentally healthy states that are characterized by the appearance of one or very rarely two psychotic symptoms.

Deviancy that is Not Caused by Mental Disorder

There are many forms of social deviancy that are not caused by mental disorder. Social pathology deals with them.

There are two features of mental disorder that are not specific to any form of social deviancy other than that caused by mental disturbance: first, the impairment of mental functions that is preceded or followed by psychological dysfunction, and second, the impairment of mental functions as well as psychological dysfunction is beyond an individual's control.

Unlike mental disorder, social deviancy is, as stated, under an individual's control. No matter how strong social pressures are, one can resist them, and not become a social deviant. On the other hand, if due to a set of biological, psychological and sociocultural circumstances, one falls ill from any kind of mental disorder, they cannot by themselves delay or prevent the appearance of mental symptoms.

Briefly, people are free not to become social deviants. They are not free not to go down with mental disorder.

If social deviants other than mentally disordered people mentally suffer they do it due to being in more or less on-going conflict with the given social environment; or, more precisely, due to punitive measures that society undertakes against them. Mental suffering of those who suffer from various kinds of mental disorder is of different origin.

Sociopathological phenomena—as well as other phenomena sociology deals with—are by definition determined by social circumstances. That is not the case with mental disorders.

Mental disorder is a form of social deviancy unlike any other form of social deviancy. Social deviancy is virtually the only feature mental disorder shares with other kinds of social deviancy.

Normal Reactive State

The question of how to differentiate a normal reactive state from a genuine mental disorder has been a contentious issue for a long time. Allan V. Horwitz and Jerome C. Wakefield have recently devoted an entire book to this topic. They picked sadness after loss as an example of nondisordered response to a traumatic event. They dubbed "normal sadness" such kind of sadness, and enumerated its three major characteristics: "it is context-specific; it is of roughly proportionate intensity to the provoking loss; and it tends to end about when the loss situation ends, or else it gradually ceases as coping mechanisms adjust individuals to new circumstances and bring them back into psychological and social equilibrium" (2007: 27-8).

If we take Adjustment Disorder and Post-Traumatic Stress Disorder as the examples of reactive psychic disorders, it is easy to see that either does not meet the last two criteria of a normal reaction. As far as their intensity is concerned the symptoms of Adjustment Disorder as well as the symptoms of Post-Traumatic Disorder are disproportionate to the traumatic event. Moreover, the symptoms of these disorders, in particular their chronic type, do not cease when the traumatic situation ends.

Indeed, the notion of proportionality is critical in decision making about whether a reaction is pathological or not. What does *proportional* mean? The disproportionality of a reaction should be rated, that is, quantified. Reaction is proportional in terms of duration and intensity up to a certain point; from that point on it is disproportional. However, such kind of quantification can be practiced only within the borders of a specific cultural environment. Being made in the context of a particular culture, the measure of proportion is invalid in some other cultural context. Hence, any assessment of the (dis)proportionality of a reaction is culture-bound, i.e., relativistic. In other words, it is baseless to prescribe a universal measure of normal or pathological mourning duration.

The same holds for the intensity of a reaction, or, more accurately, the intensity of its (external) expression. What is a proportional, meaning normal and comprehensible reaction in terms of intensity? A Scandinavian can hardly understand the hustling and bustling of a Palestinian mother who mourns the loss of her six-year-old son. On the other hand, her compatriots would think that she went nuts if the expression of her sorrow was constrained and measured.

Thus, a normal, non-disordered mental reaction to an unfortunate event (life event) is in terms of duration and intensity proportional to the cultural conventions (habits) governing people's behavior following a traumatic event. A pathological reaction is not proportional (Kecmanovic, 2009a). It is of note that most mental disorders are not perceived as reactions to a particular life event.

Psychotic Symptoms in Mentally Healthy Individuals

The phenomenon of psychotic symptoms, primarily auditory hallucinations or delusions, will be discussed below in the text. Here, I only point at two key differences between a mentally disordered person and a person with either auditory hallucinations or delusions as isolated symptoms.

A person with either auditory hallucinations or delusions has impaired mental functions (perception or thinking), but does not have internal psychological dysfunction. Auditory hallucinations or delusions are not component parts of a psychopathological context. The psychopathological context is missing. Besides, such a person is said not to mentally suffer due to auditory hallucinations or delusions. It is not the case with mentally ill people. They do suffer.

To date there have been numerous attempts to define mental disorder. The authors of every such attempt criticized the previous definitions, considering them erroneous or insufficiently precise because, in their view, they could not clearly distinguish the mentally disordered from the non-disordered.

Two attempts to define mental disorder are particularly important: the definition of mental disorder in DSM-III (1980) that appears in slightly altered form in DSM-IV (1994), and the definition of mental disorder presented by Jerome C. Wakefield in his numerous texts ranging from the early 1990s to today.

Definition of Mental Disorder
in the American Classification of Mental Disorders

The operational definition of mental disorder as such is given in the "Introduction" to DSM-III. This was something new, since the first two editions of DSM did not give a definition of mental disorder *per se*.

Since the definition of generic mental disorder is used in formulating the operational definitions of the individual disorders, the definition of mental disorder found in DSM-IV should be cited in its entirety.

"In DSV-IV, each of the mental syndrome or pattern is conceptualized as a clinically significant behavioral or psychological syndrome or pattern that occurs in an individual and that is associated with present distress (e.g., a painful symptoms) or disability (i.e., impairment in one or more important areas of functioning) or with a significantly increased risk of suffering death, pain, disability, or an important loss of freedom. In addition, this syndrome or pattern must not be merely an expectable and culturally sanctioned response to a particular even, for example, the death of a loved one. Whatever its cause, it must currently be considered a manifestation of a behavioral, psychological, or biological dysfunction in the individual. Neither deviant behavior (e.g., political, religious, or sexual) nor conflicts that are primarily between the individual and society are mental disorder unless the deviance or conflict is a symptom of a dysfunction in the individual, as described above" (1994: XXI-XXII).

The DSMs' definition of mental disorder has been criticized from many angles (Sadler, 2002; Horwitz, 2002a; Eriksen and Kress, 2005).[11]

I will focus on one of the numerous deficiencies of DSMs, and not only of DSM's definition of mental disorder: its imprecision, in particular in regard to the grade of intensity of mental disorder indicators, and the failed attempts to decrease or possibly remove it. I have chosen this issue because it exemplifies one of the controversies and dilemmas in contemporary psychiatry.

No Grading of the Intensity of Mental Disorder Indicators

Let us start with my definition of mental disorder. Everyone who has carefully read it might wonder: how much deviation should there be from the behavior and belief standard and how much impairment in mental functions should there be and how much mental disorder should be beyond and individual's control and how much that particular individual should suffer for grounds to speak about mental disorder or suspect that a specific individual is mentally disordered?

Obviously, the question is as to how high *degree of deviation* or *degree of impairment* or *degree of control* or *degree of suffering is required* that someone may be mentally disordered. As soon as there is a grading and not a "yes" or "no," this is a dimensional and not a categorical definition. A specific characteristic extends from the lowest to the highest degree of intensity.

The dimensionality in four of the defining elements of my definition of mental disorder contains one of the important sources of the *arbitrariness* that is an integral part of a psychiatrist's evaluation that someone is mentally disordered. The element of arbitrariness results from the fact that no specification is given as to how much someone should deviate from the behavior and belief standard and how much their mental functions should be impaired, and how much their disorder should be beyond their control and how much they should suffer in order to say that they are (probably) mentally disordered. The problem therefore lies in the fact that no specific *degree of intensity or degree of scope* is mentioned for the individual characteristics of mental disorder that is *required* so as to diagnose someone who presents them in that specific degree as someone who is (probably) mentally disordered.

The definition of mental disorder set out in the "Introduction" to DSM-III and DSM-IV is imprecise in the same sense. It does not specify the degree of distress and impairment in one or more areas of functioning that is specific to mental disorder and the impaired functionality of mentally disordered people.

The authors of the DSMs were conscious of the limitations in the definition of mental disorders they formulated; its imprecision, among other things. So what did they do to decrease or possibly remove the imprecision? First, when defining generic mental disorder and a large number of individual types of mental disorder, they stressed that the symptoms and forms of behavior are *clinically significant*. Second, they introduced the category of *subthreshold disorders*. Both are intended to decrease the imprecision of the definition of mental disorder so as to establish the clearest possible boundary between mentally disordered and non-disordered.

How Significant is "Clinically Significant"?

The very beginning of the definition of generic mental disorder set out in DSMs reads that it is a *clinically significant* syndrome.

What did the authors of the definition want to say when they defined mental disorder as "clinically significant"? Although DSM-III is the result of teamwork, it is well known that Robert L. Spitzer, Professor of Psychiatry at Columbia University, formulated the definition of mental disorder in DSM-III. Spitzer acknowledged in a paper that he wrote with

Jerome C. Wakefield (1999) that the goal of introducing the syntagma "clinically significant" to the definition of mental disorder was to "raise the threshold," making the distress and functional impairment *clinically significant* in order to prevent mentally healthy people from being diagnosed as mentally disordered (the false positive). Did they achieve their goal by stating that distress and impairment in the functioning of one or more areas had to be *clinically significant*?

Before answering this question, I would like to draw the reader's attention to the imprecision of the syntagma *clinically significant*. What criteria can a psychiatrist use to say that someone's distress or impairment in one or more areas of functioning is clinically significant? What does *clinically significant* actually mean? What is the threshold of intensity that should be crossed by someone's distress or impairment in order to be clinically significant? And what about those cases where a psychiatrist is too anxious to be helpful, and as a result finds distress and functional impairment clinically significant in almost everyone who turns to them for help? And what is the probability that two psychiatrists with the same knowledge and experience, who advocate different general concepts about the onset and nature of mental disorders, will evaluate the same symptoms of the same client as clinically significant enough to declare them mentally disordered, and consequently, apply the proper psychiatric therapy? After all, is it at all possible to operationalize something like *clinically significant*?

Finally, can an additional non-operationalized characteristic ("clinically significant") increase the usability of the operational characteristics of individual mental disorders?

All these questions have no reliable answer. This is because in order to get close to the answer we would have to have a criterion to evaluate the accuracy of the answer given by those psychiatrists who evaluated someone's mental disorder using the operational definition of mental disorder with the added criterion of *clinically significant* and the accuracy of answer given by those psychiatrists who used the same operational definition without the added criterion.

Having a criterion of the accuracy of the answer would mean having an instrument to validate the answer. Yet there is no such instrument to validate the definition of mental disorder. The validity of any definition of mental disorder cannot be determined based on the symptoms that someone exhibits or based on other characteristics that are most often mentioned in different definitions of mental disorder, such as: deviation from the individual and the social standard; dysfunction; disability; impairment; unwanted state; deficiency; biologically inferior state; failure to perform naturally selected functions. All these assumed characteristics of mental disorder are difficult to measure. Too many subjective factors take part in the evaluation of whether or not these characteristics are present and how strongly to be able to use them to evaluate the validity of any definition of mental disorder.

Only an objective organic-pathological finding, i.e., a reliable structural-functional correlate can be used to evaluate the validity of a specific definition of mental disorder. But unlike most physical diseases, there is no such objective indicator to validate the definition of mental disorders. As Allen J. Frances put it: "Although there have been many tantalizing putative biological findings for particular disorders, all reflect no more than group mean differences and none has achieved anything close to the needed sensitivity and specificity to qualify as a diagnostic test" (2009b).

This critical discussion of the purposefulness of introducing the element *clinically significant* to the definition of mental disorder has brought us to the point of making any definition of mental disorder (even more) problematic. The reader might now wonder: does the fact that no valid definition of mental disorder exists mean that mental disorder does not exist? The answer is no.

Mental disorders are associated with distress, dysfunction, disability, impairment in one or more areas, deviation from the individual and social standard, and other characteristics, but *cannot be reduced to them* as noted by Allen J. Frances, Thomas A. Widiger and Melvin Sabshin (1991: 15). All these characteristics are simply imperfect indicators of mental disorder and not essential elements of its operational definition. They do not define what is meant by mental disorder but indicate that a specific individual is *probably* mentally disordered, but not for certain.

The introducing the element of "clinically significant" into the operational definition of mental disorder has not helped establish its usefulness nor has it helped decrease the number of mentally non-disordered people who are diagnosed as mentally disordered (the false positives). Therefore, asserting that a specific behavioral or psychological syndrome or pattern must be clinically significant, along with the other characteristics, in order to be a mental disorder should be understood as one more *failed attempt* to remove the element of subjectivity or, if you will, arbitrariness from the evaluation of who is mentally disordered.

Quite to be expected, dilemmas regarding whether someone is mentally disordered primarily or mostly arise when deviation from the *individual* and the *social* and impairment of mental functions is milder.

Harold A. Pincus notes (1998) that he received a letter from Robert L. Spitzer, executive editor of DSM-III, in which he asks whether colleagues from the American Psychiatric Association were pleased that the criterion "clinically significant" was added to the operational definitions of many disorders. We answered him, says Pincus, that we were both pleased and displeased. We were not pleased, explains Pincus, because this diagnostic criterion is imprecise and cannot be determined in the standard way. But, all things considered, we were pleased, continues Pincus, since the criterion "clinically significant" puts the decision as to whether an individual is disordered into the hands of each and every clinician.

I would say that the reasons to be pleased and displeased are both justified. They clearly speak of the arbitrariness involved in deciding that a person is mentally disordered. This arbitrariness, as I have shown, mostly stems from the imprecision of the term *clinically significant*.

Was it at all necessary to additionally characterize a specific syndrome or form of behavior as *clinically significant*?

When it is said that such and such symptoms that have lasted for such a period of time comprise this or that mental disorder, is it necessary to add that this is a clinically significant syndrome or form of behavior? Aren't such symptoms clinically significant by the very fact that they are sufficient to diagnose a specific mental disorder? It is not very likely that someone using the operational definition of a specific mental disorder in the diagnostic procedure thinks that a syndrome or psychological pattern is *clinically insignificant*.

The degree of significance is already contained in the characteristics of both my definition of mental disorder and DSM's definition, which means it is understood that only a more *significant* degree of the intensity of some or all characteristics indicates mental disorder. In a word, it goes without saying that only someone whose symptoms are *significantly* intensive may be mentally disordered. As rightly noted by Massimiliano Aragona: "Clinical significance cannot be a solution in the search of a demarcation criterion; it means nothing *in se*, being only another way to express the mere fact that clinicians have to judge whether a subject is healthy and does not need any treatment or pathological and in need of treatment" (2009).

It is hard to suppose that the authors of those operational definitions of particular mental disorders that start by mentioning that it is a "clinically significant" syndrome, believed that psychiatrists and clinical psychologists would use their operational definitions when diagnosing different types of mental disorders, and at any moment think that an individual's distress and disability should be (clinically) *insignificant*, i.e., *insignificantly* expressed in order to diagnose a specific mental disorder.

Conscious of the fact that adding the syntagma *clinically significant* did not decrease the number of false positive diagnoses, i.e., did not decrease the number of mentally non-disordered diagnosed as mentally disordered, Spitzer himself, in a paper he wrote with Jerome C. Wakefield, entitled "A re-analysis of the reliability of psychiatric diagnosis," critically discusses this attempt to make the diagnosis of a large number of disorders more reliable, and writes: "DSM-IV clinical significance criterion was an attempt to deal with a real and difficult problem with the DSM diagnostic criteria—the potential for false positive diagnoses. However, its wholesale application in DSM-IV is *problematic* and has *no empirical support*" (1999, my emphasis). Robert E. Kendell characterized the introduction of "clinically significant" as a component part of the diagnostic criteria of different types of mental disorders as a "cumbersome strategy that has proved only partially successful in eliminating false positive" (2002: 5).

Are "Subthreshold Disorders" Actually Disorders?

The distinguishing feature of a good classification is that it includes the maximum number of units of the phenomenon being classified. No such ideal classification exists that is comprehensive in the sense that it "covers" all the entities of a specific phenomenon.

Neither DSM-III nor DSM-IV are ideal classifications and so it is quite to be expected that a number of mental disorders are not mentioned in them. I said mental disorders; yet the essential question here is whether disorders that are not under specific names included in the classification as is the case with "not elsewhere classified" or "subthreshold disorders" are actually disorders?

Authors do not agree on the criteria—whether it is the criteria of clinically significant distress and functional impairment or the number of symptoms or how long the symptoms last—that disorders do not satisfy to thus be called *subthreshold.*

Most authors, however, agree that not fulfilling the criteria of "real disorders" primarily refers to the number of symptoms. This means that subthreshold disorders are subthreshold primarily owing to the fact that patients who exhibit them have a smaller number of symptoms than are needed, according to the definition of the corresponding disorder, to be diagnosed as suffering from a "real" mental disorder. For example, Pincus, Davis and McQueen (1999) say that "subthreshold depression" is depression that presents with fewer than five symptoms, and causes clinically significant distress and clinically significant functional impairment. According to DSM-IV, a patient must exhibit five of the nine symptoms mentioned in the classification in order for their psychic disturbance to be diagnosed as *Major Depressive Disorder*. With subthreshold depression, therefore, the patient may exhibit less than five symptoms of depression.

If all the symptoms that are required for the diagnosis of a specific disorder are not exhibited and do not cause clinically significant distress or lead to clinically significant impairment in one or more areas of functioning, then this is a so-called *subclinical disorder*.

Unlike "real" mental disorders, as I have conditionally called those disorders that satisfy all the criteria set out in their operational definition ("suprathreshold disorder" would be a more accurate name, but it, as well as "subthreshold," is rather clumsy), subthreshold mental disorders are not operationally defined. They are defined more negatively than positively. What they have in common is the fact that they *do not* satisfy the symptomatic criteria of a specific "real" mental disorder.

An analysis by Pincus, Davis, and McQueen (1999) of papers dealing with subthreshold depression published in psychiatric journals from January 1, 1991, to the end of December 1995, shows how broad is the spectrum of conditions covered by the concept.

The names given to the same set of symptoms changed from one author to another and the same name was used to designate different sets of symptoms. For example, here are some names used for *subthreshold depression*: minor depression, subthreshold depressive disorder, minor depression with or without mood disorder, subthreshold depressive symptoms, etc.

Furthermore, regarding the number of symptoms needed for a diagnosis of subthreshold depressive disorder, it was most often said that it was enough for the patient to exhibit two symptoms to be diagnosed with this disorder.

Regarding the mandatory duration of the symptoms, some authors did not even use this criterion; others said that the symptoms had to be expressed at least ten days, two weeks, or a full month.

Psychiatrists agree that subthreshold disorders exist but do not agree as to how many symptoms are required, which ones and how long they should be exhibited to say that a patient has this or that subthreshold disorder. They also do not agree on the name of the subthreshold disorder of a "real" disorder.

If we bear in mind this great disagreement about subthreshold disorders, several questions arise that are difficult to answer.

- If there are as many different subthreshold disorders of the same "real" disorder as there are authors who use their own definition of subthreshold disorder, how can we know what subthreshold disorder is?

- How can we tell that a subthreshold disorder is not an insufficiently developed episode or incomplete remission of a basic, i.e., "real" disorder?

- How can we tell whether subthreshold disorders are *sui generis* or attenuated (milder) forms of "real" disorders?

- How can we tell whether a diagnosis of subthreshold disorder only reflects numerous difficulties that could have hindered the diagnosis of the corresponding "real" disorder (the diagnostician's lack of experience, knowledge and skill; insufficient time to make the diagnosis; medication that the patient previously took that "blurred" the clinical picture)?

- How can we tell whether subthreshold disorders are not at all disorders but mental difficulties, mental impediments, "living problems"?

- If subthreshold disorders are the same as what are generally called mental difficulties, mental impediments, mental problems that are usually not denoted as pathological, how can we know which subthreshold disorders or non-pathological mental impediments are produced by a "real" mental disorder?

- How can we know which subthreshold disorders or mental impediments, if not caught on time and properly treated, could result in the corresponding "real" mental disorder (with a certain probability)?[12]

- Bearing in mind the above unresolved issues related to essential aspects of subthreshold disorders, how is it possible to assert, as some authors do—e. g. Wittchen *et al.*, 1998; Judd *et al.*, 1998; Olfson, 1996—that subthreshold disorders are two to four times more numerous than "real" disorders?

I have shown that the additional designation of a disorder or syndrome as *clinically significant* is clinically insignificant at heart. *Clinically significant* is also part of the definition of subthreshold disorder. What was said regarding this addition to the definition of "real" mental disorders, i.e., that it does not contribute to their more precise definition, also holds for subthreshold disorders. This practically means that a diagnosis of subthreshold disorder, or specifically subthreshold depression, could be made based on only two symptoms that last ten days or two weeks; for example, based on the fact that someone is depressed and has lost interest in things that previously interested them, or that someone is depressed and does not sleep as well as they used to.

When the reader reads this "minimalist" definition of subthreshold depression, I am sure they wonder: according to these criteria, hasn't almost everyone had subthreshold or mild depression once or even more times in their life?!

It is widely believed that subthreshold disorders appear only within the classification of categorically defined disorders. Categorically or operationally defined disorders have a *defined* mandatory number of specific symptoms, mandatory length of duration of the symptoms, and defined diseases or circumstances that must be excluded as the possible cause of these specific symptoms. Disorders that are *below the defined threshold* in one or more of these characteristics are *subthreshold*. But even when disorders are dimensionally defined, there must be a cutoff point for each of the dimensions used to define a specific disorder. Above that point a characteristic is considered pathological and below that point it is considered normal, mentally non-disordered. Therefore, it is to be assumed that if a classification were made with dimensionally defined mental disorders, it would have *subthreshold disorders* too.

Subthreshold disorders belong to the rather wide gray zone between mentally disordered and mentally non-disordered states, in a word, between (mentally) normal and pathological. More than one hundred years ago Emil Kraepelin acknowledged this murky zone. He wrote: "Whenever we try to mark out the frontier between mental health and disease, we find a neutral territory in which imperceptible change from the realm of normal mental life to that of obvious derangement takes place" (1917: 296).

Psychiatrists have always shown interest in this undefined area. When they go into this area, they cross the boundary of their competence, knowledge and skill, and ultimately psychiatrize distress, mental adversities, problems in living that are not pathological and do not reflect mental disorder. That is one view. The other view is that psychiatrists should broaden their areas of interest and professional intervention because by doing so they can relieve people from distress, prevent the possible development of "real" mental disorders and assist them to get back on their own feet.

Numerous arguments can be cited for each of these two positions. Regardless of the side they come from all arguments, directly or indirectly, reveal how imprecisely defined is this broad field between mentally non-disordered and disordered.

It should come as no surprise that this "mid-area" is even less clearly defined than the area of the pathological and the area of the normal. When the insufficiently precise definitions of two subjects are used to define a third, the result can only be even fuzzier.

Wherever there is great disagreement regarding the nature and boundaries of a phenomenon, the door is wide open to arbitrariness, improvisation, and a wide variety of abuse with a wide variety of goals.

Issues related to subthreshold disorders have been extensively discussed over the last few years. The ever stronger interest in subthreshold disorders reflects the growing awareness of the imperfections of DSMs, and of difficulties in demarcating the individual mental disorders in particular. It is also in tune with emerging ideas that early intervention in psychosis might be feasible and beneficial.

I have gone into the definition of mental disorders as *clinically significant* and *subthreshold* mental disorder in order to show, first, how difficult it is to precisely define ("demarcate") mental disorder and non-disorder, and second, how past attempts by the authors of DSMs to define individual mental disorders as precisely as possible have not produced the expected result.

Acknowledging the arbitrariness of *any* specification of the degree of an individual's deviation from the behavior and belief standard of a given environment and the degree of impairment in mental functions as well as the degree of distress and of not having control over one's mental disorder of that particular person that is needed to suspect that they are mentally disordered, I have not tried, like the authors of DSMs, to determine any additional criteria that would increase the precision of "degree of deviation" and "degree of impairment," and thereby that of my definition of mental disorder.

Allen J. Frances, in the preface to *Philosophical Perspectives on Psychiatric Diagnostic Classification* (1994: VI), notes that although many have tried (including the authors of DSM-III), no one has succeeded in developing a list of infallible criteria to define mental disorder. Frances is not alone in claiming that there is no satisfactory definition of mental disorder and that most likely there never will be. For example, Dominic Murphy (2006: 6) feels that there is no satisfactory definition of mental disorder in contemporary literature on mental disorder. Derek Bolton, author of a monograph on mental disorder, on his part, states that "we might never get a completely coherent theory about mental disorder that could be used to say when mental life is 'ordered' and when it is 'disordered'" (2008: 35).

Not for a moment do I think that my definition of mental disorder is above criticism. I understand it as one more attempt to define what distinguishes mental disorder from similar or only seemingly similar phenomena.

As stated, Jerome C. Wakefield is the author of a definition of mental disorder that has attracted considerable attention in the past dozen years from those involved in defining mental disorder. Wakefield's definition is one more attempt to demarcate mental disorder (as clearly as possible) from non-disorder. The reader will see on the following pages just how (un)successful he was.

Mental Disorder as Biological Disadvantage and as Not Performing Naturally Selected Functions

The idea that biological weakness or disadvantage is an important characteristic of mental disorder, and the idea that impairment in functions selected naturally by evolution is one of the basic characteristics of mental disorder are not far from each other.

The most vocal advocates of the first idea are Glenis J. Scadding (1967) and Robert E. Kendell (1975b), and of the second, Donald F. Klein (1978), Christopher Boorse (1975, 1976) and Jerome C. Wakefield (1992, 1996, 1999a, 2007).

Scadding, a doctor (not a psychiatrist) who has written numerous praiseworthy papers on nosology, asserts that "in medical discourse, the name of a disease refers to the sum of the abnormal phenomena displayed by a group of living organisms in association with a specified common characteristic, or set of characteristics, by which they differ from the norm for their species in such a way as to place them at biological disadvantage" (1967, my emphasis). Scadding himself did not specify what he meant by "biological disadvantage."

In addition to including deviation from the norm (abnormal phenomena), Scadding's definition includes two new elements as characteristics of disease or disorder. First, Scadding says that it is deviating from the norms of the species to which the living organism belongs, and second, it is deviating from the norm that puts the organism at a biological disadvantage. Both these findings are correct. First, an individual always deviates from the norms of the species to which it belongs and not some other species, and second, it is a fact that disease puts a sick individual at a disadvantage.

standard. "I propose that evolutionary theory allows us to infer such a standard—suboptimal functioning—and further allows us to objectively specify the optimum." Klein continues, "this often allows us to state that something is biologically wrong, not simply that is rare or objectionable" (1978).

When discussing definitions that see disease as a biological disadvantage, what draws attention in Klein's definition is the assertion that the definition of disease is derivable from the idea of optimal biological functioning within the concept of evolution. My remarks on Klein's definition of disease follow.

First, it is very difficult to define optimal biological functioning. (This remark also refers to Talcott Parsons' definition of disease, since he defined disease before Klein as a suboptimal level, although primarily of social functioning.) Is it the optimal biological functioning of individual organs, organic systems or of the entire organism? If *optimal* denotes the best level of biological functioning, then for the liver or kidney this would be the structural-functioning status of these organs that is found in the greatest number of people in a given environment. This would also be the average level of biological functioning. And is average the same as optimal? And isn't the concept of *optimal* in this case defined by what we currently know to be the optimal values of tests of the functional work of individual organs or organic systems. In other words, optimal would be what we currently think is optimal. In several years, today's optimal might become non-optimal.

The change in optimal blood pressure values is a good example of this last assertion. Until several years ago, 140 millimeters of mercury was the optimal upper value of blood pressure for people over forty. Today the optimal upper blood pressure value for people of the same age is not 140 but 120. (It is hard to tell how much influence pharmaceutical companies had in changing this value, because every decrease in the desired blood pressure is accompanied by greater sales of medicine to lower blood pressure.)

Or the example of what is optimal for the entire organism. Parameters can be used to establish whether there is a difference between someone's (calendar) age and biological age. Calendar age is how old one is and biological age is expressed by average values of the functional tests of a large number of people of a certain age in a certain environment. Most people's calendar and biological age are approximately the same. Simply put, most people are as biologically old as their number of years. In this case as well, what is average equals what is ideal.

The question now arises as to what is the optimal biological age of an organism compared to its calendar age? There is no answer to this question and it is therefore hard to derive the concept of disease from the concept of optimal or suboptimal biological functioning.

Christopher Boorse by his interpretation of the terms "illness" and "disease" is closest to the Wakefield's definition of disease (disorder). For this author, "illness" depends on value judgment about suffering or deviance, whereas "disease" is something objective in so far as it indicates how much one fails to conform to the "species-typical design" of humans. Such kind of design, as Murphy (2005) put it, specifies the component parts of the body and the functions they perform. And "function" is understood in evolutionary terms as failure to contribute to survival and reproduction.

Wakefield's Definition of Mental Disorder

The most cited of the above-mentioned authors is certainly Jerome C. Wakefield, Professor of Social Work at New York University, New York City. He opened wide the door to the concept of evolution in defining disease in numerous papers in the past twenty years. The fact that an entire issue of the *Journal of Abnormal Psychology* (1999) was devoted to a critical review of Wakefield's approach indicates, *inter alia*, the importance of Wakefield's concept among psychologists and psychiatrists who have dealt with the definition of mental disorder.

Wakefield feels that mental disorder cannot be defined independent from the definition of somatic disease. "Any proposal to define 'mental disorder' in a way unique to psychiatry that does not fall under the broader medical concept of disorder fails to address this issue" (2007).

He contends (1992) that disease is *harmful dysfunction* (*HD*) and defines dysfunction as the failure of internal mechanisms to perform their naturally-selected functions, i.e., functions that evolution intended for them to perform. This *harmful* in the syntagma *harmful dysfunction* indicates that this dysfunction harms the individual. "A condition is a mental disorder if and only if (a) condition causes some harm or deprivation of benefit to the person as judged by the standards of the person's culture (the value criterion), and (b) the condition results from the inability of some mental mechanisms to perform its natural function, wherein a natural function is an effect that is part of the evolutionary explanation of the existence and structure of the mental mechanism (the explanatory function)" (1992).

Wakefield maintains that using the criterion of evolutionary dysfunction can successfully differentiate diseases from states that are not diseases. For example, if the heart cannot pump blood, then this is disease because the heart's inability to pump blood expresses the heart's inability to perform one of its natural functions. "Pumping is a natural function of the heart because it is clear from the nature of the mechanisms involved and the role of pumping in broader vital processes that the pumping cannot be an accidental by-product of having a heart but rather must somehow be part of the explanation of why the heart exists and how it is structured" (1999a).

Such an analysis inevitably leads to the question: what type of process could be responsible for this ostensible design in natural processes without someone to create such a design. Wakefield gives the following answer. "Evolutionary theory provides the only plausible scientific account that presently exists of how the natural functions of a mechanism can explain the existence and structure of the mechanism (earlier accounts of the same phenomenon include Aristotle's 'final causes' and Aquinas's 'God's intentions'). According to the evolutionary theory, some effects of a mechanism were beneficial to past organisms and thereby caused the natural selection of the mechanism." Therefore, Wakefield argues, those effects are part of an explanation of the existence and structure of the mechanism in present-day organisms. Such naturally selected effects are the natural functions of the respective mechanisms." And where does this argument lead to? "This (…) theoretical argument leads to the conclusion that disorders are failures of mechanisms to perform functions for which they were naturally selected" (1999a).

As stated, Wakefield feels that the definition of mental disorder is a component part of the definition of every disease. In this regard, he asserts that when a mechanism that deals with motivation, perception, thought, emotion, language, learning, socialization and other basic psychological functions fails, i.e., when it fails to perform the function that natural selection has determined it should perform, mental dysfunction appears. If this mental dysfunction harms the individual, we have mental disorder, writes Wakefield (2005: 84).

Wakefield's attempt to link two concepts in the definition of disease: the scientific judgment of the inability of internal mechanisms to perform their naturally-selected functions, on the one hand, and the socially determined valuation of the harm to the organism, on the other, is praiseworthy.

There has been considerable discussion of Wakefield's definition of disease in recent years. Many remarks have been made. Some authors (for example, Fulford, 1999; Lilinfield and Merino, 1999; Richters and Hinshaw, 1999) have appraised Wakefield's definition of disease as simply unacceptable. Some (for example, Spitzer, 1999) have positively valued Wakefield's linking the concept of dysfunction with the theory of evolution in the definition of mental disorder.

Wakefield had three goals in mind with his definition of mental disorder: first, to firmly ground the concept of mental disorder in a universal, established, biological theory and thus make the definition of mental disorder less vulnerable to attack by psychiatric critics who state that the definition of mental disorder used by psychiatrists can be applied to many forms of socially deviant behavior that is therefore pathologized; second, to define the concept of dysfunction which is key to many definitions of mental disorder; and third, to leave one part of mental disorder linked to the current social environment and its values.

He reached the first goal by basing his definition of mental disorder on the law of natural selection, i.e., the failure of biological and mental mechanisms to perform functions selected for them by evolution. The second goal was reached when he linked dysfunction, as a key category in defining mental disorder, to natural evolution which has a universal nature. The third goal was reached when he said that mechanisms' failure to perform functions established by evolution is not sufficient to result in behavior (in the broadest sense) that would be evaluated as mentally disordered. Such behavior had to harm the individual and, consequently, society. In a word, it had to harm the individual in the specific sociocultural environment.

Wakefield started from an assertion shared by many authors concerned with defining disease, and that is that an individual's dysfunctionality (or lesser functionality) is an essential characteristic of disease (disorder). The following question always arises in this regard: what is function and what is dysfunction? More specifically, what functions are disordered? One of the serious criticisms to the definition of mental disorder set out in DSMs is that there is no explanation of "dysfunction" that holds an important place in the definition of mental disorder. Let us recall that DSM-IV states: "Whatever its original cause, it must currently be considered a manifestation of a behavioral, psychological, or biological dysfunction *in* the individual" (1994: XXI-XXII, my emphasis). This sentence is not followed by an explanation of dysfunction or what the authors mean by dysfunction.

In order to find a reliable and stable criterion to establish good, "normal" functions, Wakefield linked the concept of normal function to a stable, independent entity, and that is natural selection or evolution. He feels that normal function is one that results from natural selection; it is the function that was selected in the evolutionary process. Dysfunction is the inability to perform a naturally selected function.

Briefly, Wakefield links dysfunction, which is not an essentialist concept, to an essentialist concept—natural selection, which comes from evolutionary biology.

Critique of Wakefield's Concept of Mental Disorder

Many questions arise regarding Wakefield's definition of mental disorder. I will set out but a few of them.[13]

First, Wakefield did not succeed in completely freeing the first part of the definition of mental disorder from value judgment. This part (the failure of a mechanism to perform functions defined by evolution) was to guarantee the scientific, objective, value-neutral nature of the definition of mental disorder. Here is why. The theory of natural selection is one of many possible theories that can be used to explain the origin and nature of mentally disordered behavior. If natural selection is chosen from among many theories when trying to define the origin and nature of mental disorder, then this means it is considered better, more suitable than other theories and this is nothing other than making a value judgment that such and such a theory is better, more suitable, and more accurate.

Second, the entire construct of Wakefield's definition of mental disorder is based on a hypothesis. We assume that a specific behavior, way of thinking, feeling, reasoning and so on results from and is the manifestation of the failure (dysfunction) of one or more naturally selected functions. Therefore, the essence of such a definition of mental disorder is not found in specific symptoms, a specific behavior, something visible and observable that can be described, but is something invisible, inaccessible to the senses, simply a theory, a hypothesis.

This practically means that using Wakefield's definition cannot increase the reliability of the diagnosis of mental disorder, which was the basic goal of the theoretical definition of mental disorder set out in DSMs. This drawback disqualifies Wakefield's definition of mental disorder, particularly in the eyes of research psychiatrists (Bolton, 2008: 132-134).

Bearing that in mind, it is rather surprising that Robert L. Spitzer, who has done so much to increase the reliability of psychiatric diagnoses, considers (1999) Wakefield's concept of mental disorder as harmful dysfunction so important that it should be included in DSM-V. It is no less surprising that Robert E. Kendell, asserts that it would be "worthwhile revising the basis DSM definition of mental disorder in light of Wakefield's (1992) cogent analysis of the concept" (2002: 5) .

Third, Wakefield himself (2005: 84) rightly says that we still know so little about the psychological mechanisms (only psychological? D.K.) that have to do with mental functions (motivation, perception, thought, emotions, language, learning, socialization, etc.), but that "through observation of human capacities we can infer that they exist."

The question that arises is how we can know that a mechanism having to do with specific mental functions has failed and that there is dysfunction, if we do not know the mechanism itself or do not know very much about it?

Fourth, how can we know whether a specific clinical syndrome results from the failure of specific mechanisms to perform their naturally selected functions or results from an inherited or acquired response to specific circumstances in the given social environment, or is even an adaptive response formed by evolution? (Bolton, 2008: 131)

How could we manage to provide the right answer? (If there is only one right answer?) According to Wakefield, we only talk about mental disorder when mechanisms do not perform functions set out for them by evolution. Yet, how could one rule out other options? Why couldn't mental disorder be perceived as an inherited dysfunctional response to stimuli coming either from within the organism or from outside? Or as an evolutionary determined adaptive response? How could one screen out unsubstantiated claims that, for example, claim schizophrenia or depression is meaningful when looked at from an evolutionary perspective? And how could one empirically test these options?

Fifth, is it possible to separate the biological from the social-psychological as Wakefield does in his definition of mental disorder? The environment is a component part of the concept of natural selection and evolution. But the environment has never been only natural. It has always been primarily social, and also variable, and is particularly so today. This statement has to do with the environment of people who live for a longer period in one place or one country and especially those who frequently change their place of residence and move from one end of the planet to another. There are many such people today and there will be even more in the years to come.

Biological changes and psychological changes that are based on biological changes arise from mutation processes that are mostly random. Kept are the characteristics caused by biological changes that enable the best adaptation, coping and survival in a given environment. When this environment quickly changes, it is very difficult to say whether there is enough time to test the adaptation potential of changes caused by mutation, to see whether and how much they help in "survival of the fittest." Consequently, it is hard to say which functions are designed by evolution.

Sixth, it is also difficult to tell which of the functions of different mental abilities (mental mechanisms), are completely determined by the evolutionary process and which are only partially determined by it. A separate issue is whether and how much complex psychological systems, such as attachments to other people, acquiring a reputation in society, and gaining new experience, are determined and formed by evolution. Who can say for certain when these motivational or functional systems fail, when they are over-expressed and when they are under-expressed?

For example, when does the anxiety system fail? When it does not perform the function that was naturally selected, i.e., when it is activated in the absence of danger or when it is too strongly activated when danger appears? And one should not neglect that what people in one environment perceive as danger, is not considered danger for people from another environment.

In fact, mental functioning is never only an evolutionary-genetic matter. It is simultaneously determined by environmental, sociocultural and individual factors. This is why it is wrong to look at it from the aspect of its evolutionary specifications alone.

There are no grounds to separate functions formed by natural selection from those that are socially constructed, as Wakefield did in his definition of mental disorder. His design to find solid, value-neutral support in natural selection as something that is biological and universal is therefore questionable.

Seventh, a specific trait or characteristic could have been formed by our ancestors as a result of evolutionary events. But in changed natural-social conditions it did not have to fail even if it lost its potential to adapt. It has remained to the present because it was not harmful. (Gold and Kirmayer, 2007) The specific trait used to be an adaptational advantage in the fight for survival. Today it has lost that property.

In light of the above, how can we tell whether the function of that specific trait or mental ability is dysfunctional or whether the function has lost its adaptational advantage but has been preserved because it is not harmful? To recall: for Wakefield, a specific somatic or mental function is normal when it performs the way it was evolved to perform and is abnormal when it does not perform the way evolution intended it to perform.

Eighth, when I set out my concept of mental disorder, I said that the degree of intensity of the individual elements of the definition of mental disorder was an open question. This same question, within the context of Wakefield's definition of disorder, would read: *how big* does the disorder of naturally selected functions have to be and *how much* should this or that dysfunction harm the individual?

Ninth, generally speaking, an extremely large number of mechanisms and circumstances take part in generating and shaping mental disorders. Many of these mechanisms are not based on the biological systems that Wakefield primarily had in mind when he formulated his concept of disease as "harmful dysfunction," and defined dysfunction as the failure of mechanisms to perform their naturally selected functions.

It seems to me that Perring (2005), author of the unit on "mental illness" in the Stanford Encyclopedia of Philosophy best summarized the remarks that can be made about Wakefield's concept of disease as "harmful dysfunction." First, in most of medicine, and particularly in psychiatry, we simply do not know what can be considered natural from the evolutionary viewpoint. Second, even if we had a comprehensive theory of evolutionary psychology, is it appropriate to use this very theory when evaluating whether certain states are normal? The question is completely open as to whether medical experts should base their judgments on the view that states are natural so long as they help advance the species. Third, evolutionary biology and psychology do not provide the only possible model on which to base an evaluation of what is health and what is disease. Therefore, when choosing between two or more models, we must use values. This means that if we decide to use evolutionary psychology as a basis for judging what is healthy and what disordered, our choice will not be based on purely scientific, objective criteria, but will have a value or normativity element.

These are reasons why Wakefield's assertion cannot be taken at face value that only evolutionary theory makes it possible to define dysfunction in a value-neutral, objective ("scientific") manner.

How to Make Demarcation between
Mental Disorder and Non-Disorder More Unclear

To date, demarcation between mental disorder and non-disorder has been questioned in various ways. Indeed, not all of those who made the line between mental disorder and non-disorder more unclear did it intentionally. In some cases, that was the initial idea. In others, the blurring of the difference between disorder and non-disorder was a fall-out of a concept that did not initially target demarcation between disorder and non-disorder.

Psychosis has been used as an epitome of mental disorder in virtually all cases of clouding the disorder—non-disorder difference. In other words, in the first place the demarcation between *psychosis* and mental health has been disputed. As if fuzziness of the demarcation between non-psychotic states, on the one hand, and mental health, on the other, went without saying.

As the reader will see in the text below, the disputing of the dissimilarity of psychosis and mental health has been performed in numerous ways: by the inversion of the meaning of mental disorder and non-disorder; by drawing on the findings that show that, contrary to what is believed, psychotic symptoms such as auditory hallucinations and delusions are not rare in non-psychiatric populations; by denying the specificity of psychotic experience; by arguing that the difference between psychotic behavior and experience, on the one hand, and behavior and experience of mentally sound people, on the other, is just a matter of degree, and by showing how psychiatrists are inept at differentiating those who are genuinely disordered from those who pretend to be disordered but are in fact mentally healthy.

I will focus on the following most relevant forms of disputing demarcation between mental disorder and non-disorder that have been articulated in the last half a century.

- Laing's way of deconstructing madness;
- The use of the existence of auditory hallucinations and delusions in non-psychiatric populations for the purpose of deconstructing madness;
- Devereux's way of deconstructing madness;
- Psychiatrists are not able to differentiate between those who pretend to be mentally ill and those who are genuinely disordered.

Laing's Inversion of the Relation between Mental Health and Illness

Ronald D. Laing, a Scottish psychiatrist, is a passionate critic of psychiatry. He questions fundamentals of psychiatry such as diagnostics, treatment, and mental institution. His name is associated with antipsychiatry. As Laing from one book to another modifies and even changes his view of various phenomena related to mental disorder and psychiatry, it is not easy to say how he actually conceptualizes mental health and illness and the relation between them. I will focus on his book *The Politics of Experience* (1967) in which he most concisely defines his concept of mental disorder and non-disorder.

Laing argues that psychosis is an individual's survival strategy in an inhuman social environment. "The experience and behaviour that gets labelled schizophrenic is *a special strategy that a person invents in order to live in an unlivable* situation" (1967: 95, emphasis in original). In other words, a person who lives in an inhuman society preserves their mental health by becoming psychotic. Those who are held sane are, in fact, insane. "The 'normally' alienated person, by reason of the fact that he acts more or less like everyone else, is taken to be sane" (1967: 24). Yet their sanity is a far cry from an authentic human life. Therefore, psychotic people who break contact with such a reality, Laing argues, should be viewed as healthier than those who are widely considered mentally sound. "Madness need not be all breakdown. It may also be breakthrough. It is potentially liberation and renewal as well as enslavement and existential death" (1967: 110).

Such a view of looking at madness raises many questions which Laing is short of answering.

First, there are only a small number of people who are psychotic in a society. The question arises as to why only these people react by psychosis to an inhuman social milieu, while the rest of the population does not? Do they have a proclivity to psychosis or psychosis *diathesis*? If that is the case then their psychosis could be accounted for at least partly by an internal condition that has nothing to do with the character of the social-political ambience. Or maybe they develop psychosis because they are more vulnerable to imperfections of the existing social milieu. And how could we know which of these two options in regard to causality is more valid, if valid at all, in each particular case?

Second, is the reaction to an inhuman social milieu the only mechanism underlying the development of psychosis, or can people become psychotic for other reasons, as well? If the latter is the case, would it be clinically possible to distinguish psychosis which is instrumental in preserving one's mental health from psychosis that robs a person of their capacity to change themselves and the miliey they live in?

Third, is the flight into madness the result of an individual's (conscious) decision or does it occur spontaneously? If it is the result of a decision, this means that one can go mad when they want to go mad. However, that is not how one goes mad. Madness occurs beyond one's will. It has nothing to do with whether we want or do not want to go mad. On the other hand, if one goes mad spontaneously, i.e., as a reaction to an inhuman social ambience, then madness, which Laing talks about, is a reactive madness. If that is the case then Laing introduces a dichotomous concept of madness (schizophrenia): reactive and non-reactive schizophrenia. And would it be possible to clinically differentiate them? And would the change of the existing social milieu, i.e., humanizing and de-alienating it be the treatment of choice for the putative reactive schizophrenia?

Laing's inversion of health and illness does not rest on solid conceptual grounds. The least of all it is clinically befitting.

One thing is for sure, his vision of mental disorder and non-disorder completely blurs the frontier between them. In fact, it confers a different value to each one. What is regarded as positive (health) gets a negative connotation, and what is regarded as negative (illness) becomes positive, to some degree at least.

After reading *The Politics of Experience* one cannot help but ask themselves, who is mad, after all; and is there such a thing as madness? That is the result of the deconstruction of madness the Laing way.

Mentally Healthy People Have Auditory Hallucinations

There have been reports of mentally well people having auditory hallucinations.[14] Lately, these findings have been exploited to make the frontier between mental disorder and non-disorder even more unclear and, in the last instance, to deconstruct madness.

There are two streams of interest in auditory hallucinations that have mentally well people: one is *popular* and another *scientific*.

Let us first have a look at the origin and development of popular interest in auditory hallucinations. A television presentation of non-psychiatric patients who talked about hearing voices is said to have incited a huge response of the TV auditorium, first of all of people who hear voices. This TV program was screened on Dutch television in the mid-eighties. Marius Romme, a Professor of Social Psychiatry, and Sandra Escher, a science journalist, were the presenters. These two persons established the Hearing Voices Movement in 1987. Since then same or similar movements were formed in all western countries. Today, a network called INTERVOICE (The International Network for Training, Education and Research into Hearing Voices) coordinates the activities of, and provides support to, a great many individual organizations and networks designed for hearers of voices.

There are several main guiding principles of hearing voices movements. First, the frequency of hallucinations in mentally healthy people demands due weight to be assigned to this phenomenon. Between 6 percent and 9 percent of mentally non-disordered people are said to hear voices. This is much more than the number of people suffering from Schizophrenic Disorder or Manic-Depressive Psychosis. Up to half a percent of the population suffers from Schizophrenic Disorder and up to half a percent from Manic-Depressive Psychosis. About two-thirds of the former are said to have auditory hallucinations, and about 15 percent of the latter to have the same kind of perceptual disturbance.

Second, hearing voices is not a pathological phenomenon. Therefore, psychiatrists and clinical psychologists should not deal with people who hear voices. If voices hearers approach mental health workers, they will pathologize voices, consider them as the manifestation of an underlying mental disorder, and consequently treat them with drugs. And that is the last thing that hearers of voices need.

Third, those who hear voices should not regard voices as something bad that they should be ashamed of, as something they should try to get rid of. On the contrary, hearers of voices should heed voices. Voices are a part of their personality, of their personal history, and therefore they should be preserved and nurtured. The more so as voices, like dreams, carry a specific message. Voices hearers should analyse their voices. Efforts should be made to decode their meaning, and the deciphered meaning should be used for the benefit of psychological development and mental health of the respective individual. Dialogue should be established even with threatening voices, i.e., voices that command an individual to harm themselves and/or other people. The reason for their threatening tone should be revealed, and then strategy invented how to cope with such voices.

I want to draw the reader's attention to two aspects (and consequences) of the ideology of hearing voices movements. First, even though it is of utmost importance to make an as clear as possible distinction between auditory hallucinations in mentally sound and mentally disturbed people, the ideologues of hearing voices movements do not pay due attention to it.

Needless to say that psychiatrists and clinical psychologist are the only persons who are qualified to make such distinction. And how will they be able to do this job, if hearers of voices have been advised to shun mental health workers, to keep distance from them? Yet the consequences of not providing proper psychiatric assistance to those who besides having voices are mentally ill are realistically and potentially serious.

Fourth, the leaders of the hearing voices movements do not restrain from asserting that the fact that such a large number of ("otherwise") normal people hear voices, that is, have a psychotic symptom, indicates that psychosis (madness, mental disorder) is not as different from mental health as it is widely believed. Thereby they tend to blur the demarcation between mental disorder and non-disorder, or to make it even more fuzzy, to say the very least.

The scientific approach to the phenomenon of mentally sound people having voices differs from the popular one in that its protagonists use methodologically sound methods to assess how frequent auditory hallucinations are in non-psychiatric populations, and to trace down the origin of hallucinations in mentally sound people. Scholars who deal with the phenomenon of normal people hearing voices usually tend to draw (more) explicit and far-reaching conclusions from the finding that a portion of the non-psychiatric population hears voices than the leaders of hearing voices movements do. Also, they are seemingly more interested in antagonizing "traditional" psychiatric views of hallucinations as, in most cases, pathological, and in urging psychiatrists to change their "outdated" views of hallucinations.

Mentally Healthy People Have Delusions

There are fewer texts dealing with delusions in non-psychiatric populations than texts dealing with hallucinations in this kind of population. Yet the former are not rare, either.[15]

On the basis of the analysis of 15 research papers Daniel Freeman, a Consultant Clinical Psychologist in the South London and Maudsley NHS Foundation Trust, maintains that there is conclusive evidence that delusions in the general population by far outnumber psychotically disturbed people. About 1 to 3 percent of the general population have delusions of such a degree of severity that make them comparable to delusions that psychotic patients have. Another 5 to 6 percent of the general populace have delusions of less severity. "Although less severe, these beliefs are still associated with a range of social and emotional difficulties." Finally, "a further 10 to 15 percent of the non-clinical population have fairly regular delusional ideation" (2006).

Michelle L. Esterberg and Michael Compton (2009), on their part, maintain that, in spite of variations in the assessment of the frequency of psychotic experiences in the general population, that occur most likely due to difference in samples, definitions, and diagnostic instruments, "the estimates lend credibility to the notion that psychotic symptoms occur among a much broader segment of the population than just those with traditionally defined psychotic disorders."

In *Paranoia. The 21st Century Fear* (2008) Daniel Freeman and Jason Freeman write (2008: 10-11) that paranoia is so widespread "that around 15-20 percent of the population have frequent paranoid thoughts." Then they add: "But a further 3-5 percent have severe paranoia—what psychologists call persecutory delusions."

It is worth noting the way in which Freeman and Freeman use the notions of "paranoia" and "severe paranoia." Paranoia is common, they claim. "Paranoia is so prevalent that there is a very good chance that, at some point in your life, you will be among the 25 percent" (2008: 11). On the other hand, severe paranoia "is serious enough to need medical treatment." Thus, it turns out that the only difference between the former and the latter is that the latter is severe. In other words, the only difference between paranoia of every fourth citizen and paranoia as a mental disorder is the degree of severity (of paranoia).

Since the term "delusion" appears as the key notion in the further deliberation it would be worthwhile to define it. Delusion or a delusional idea is an unfounded belief or conviction, which is personally important to those who have it. They are not ready to renounce it in spite of the evidence to the contrary. Delusional ideas have an impact on other mental functions of those who harbour them. A delusional idea is not shared by other community or society members.

This kind of definition of delusion is close to the definition of delusion that Karl Jaspers specified.

In the context of discussing implications and consequences of the appearance of delusions in the non-clinical population, the question as to whether the delusion should be conceived of dimensionally or categorically is of utmost importance.

The question is as follows: is delusion something new in an individual's mental life, something that is qualitatively different from other mental occurrences and phenomena, or is delusion but an accentuated form of something that occurs in normal psychic life. In the latter case, there is only a quantitative difference between normal psychic phenomena and delusion.

In order to make clear what a dimensional definition of delusion looks like I will set out how delusion is graded (ranged) in instruments designed for the assessment of delusion(s). I will give three examples.

Jim van Os, Manon Hansen, Rob B. Bijl et al. (2000) use *Composite International Diagnostic Interview* (CIDI) to classify members of a sample of 7,076 people, aged between 18 and 64, into those who are psychiatric patients and those who are not psychiatric patients.

The authors name three types of delusions: "'True', psychiatrist-related delusion"; "Not clinically relevant delusion (not bothered by it and not seeking help for it)"; "Secondary Delusion (result of somatic disease or ingestion of drugs)," and "No delusion—plausible explanation is the fourth option." ("Symptom is not really a symptom because there appears to be some plausible explanation for it.")

Hallucinations have been graded in the same way.

The first type of delusion—and of hallucination, for that matter—is supposed to be *more intense* than the second one.

Here is the second example of delusion rating. Louise C. Johns, Mary Canon, Nicola A. Singleton et al. (2004) use *Psychosis Screening Questionnaire* (PSQ) to assess the presence and the degree of expression of individual psychotic symptoms. The authors rate paranoia as follows: "Over the past year, have there been times when you felt that people were against you?," "Have there been times when you felt that people were deliberately acting to harm you or your interests," and "Have there been times when you felt that a group of people were plotting to cause serious harm or injury."

The *intensity of paranoia* is supposed to rise from the first to the third question.

Finally, here is how Daniel Freeman (2007) conceptualizes the multidimensional nature of delusions. He differentiates seven characteristics of delusions: unfounded; firmly held; resistant to change; preoccupying; distressing; interferes with social functioning, and involves personal reference. I will set out variability in individual characteristics, as described by Freeman. The mention of the variability in the three first characteristics of delusions will suffice to give the reader an idea of how the author rates the *intensity of characteristics*.

- *Unfounded.* "For some individuals the delusions reflect a kernel of truth that has been exaggerated (e g. the person has a dispute with the neighbour but now believes that the whole neighbourhood is monitoring them and will harm them). It can be difficult to determine whether the person is actually delusional. For others the ideas are fantastic, impossible and clearly unfounded (e. g. the person believes that s/he was present at the time of the Big Bang and is involved in battles across the universe and heavens)."

- *Firmly held.* "Beliefs can vary from being held with 100 percent conviction to only occasionally being believed when the person is in a particular stressful situation."

- *Resistance to change.* "An individual may be certain that they could not be mistaken and will not countenance any alternative explanation for their experience. Others feel very confused and uncertain about their ideas and readily want to think about alternative accounts of their experience."

(This is from the table titled "The multidimensional nature of delusions," in the original paper.) Indeed, the debate about "continuity" of psychosis vs. discrete categories, i.e., about "dimensions" vs. "syndromes" has not yet provided definitive answers (Rossi and Daneluzzo, 2002). However, regardless of which option one lends more credibility to, even those clinicians who favour "continuity" and "dimensions" use the term *psychosis*—when they estimate it appropriate—to describe the mental condition of the given patient. By doing so they imply that there is a cut-off point on a continuum of more or less similar behaviours and experiences where a new quality emerges in the way a patient relates to themselves, the world and other people which prompts a clinician to diagnose the patient as psychotic; just *psychotic* without specifying as to whether that particular patient is "a little bit," "partly" psychotic, or psychotic "to the full."

Here are the notions that use those who favor the dimensional approach: *a certain degree of psychosis, not clinically relevant delusion, subclinical form of psychosis, severe paranoia, less severe paranoia, mild paranoia, low-level paranoia, and occasional paranoid moments.*

Those who prefer the categorical model find these notions misleading and confusing. They cannot help but ask: is "paranoia" as opposed to "severe paranoia" still paranoia; is a "clinically not relevant delusion" still a delusion?

It seems that those who support the dimensional definition of delusion, in fact, decompose the notion of the delusion as something that is discrete and distinct, and different from for example (more or less severe) suspiciousness that is common in the non-clinical population, or from ideas of reference which can appear in people with Schizotypical Personality Disorder. (It is worth reminding the reader that *delusions of reference* are not the same as *ideas of reference* due to the mere fact that the former are delusions, and the latter are not.)

One of the most serious consequences of grading and thereby decomposing delusion, of disputing its specific quality, is the inability to determine whether someone is delusional. And how could it be possible to distinguish delusion from non-delusion when the difference between *low* or *lowest degree* of delusion and non-delusion is virtually imperceptible, unspecified and of no practical significance; and clinically unbinding, of course. Such a concept of delusion, advocated by those who are determined to dissolve it, prevents psychiatrists and clinical psychologists from distinguishing not only delusional from non-delusional, but also, in the last instance, disorder from non-disorder.

Continuity between Madness and Mental Health

Richard Bentall, Patrick Bracken, and Philip Thomas are among the most distinguished scholars who exploit psychotic symptoms such as hallucinations and delusions in mentally healthy people for arguing that there is a continuum between madness and mental health. This idea actually underpins the dimensional concept of delusion.

I will set out their views because they exemplify the way in which the deconstruction of madness is performed.

Bentall, Professor of Clinical Psychology at the University of Bangor, in Wales, UK, presented his views in numerous papers, and in particular in his books *Madness Explained. Psychosis and Human Nature* (2004), and *Doctoring the Mind* (2009). Bracken and Thomas also published extensively. The book they wrote together is entitled *Postpsychiatry* (2005).

Let me start with Bentall. This scholar writes that "it seems reasonable to assume, as a general principle, that abnormal behaviours and experiences exist on continua with normal behaviours and experiences" (2004: 115). (Bentall uses the term "abnormal" to designate "pathological.")

And how does this clinical psychologist define the principle of continuity? "Abnormal behaviours and experiences are related to normal behaviours and experiences by continua of frequency (the same behaviours and experiences occur less frequently in non-psychiatric populations), severity (less severe forms of behaviours and experiences can be identified in non-psychiatric populations), and phenomenology (non-clinical analogues of the behaviours and experiences can be identified as part of normal life" (2004: 115).

Bracken and Thomas express the same view in a slightly different form. They write: "There is increasing evidence to support a dimensional view of psychosis." And then they add: "Those diagnosed as schizophrenic are simply those who present with the most severe expression of traits that are to be found subclinically in the community" (2005: 42).

In regard to the continuity of frequency Bentall as well as Bracken and Thomas refer to the findings of empirical studies that show that mentally healthy people have psychotic symptoms, first of all hallucinations and delusions.

As for the severity of symptoms continuity Bentall adduces the results of several studies that show that speech disorders like incoherent speech, as well as mood swings and hypo manic affect are not rare in people who are not mentally disordered.

Finally, so as to back the phenomenology continuum Bentall mentions the similarity of the clinical picture of schizophrenic patients, on the one hand, and Schizotypical Personality Disorder, on the other, and draws the conclusion that "psychosis might be thought of as extreme end of a normally distributed spectrum of personality traits on which we impose an arbitrary cut-off point to separate those who are mentally ill from those who are not" (2004: 107-8).

Is There a Continuum between Psychotic Symptoms in Non-Psychiatric and Psychiatric Populations?

The following is my critique of the conclusion by Bentall, that I cited a few lines above.

First of all, there is a difference between hallucinations and delusions as symptoms of a psychotic disorder, primarily Schizophrenic Disorder, and hallucinations and delusions in mentally healthy people. Unlike in mentally sound people, hallucinations and delusions are virtually never the only symptoms in psychotic people.

One might remark that Delusional Disorder is the example of psychotic disorder characterized by only one symptom—delusion(s). The one who makes such a comment should reread the DSM-IV operational definition of Delusional Disorder. Diagnostic criteria of this disorder have five elements (A, B, C, D, E). The "C" criterion runs as follows: "Apart from the impact of the delusion(s) or its ramifications, functioning is nor markedly impaired, and behaviour is not obviously odd or bizarre" (1994: 301).

The authors of DSM-IV say, in a bit awkward form, that delusion(s) is not the only symptom of Delusional Disorder. Those with this disorder have disturbed some other mental functions too as the result of either the impact of delusion(s) or its ramifications.

Why should we pay attention to the fact that those with Delusional Disorder, apart from delusions, have impaired a number of other mental functions and that consequently they suffer from internal psychological dysfunction? Because it shows that there are actually no monosymptomatic mental disorders. Each and every mental disorder implies a *psychopathological context*. Mental disorder consists of a particular psychopathological context. And that is just the psychopathological context that lacks in mentally normal people who have hallucinations or delusions.

Impairment of one or more mental functions that precedes or follows internal psychological dysfunction constitutes the psychopathological context or internal psychological dysfunction. Mentally healthy people can have hallucinations or delusions, but they do not have the internal psychological dysfunction.

Besides the psychopathological context, *mental suffering* (distress) is the second main difference between mentally healthy people with hallucinations or delusions and mentally disturbed people who have hallucinations or delusions. The former are *not* distressed due to hallucinations or delusions. They are doing well. They are "otherwise well-adjusted people" (Bentall, 2004: 96). Those who have hallucinations or delusions "have accepted those experiences, are *comfortable with them and live their lives alongside them without difficulty*" (Bracken and Thomas, 2005: 43, my emphasis).

That is not the case with mentally ill people in general, and psychotic patients in particular. Mental suffering (distress) is one of the four key characteristics of my definition of mental disorder. (See my definition of mental disorder in the text above.) After all, distress is one of the substantial characteristics of mental disorder in DSM's definition of mental disorder, as well.

I this context, it is worth mentioning that Tanya M. Lincoln looking for any difference between delusional beliefs of those suffering from Schizophrenic Disorder and those with no Schizophrenic Disorder found "the distress as well as beliefs involving persecution and loss of control to be the most relevant aspects in distinguishing persons with schizophrenia from persons without schizophrenia" (2007).

The point I want to make is as follows: since hallucinations and delusions of mentally healthy and mentally disturbed people significantly differ, they cannot be put on a continuum. Therefore, the principle of continuity should be disputed.

It is not the case that "the same behaviours and experiences occur less frequently in non-psychiatric populations," as Bentall claims. Pathological behaviors and experiences are not related to normal behaviour and experiences by continua of frequency because the former are part of a psychopathological context, and they, among other things, cause mental suffering of those who have them, whereas the latter are isolated symptoms; they do not occur within a psychopathological context, and do not cause distress.

The same argument against the validity of the principle of continuity can be utilized in regard to the alleged continuum of severity and phenomenology.

The other question is whether hallucinations and delusions are to be considered as vulnerability to schizophrenia, as a potential whose realization depends on a host of biopsychosocial circumstances. However intriguing and important this question is, especially in light of early intervention in psychosis, which is today getting ever more currency, it is not in the focus of attention of those who deconstruct madness (psychosis). Thus, Bentall does not mention the continuum of evolution from hallucinations or delusions in non-psychiatric populations to pathological behaviours and experiences in psychiatric-populations. And Bracken and Thomas, after posing a rhetorical question "How are we to regard people in the community with non-clinical voices or delusions? Should we consider them to be 'pre-schizophrenic'?", reply: "We argue that this position is problematic" (2005: 43).

The Integration of the Pathological into the Normal

I will cite two passages, one by Bentall, and another by Bracken and Thomas, to show how they efface the difference between the normal and the pathological.

First, Bentall: "If people can sometimes live healthy, productive lives while experiencing some degree of psychosis..., if the boundaries between madness and normality are open to negotiation..., and if out psychiatric services are imperfect and sometimes damaging to patients, why not help some psychotic people just to *accept* that they are different from the rest of us" (2004: 511, emphasis in original).

Now, Bracken and Thomas: "How should we think of those people in the community who have psychotic experiences and who meet the criteria for psychosis? Are we to think of them as undiagnosed patients in need of panoply of NSF (National Service Framework) and NICE (National Institute for Clinical Excellence) guidelines, including assessment, treatment, and care plans? Or are we to think of them in some other way, perhaps as people who have unusual experiences, but who have accepted those experiences, are comfortable with them and live their lives alongside them without difficulty?" (2005: 43).

What are the points the cited authors want to make? First, psychosis is not pathology. Psychosis is just unusual experience, especially in people who "experience some degree of psychosis." After having cited the findings that show how hallucinations and delusions are common in non-clinical populations, Bentall comes to the following conclusion: "The results from these and other studies suggest that there is no clear dividing line between severe mental illness and normal functioning. Rather, there seems to be continuum running from ordinary personality traits, through eccentricity, to the full-blown psychosis" (2009: 108).

Second, those who are psychotic can live healthy, productive lives. They are happy with their psychotic experiences. There is no mention of psychosis as a serious disorder that causes people's suffering and impairment "in one or more important areas of functioning."

Third, since psychotic people are *just* different from the rest of the population, psychiatrists should think twice before treating them with psychiatric therapeutic methods.

In concluding, I want to point out that there is a growing body of evidence showing that some normal people have psychotic symptoms such as (auditory) hallucinations and delusional beliefs. Some authors use this finding to show that sanity and madness can hardly be distinguished.

However, psychotic symptoms in non-psychiatric and psychiatric populations differ. The psychopathological context (or the context of psychosis) gives a specific pathological meaning to symptoms of those with psychosis. Moreover, the cluster of symptoms that constitute a psychopathological context causes mental suffering of mentally disordered persons. In other words, since they have different meaning, symptoms which appear in the context of psychosis cannot be compared to psychotic symptoms which are experienced by otherwise healthy people.

Those who put these two kinds of phenomena on the same footing cloud the boundary between madness and sanity and, in fact, make it even more unclear. They do not see psychosis as an illness, i.e., as a negative condition, which is opposite to health. Thereby they deconstruct madness.

One final point. Josef Parnas, Pierre Bovet, and Dan Zahavi (2002) point at the serious deficiency of the contemporary operationalist psychopathology—"a lack of descriptions of subtle pathology…."

In tune with the spirit of clinical phenomenology, and of the works by Eugène Minkowski and Wolfgang Blankenburg in particular, they analyzed autism which "reflects a profoundly changed existential pattern" of schizophrenic patients. As it is known, autism is considered one of the main features of Schizophrenic Disorder.

They stress out that autism encompasses three key characteristics: a disturbance in the realm of self, a unique disturbance of intentionality, and an impaired dimension of intersubjectivity. Briefly, "I," "the world," and "We," as three inseparable instances, are affected in the schizophrenic autism.

The changes that occur in a schizophrenic patient are profound and disturbing indeed. The world is no longer "*pregiven* as a tacit, *unnoticed* and unquestionable foundation of experience." The patient perceives it as strange. "Everything may become a matter of deliberation … there is no evident and easy way to choose a dress, or to be sure of one's own opinion during a conversation or a dispute." The patient does not perceive themselves as the protagonist of their own actions, thoughts, and even movements. "There is an increasing gap or distance between the sense of self and experiencing" (2002). The patient feels as if they were someone else; also, the world looks strange to them. Familiar situations, objects, and people get a new, often extremely odd meaning.

There is no doubt that those who are mentally undisturbed, irrespective of whether they have or do not have hallucinations or delusions, do not experience the mentioned symptoms, i.e., do not undergo such a "profound reorganization of subjectivity." Briefly, the experience of psychosis is unique and in so far incomparable. And it is not shared by mentally healthy people.

One can look for similarities and continua between mentally healthy and mentally disturbed people, but should never lose of sight the fact that the dissimilarities and discontinua between these two populations by far outweigh their apparent resemblance.

Devereux's Concept of Ethnic Psychosis

Georges Devereux's "Schizophrenia: An Ethnic Psychosis or Schizophrenia Without Tears" is a contribution to the deconstruction of madness and blurring of the line dividing mental disorder and non-disorder. The text was initially published in *L'evolution psychiatrique* (1965), a French psychiatric journal. It was reproduced in the book *Essais d'ethnopsychiatrie générale* (1970: 248-274), that was translated into English ten years later (*Problems in Ethnopsychiatry*, 1980: 214-236)

Before I explain the way in which Devereux deconstructs madness it is worth asking where the notion of *ethnic psychosis* come from. After all, this notion is the key element in the title of the above mentioned paper.

According to Devereux, ethnic psychosis is characterized by the following features. First, "the underlying conflict of the psychosis or neurosis is also present in the majority of the normal people." The only difference is that "the conflict in the neurotic or psychotic is simply *more intense* than it is in other peple" (1980: 216-7, emphasis in original). Second, the patient does not invent the symptoms of the clinical picture. They have been created by the culture the patients live in. Thus, they are culture-made. One can be mentally disturbed only in those ways which are culturally prescribed. If one does not express their disturbance in accordance with a culturally defined image of a mentally disturbed person, they run the risk of being labelled a heretic, a criminal, or a witch.

Devereux contends that the Occidental man of today is "conditioned by his own culture to react to any state of stress by schizophrenia-like behavior (symptoms) even when his *real* idiosyncratic conflicts are not of the schzophrenogenic nature" (1980: 218, emphasis in original). Today's people react by schizophrenic symptoms because the ethnic segment of their personality contains culturally structured schizophrenogenic conflicts. Briefly said, schizophrenia best fits ethnic conflict, and it is schizophrenic symptoms that we expect from them, "socially as well as psychiatrically."

"The ethnic personality of modern man is basically schizoid," Devereux writes, "even when he happens to become a hysteric or a manic-depressive" (1980: 219).

Yet why is the ethnic personality of modern people schizoid? Why they are said to be schizoid?

I will set out basic characteristics which Devereux recognizes as typical for today's Occidental people. These characteristics are usually called *schizoid*.

Withdrawal, aloofness, hyporeactivity. Those features are held in esteem in today's world; they are highly saught after. If you want to climb the social ladder you have to be unemotional.

Absence of affectivity in sexuality. People are advised not to get emotionally committed to other people. That holds for the sphere of sexuality, as well. The affective sides of sexuality should be strictly kept under control.

Segmentalism and partial involvement. Interpersonal communication are superficial. They do not involve any genuine interest in other people's needs.

Dereism. The distortion of reality is widely spread. It is distorted so as to make it fit an illusory model "evolved in accordance with purely subjective or else cultural needs and demands" (1980: 226). People believe what they want to believe, what they need to believe.

The blurring of the frontier between reality and the imaginary. Today's people are in the pragmatism of technical civilization with one foot, and in superstition and religion with another.

Infantilism. People lack a critical view of what is going on in the society. They trust politicians who are interested only in their own business, in how to stay in power as long as possible. Since they are immature and infantile, people can easily be manipulated.

Fixation and regression. Fixation and regression support infantilization. People are not able to see beyond the horizon of their immediate needs, their greediness and their sense of insecurity.

Depersonalization. Depersonalization is an integral part of segmentalism and infantilism. Depersonalization is the result of inauthentic relations among people, of people's urge to intrumentalize their fellow citizen, to abuse them for the sake of their own selfish needs. Depersonalization does not affect only those who are instrumentalized but also those who resort to instrumentalization. "In modern society, true individuality—that most precious and socially most valuable of all aspects of the human being—is a source of trouble rather than gratification, far from being rewarded, it is penalized.... Therefore, hardly anyone dares to be himself" (180: 234).

Concluding his consideration of schizophrenia as a typical and "culturally privileged psychosis of modern western society" Devereux stresses out that it is no wonder that modern western culture, as any other culture, has its own psychosis. The problem is that, today, the ethnic psychosis happens to be schizofrenia "rather than some relatively benign psychic disorder such as hysteria, so prevalent in the nineteenth century and still prevalent among many primitive groups" (1980: 235). And Devereux adds: "Our society must either stop fostering mass schizophrenia or it will simply cease to be" (1980: 236).[16]

*A Critique of Devereux's View of Schizophrenia
as an Ethnic Psychosis of Modern Western Societies*

First, it is difficult to guess why Devereux uses the term *ethnic psychosis*. It is more difficult to do so because, apart from being a psychoanalyst, Devereux is an anthropologist. And as an anthropologist he should know that it is not possible to equate an ethnic group (*ethnie*) and modern western societies. The latter includes a great many nations, i.e., nation-states, and a huge number of ethnic groups. An ethnic group has a proper name, common myths of ancestry, shared memories, and culural specificities. Ethnics have a link with homeland and nurture mutual solidarity (Smith, 2001: 13). Thus, modern western societies cannot be reduced to an ethnic group, and thereby the type of psychosis which is said to be dominant in today's western world cannot be dubbed *ethnic psychosis*.

Second, Devereux establishes a link between, as he put it, the underlying conflict of the psychosis and the conflict that is present in the majority of normal people in modern societies. However, when he describes the attributes of people's psyche in today's world he talks about their pattern of behavior and experience rather than of a conflict underpinning their way of behaving and experiencing. As for schizophrenia, if any conflict underlies symptoms which schizophrenic patients present with, we can only make hypotheses about it and about how it gives rise to schizophrenic symptoms. In fact, Devereux finds normal behaviors and experiences and pathological behaviors and experiences similar. He does not identify a common conflict underpining the former and the latter.

Third, apart from pointing at characteristics of the psychological profile of people in today's world, which he recognizes as schizoid, Devereux does not provide any evidence that schizophrenia is a psychosis which is typical for modern western societies.

Furthermore, if it is true that the "Occidental man of today is conditioned by his culture to react to any state of stress by schizophrenia-like behavior (symptoms)," as Devereux claims, then, there should be more schizophrenic patients today than there were schizophrenic patients in previous epochs. There are no such indications. Quite the opposite. Data show that there are decreasing rates of incident schizophrenia cases in psychiatric services (Munk-Jorgensen, 1995).

Fourth, if each epoch has its own "ethnic psychosis," then one can speculate that, if the dominant type of personality was ever cyclothymic, manic-depressive psychosis should have been the ethnic psychosis at that time. There is no evidence to support such an assumption. (Of course, so-called culture-bound psychoses, like koro, windigo, amok, latah, are ruled out. So are so-called mass psychoses which were not so rare in the Middle Ages.)

Fifth, in the paper entitled "Ethnopsychiatry as a frame of reference in research and clinical practice" (1980: 72-90) Devereux rightly notes that psychosis *decultures culture*. Psychotic individuals do not deculture a specific culture but the culture because they to not relate towards it as normal people do. They ignore cultural instruments or use them in an idiosyncratic way. The culture presuposes commonality of the meanings of objects, events, rituals, symbols. Psychotics look at the culture from an autistic viewpoint and thereby the culture stops existing as the culture. Culture stops being cultural, to put it that way.

Bearing in mind the above mentioned deculturing effect of psychosis the question arises as to how there could be a correspondence between culture-shaped behaviors and experiences of normal people and behaviors and experiences of psychotic people? And such a correspondence is, as stated in the text above, at the basis of Devereux's arguments about "ethnic psychosis."

Finally, the idea underlying the notion of *ethnic psychosis* is that behaviors and experiences of normal people and behaviors and experiences of psychotics are not as far away as they are believed to be. Quite the opposite. They are nearly the same. ("The patient is *like* everyone—but *more* intensely so than anyone else" (1970: 251) (emphasis in original)).

By normalizing experiences and behaviors of psychotic people Devereux first negates that psychosis is a unique personal experience, and second, he makes the demarcation between mental disorder and non-disorder even more unclear, and deconstructs madness as well.

In order to show that there are grounds to suspect psychiatrists' ability to distinguish the mentally disordered from the non-disordered, a number of researchers resorted to a slightly unusual procedure to verify psychiatrists' knowledge: they tried to deceive them.

A very simple—and I must say underhanded—way to verify psychiatrists' knowledge and their ability to distinguish mental disorder from non-disorder is to try to deceive them by having mentally healthy people present themselves as disordered. The idea is as follows: if psychiatrists are able to detect the deception, i.e., that those who present themselves as mentally disordered are not mentally disordered, then they know how to distinguish the mentally healthy from those who are not. If they are unsuccessful, then the lack of a valid definition of mental disorder has a very unpleasant consequence: psychiatrists diagnose as disordered those who are not (false positives) and the mentally non-disordered are diagnosed as disordered (false negatives).

David L. Rosenhan's Experiment

Of all the attempts to use the method of deception to verify psychiatrists' ability to distinguish the mentally disordered from the non-disordered, the best known is the experiment carried out by David L. Rosenhan, Professor of Psychology and Law at Stanford University. This is why it will be accorded due attention.

The first sentence of Rosenhan's text entitled "Being sane in insane places" (1973), one of several most-cited texts of all those published in psychological journals, indicates that it deserves attention in the context of defining mental disorder: "If sanity and insanity exist, how shall we know them?"

The results of Rosenhan's experiment allegedly indicate that there is no convincing proof that psychiatrists are able to distinguish the mentally disordered from the non-disordered.

Rosenhan formed a group of eight pseudo-patients, people who were mentally healthy and had no medical baggage, as the saying goes. Three members of the group were psychologists, one was a psychiatrist, one a pediatrician, one a painter, one a student of psychology, and one a housewife. The author of the study was one of the imposters.

After making an appointment for an examination by telephone, each member of the group, independent of each other, asked to be received in a mental hospital on either the eastern or western coast of the United States. The hospitals were quite different with regard to the shape they were in, when they were built and the staff/patient ratio. Only one hospital was private.

During the interview with the psychiatrist, each patient complained of the same symptoms: they heard voices that said different words, for example "empty," "thud." Except for their name, they did not change any other information about themselves and their families. They only told the mental health workers they had a different profession to avoid receiving special attention from the psychiatrist.

The psychiatrists who conducted the interview found that all the subjects were disturbed to such a point that they needed to be treated in a psychiatric institution.

It should be noted that except for changing their name and profession, all the other information given by the pseudo-patients was correct, and their personal and family anamneses, how they related to themselves, their work and friends, had nothing "suspicious" from the psychiatric viewpoint.

After they were admitted to the ward, the pseudo-patients acted quite normal: they respected the house rules and helped the staff carry out their daily work. The only thing they did that was different from most other patients was to keep some sort of diary, noting down their observations, first out of sight and then quite openly. Soon after being admitted, they even said that they no longer heard voices. They did not take the drugs prescribed by the psychiatrists and dispensed by the other medical staff. They threw them in the toilet. One fact deserves mention: they would have taken a total of 2,100 pills. That was the amount prescribed. The imposters were also encouraged to act normally on the ward. It was up to them to convince the psychiatrists and other medical staff that they no longer needed help and could be discharged.

When they were admitted, one of the imposters received the diagnosis of "manic-depressive psychosis" and all the others were diagnosed with "schizophrenia." They stayed in the hospital (each pseudo-patient in a different one) between seven and 52 days, an average of 19 days. They were all discharged with the same diagnosis of "schizophrenia in remission."

After it was shown that psychiatrists had diagnosed mentally non-disordered people as disordered, Rosenhan wanted to see if the opposite took place too, i.e., whether psychiatrists and other medical staff diagnosed mentally disturbed people as non-disturbed. In order to find out, he talked to the staff at a university hospital that had heard about the results of his experiment and doubted that something like that, such diagnostic errors, would happen to them.

So Rosenhan told the hospital staff that one or more imposters would try to be admitted to the hospital during the next three months. Each staff member was asked to note down their observations whenever a patient was admitted and during their stay in the ward, and rate how likely each case was an imposter.

Evaluations were given of 193 patients who were admitted to the hospital. "All staff who had had sustained contact with or primary responsibility for the patient ... were asked to make judgments." And what are the results? "Forty-one patients were alleged, with high confidence, to be pseudopatients by at least one member of the staff. Twenty-three were considered suspect by at least one psychiatrist. Nineteen were suspected by one psychiatrist and one other staff member." Needless to say, not a single pseudo-patient tried to be admitted to the hospital; at least not from Rosenhan's group.

After finishing the second experiment, Rosenhan concluded that a diagnostic process susceptible to such enormous error could not be reliable in the true sense of the word. We recall that Rosehan's experiments were intended to show whether it was possible to distinguish an insane person from a sane one, i.e., whether it was possible to know who was mentally disordered.

It is worth noting that Rosenhan repeated his experiments several times in 12 hospitals from 1973 to 1975 and obtained the same results each time.

Rosenhan's experiments had great repercussions among the public. Also, they have been cited in more than 1,100 journal articles (Ruscio, 2004). People had already wondered "do psychiatrists know what they are doing?" "can someone who is sound of mind be declared insane by a psychiatrist?" "can psychiatrists be trusted at all?," "is psychiatry a science or a sham?" and so on.

Critical Comments on Ronsenhan's Experiment

Rosenhan's experiment is often cited as proof that mental disorder actually does not exist. If it existed, the argument goes, psychiatrists would probably know how to tell who is mentally disordered and who is not. Since the results of the experiment cast doubt not only on the ability of psychiatrists to tell who is mentally disordered but also, indirectly, on the existence of a demarcation between mental disorder and non-disorder, the experiment deserves a critical analysis when discussing forms of questioning the difference between mental disorder and non-disorder.

First, Rosenhan does not single out the goals of his experiments conducted. I will only mention some possible goals: to establish whether psychiatrists can ascertain who is mentally disordered and who is not; to establish whether and how much the environment in which the diagnostic process takes place influences its outcome; to establish which symptoms and how many symptoms a person must exhibit or say they have for psychiatrists to state that they are suffering from this or that disease; to establish the consequences of wrongly diagnosing non-disordered people as disordered (labeling theory); to establish how staff in psychiatric hospitals act towards patients, and more broadly, what atmosphere prevails in mental hospitals.

Second, it is questionable just how much deception or attempting to deceive (the psychiatrist) is the right way to establish whether psychiatrists are able to distinguish mentally disordered people from mentally non-disordered people, which in the specific case means those who *pretend* to be disordered from those who *really are* disordered.

Third, a large number of patients in psychiatric hospitals have quite inconspicuous behavior. Motion pictures offer a distorted picture of patients' behavior in mental hospitals as a pandemonium: they make faces, stand on one leg, run in circles, crow, shout at an invisible enemy. It is quite possible that a patient who stops complaining of the symptoms that got them into the hospital and behaves completely normally will not be quickly identified as an imposter. They are usually considered to be a recovered patient and not a pseudo-patient. In this sense, it is not unusual that all the imposters were discharged with the diagnosis "schizophrenia in remission." The "in remission" means several things: there are no longer any acute symptoms of the disorder, the symptoms of disorder have withdrawn, only a small number of symptoms are presented and are visible solely to the "professional eye" or there are almost no symptoms of the basic disorder.

Fourth, doctors in the hospital ward put a certain amount of trust in the diagnostic evaluations of the psychiatrist who admits patients. This certainly facilitated pseudo-patients' "slipping in."

Fifth, the pseudo-patients behaved quite normally on the ward and no longer mentioned hearing voices. In a word, they were normal in all respects. The following question arises: shouldn't their "completely normal behavior," which means behaving like mentally non-disordered people, have included telling the staff, in particular the psychiatrist on the ward, that they were imposters, part of an experiment, and that they wanted to be discharged? What I mean to say is that Rosenhan's assertion cannot be literally accepted that after being admitted, the pseudo-patients stopped pretending that they were disordered. In fact, they continued to "play the role of being mentally disordered," which means to falsely represent themselves, by not behaving the way that every mentally non-disordered person would in the same situation.

These are some general objections that can be leveled at the Rosenhan's experiment. Yet the key question in regard to diagnosing mentally healthy as mentally disturbed, that is, the ability of psychiatrists to distinguish mental disorder from non-disorder, is how psychiatrists could admit the pseudo-patients with the diagnosis of schizophrenic disorder (except for one who was diagnosed as manic-depressive psychosis) based solely on the patients stating that they had heard voices for several weeks. Briefly, how could have psychiatrists diagnose a mental disorder on the basis of only one symptom?

Robert L. Spitzer strongly reacted to Rosenhan's experiment. He set it out in "On pseudoscience in science, logic in remission, and psychiatric diagnosis: A critique of Rosenhan's 'On being sane in insane places'" (1975). At the time Spitzer was getting ready to take on the great task of heading work on DSM-III, and he was greatly bothered, not to say irritated, by any questioning of psychiatrists' elementary knowledge: their ability to distinguish the mentally disordered from the non-disordered. Particularly since, as already mentioned, Rosenhan's experiment had considerable deficiencies from the methodological viewpoint.

Spitzer asked how psychiatrists could have made a diagnosis based on just one symptom. Specifically, he took up the differential diagnosis of auditory hallucinations.

Nothing in the pseudo-patients' anamneses indicated that the cause could have been an organic psychosis or a temporary situational disorder of psychotic intensity. Nothing in the anamneses indicated that the pseudo-patients had reason to resort to simulation in order to acquire some gain. In the given situation, Spitzer wondered what other diagnosis except for schizophrenia could have crossed the psychiatrists' minds.

Finally, it remains to be seen whether the psychiatrists diagnosed schizophrenia based on just one symptom—auditory hallucinations. The psychiatrists must have asked the pseudo-patients how they reacted to hearing voices when there was no source of sound around them. Auditory hallucinations are quite unique, unpleasant experiences, to put it mildly. It can therefore be assumed that the patients had to tell the psychiatrists how they reacted to the voices, particularly the first time they heard them: were they worried, did they become anxious, or were they depressed. No description is given of the clinical picture of each individual pseudo-patient during their first psychiatric interview. Rosenhan did not want to provide the patients' written trail left by psychiatrists after the first psychiatric interview prior to their admission to the hospital.

In the introduction to his paper Rosenhan states that he does not question the existence of anxiety, depression, or distress. What he doubts, and says so explicitly, is the existence of clearly defined entities—normal and abnormal (pathological), sanity and insanity, and clearly defined disorders within insanity (pathological).

Formulated in such a way his question is a tricky one. Here we have actually two questions: (a) are there normal and abnormal (pathological), sanity and insanity, as clearly defined entities, and (b) are there clearly defined disorders within insanity (pathological). How will one answer these questions depends on their view of whether normal and pathological, sanity and insanity, exist without mental disorders (and non-disorders, for that matter), or the difference between normal and pathological, sanity and insanity, is actually the difference between non-disorder and disorder. Briefly said, one has to make it clear: is there pathological out of context of mental disorder; could anything else be pathological (insane) except for mental disorder, i. e., a mentally disordered. If one believes that sanity and insanity, normal and pathological, exist only as non-disorder and disorder, then Rosenhan's two aforesaid questions are linked. In that case negative answer to the first question renders the second question meaningless. If there is no sanity and insanity as two different entities, how can distinct and discrete entities (mental disorders) be differentiated within insanity (pathological)?

Keen on answering the question of whether there is sanity and insanity, Rosenhan took schizophrenia as an example of pathological (insanity), as its epitome. His starting point was: if there is no difference between pathological (schizophrenia) and normal, then there is no difference between insanity and sanity, either.

Mental disorder does exist. However, it is not of the same natural kind as, for example, metals such as gold or iron. Unlike these metals, mental disorder is mutable. Yet although it differs from one individual to another, mental disorder includes impairment of one or more mental functions and a pathological context accordingly. Also, it implies mental suffering. Finally, it occurs beyond an individual's will. Although these attributes of mental disorder are apparently subjective, they are in fact objective.

Psychiatrists and clinical psychologists are supposed to be able to recognize the pathological that they have articulated. However, if one pretends to be pathological (to suffer from schizophrenia) by presenting with the symptoms that have been defined as typical for pathological (schizophrenia), and psychiatrists recognize them as pathological, this does not mean that pathological does not exist, and accordingly that there is no difference between sanity and insanity. The only thing that this does prove is that psychiatrists, like other professionals, can be swindled.

Rosenhan's experiment could not provide answer to the question of whether such entities as normal and pathological, sanity and insanity, exist; even less to the question of how would it be possible to clearly define disorders within pathological (insanity). And these are the questions that Rosenhan considered crucial.

Thirty years after Rosenhan's text was published, Lauren Slater's book *Opening Skinner's Box: Great Psychological Experiments of the Twentieth Century* (2004) came out.

Lauren Slater's "Experiment"

Slater is a psychologist with a good academic pedigree. She graduated in psychology at Brandeis University, her master's in psychology is from Harvard and her doctorate is from Boston University.

The third chapter of *Opening Skinner's Box* is devoted to Rosenhan's experiment. Slater wanted to repeat Rosenhan's experiment. It was to be her personal contribution to this famous experiment and a new test not only of psychiatrists' knowledge but also of how clearly defined is the normal and the pathological, of how perceptible is demarcation between them.

Here is how Slater's "experiment" took place. The author writes that she did not wash or brush her teeth for a day or two, then put on threadbare and dirty clothes and shoes and turned up at the emergency room in such a state. She told the nurse at the reception desk that she heard a voice that said "empty," "thud." Slater replied to additional questions in a way intended to convince the nurse that everything was fine with her "otherwise." Then the psychiatrist appeared, asked questions similar to the nurse's, asked Slater whether the voices bothered her, and said they probably did because otherwise she would not seek help and particularly not ask to be admitted to a hospital. Then the psychiatrist prescribed Risperidone, an antipsychotic. When Slater asked whether she gave the impression of being a psychotic woman, the psychiatrist replied, "Yes, to a certain degree. Besides, you are depressive. That is why I am going to prescribe an antidepressant."

Slater says that the following days she tried to be admitted to a hospital eight times. Allegedly she received the same diagnosis every time—"psychotic depression." She also said that psychiatrists prescribed a total of 25 antipsychotics and 60 antidepressants. Not a single interview with a psychiatrist lasted longer than twelve-and-a-half minutes.

Slater believes that the only reason she was not admitted to the ward, as Rosenhan's pseudo-patients were, was because in the meantime, i.e., since Rosenhan's time, the policy of treating patients has changed: today it is preferable to treat psychiatric patients in the open community wherever possible.

In the author's words, her experiment showed that she succeeded in deceiving psychiatrists, i.e., that psychiatrists in 2004 do not know how to distinguish the mentally disordered from the non-disordered, just as they were unable back in 1974. But there is something new: psychiatrists today, says Slater, diagnose someone as disordered in order to be able to prescribe medicine.

Several things will surprise the reader of the third chapter of Slater's book, particularly if they are a psychiatrist. Psychiatrists diagnosed as "psychotic depressive" someone who said they are not depressed, who denied having symptoms that are characteristic of depression, who complained only about the fact that they heard voices, who is mentally healthy in all respects except for the fact that they have not bathed or brushed their teeth for several days. Another surprise is that nine different psychiatrists diagnosed the same person the same way, which is an unbelievably high level of reliability for a psychiatric disorder. Finally, the reader will wonder why not one of the nine psychiatrists wrote in the protocol that additional information was needed about the patient, which Slater claims they did not. The surprise grows into astonishment when nine psychiatrists prescribed the same person a total of 25 antipsychotics and 60 antidepressants.

We have seen that Spitzer sharply reacted to Rosenhan's experiment 30 years ago. He reacted sharply to Slater's "experiment" too, first in a paper written with Scott P. Lilienfeld and Michael B. Miller, "Rosenhan revisited. The scientific credibility of Lauren Slater's pseudopatient diagnostic study" (2005), and then after Slater's reply (2005) in a paper whose first author is Scott P. Lilienfeld entitled "A response to a non-response to criticisms of a nonstudy. One humorous and one serious rejoinder to Slater" (2005).

Bearing in mind the fact that Slater's book belongs to so-called popular literature and her reputation in the world of psychology cannot be compared to Rosenhan's, why, then, did Spitzer consider it necessary to react, I repeat very sharply, to Slater's text? Why as well did the *Journal of Nervous and Mental Disease*, with its exceptionally long tradition and high reputation, open its pages to a discussion on the chapter of a book of highly doubtful value?

There are, by his own admission, several reasons for Spitzer's reaction and the readiness of the above journal to publish several texts on Slater's "experiment."

First, the public learns what is happening in a discipline, a field of knowledge, more from popular texts (popular science literature) than from professional and scholarly works that are most often inaccessible to laymen. This is why public opinion about a field of knowledge and a profession is formed more by popular writing in so-called lightweight publications than in the texts of prominent people from a particular field of science. The result is disastrous for both the public and the specific field of knowledge and profession. The public creates the wrong picture about a profession and the profession suffers because its "image" does not correspond to its real state. Second, as already mentioned, Rosenhan's experiment is far too important for psychiatry, thus the psychiatric community could not pass lightly over a repetition of the original experiment by a different author, particularly when the results of some of the "repeats" were given wide publicity, which was the case with Slater's "experiment." Third, in the mid-1970s, Spitzer was preparing DSM-III, intending to give psychiatry a scientific status and make it less vulnerable to attacks from those who contested it for various reasons and from various sides. This is why he sharply reacted to Rosenhan's text. The same reasons prompted him to react to an "experiment" whose results were presented to the public as proof that nothing had changed in psychiatry in the past twenty-five years after DSM-III was published, particularly with regard to the scientific status of psychiatry, i.e. psychiatry as a profession that could and should be trusted. This probable reason for Spitzer to react to Slater's text is personal, understandable and justified.

Just as Spitzer made his own investigation into some of the essential aspects of Rosenhan's experiment in order to verify and/or contest it, he did the same thing with Slater's experiment. He made a vignette of Slater's "case": he briefly described how she looked and what she complained about during her interview with the psychiatrist, i.e., what she said about herself. He sent this vignette to a number of psychiatrists and asked them to reply to several questions that were directly linked to the "experiment." He excluded all psychiatrists who were familiar with either Rosenhan's or Slater's experiments.

Here is what Spitzer received from 73 psychiatrists. In reply to the question "What diagnosis (or diagnoses) would you write in the charter," 80 percent (N = 56) of the respondents "avoided a specific DSM-IV diagnosis and instead diagnosed either psychosis not otherwise specified (56 percent; N = 39) or in some way indicated that a specific diagnosis, or any diagnoses, could not be made (24 percent; N = 17). Only six percent (N = 4) diagnosed psychotic depression. An additional 6 percent made another diagnosis but noted that the diagnosis of psychotic depression needed to be ruled out."

Spitzer did not hide his satisfaction at such diagnoses of the mental difficulties of the person presented in the vignette, ascribing the results to the influence of DSMs on the psychiatrists' education. "In our study and in contrast with to Slater's, psychiatrists generally appeared to follow the guidelines delineated in the DSM-IV, demonstrating an appropriate reluctance to offer specific diagnose in the absence of sufficient information." (This is that personal moment I mentioned earlier as one of the important reasons for Spitzer's sharp criticism of Slater's "experiment.")

In reply to the question as to whether and what medicine to prescribe, one-third (34 percent) of the respondents replied that they would prescribe an antipsychotic, but not a single psychiatrist recommended an antidepressant.

To comment on the results of Spitzer's investigation, I would point out that it shows that a great number of psychiatrists, more than half, consider auditory hallucinations sufficient indication of psychotic disorder, even when there are no other symptoms. For most psychiatrists, hallucinations and delusional ideas are pathognomonic of psychosis.

This finding shows that psychiatrists are far too eager to diagnosis psychotic disorder on the basis of only one symptom—auditory hallucinations. Such a rush cannot be defended.

From Slater's answer to the criticism she received, I would only note her insistence that her experiment was not a study in the academic sense of the word and her critics' basic mistake was to treat it as such, which means something "quite serious."

I have expanded upon the two best-known cases intended to show and prove that psychiatrists do not know what mental disorder is and therefore are unable to distinguish between the mentally disordered and non-disordered in their daily work. The first experiment, Rosenhan's, is much better known. It attracted a lot of attention among mental health workers and the public and, rightly or wrongly, played into the hands of psychiatry's critics The second, Slater's, whose author says it is nothing but a repetition of Rosenhan's, is much less known. The goal is the same in both cases: show the low validity of psychiatric diagnoses. And the method used is the same: deceive or try to deceive psychiatrists.

To conclude, I would like to emphasize that even though Rosenhan's experiment is and probably will continue to be cited as proof that psychiatrists are unable to distinguish mental disorder from non-disorder, it is based on an unusual methodological procedure. *Deception* is not the best way to show that a person who has been deceived knows very little about the subject of the deception.

Finally, I am left wondering whether the results of Rosenhan's experiment could be taken as proof that psychiatrists do not count on people turning to them for help but in fact shows that psychiatrists do not know how to properly do their job.

The Sociological Definition of Mental Disorder

Sociologists comprise by far the greatest number of those who consider mental disorder a social construction. Sociologists above all and a very small number of psychiatrists (such as Ronald D. Laing in the book *The Politics of Experience*, or Thomas S. Szasz in numerous books and papers) consider mental disorder to be exclusively a socially constructed phenomenon.

The widespread opinion is that such a view of mental disorder actually denies its existence and therefore should not be borne in mind when considering the definition of mental disorder.

As I said in the introduction, I do not agree with the opinion that this view of mental disorder actually denies it exists. Conceiving of mental disorder as a social construction is one of the possible definitions of mental disorder. It should therefore not be rejected a priori as unimportant. What we need to show, which is my intention below, is whether the sociological definition of mental disorder helps or hinders in distinguishing mental disorder from non-disorder.

Advocates of symbolic interactionism (labeling theory) are the authors of the basic sociological concepts of mental disorder.

The theoreticians of anomie (Emile Durkheim, Robert K. Merton) did not study mental disorder as a separate category. They mention mental disorder as only one of the ways of deviating from normative expectations, i.e., as one form of responding to an anomic social situation.

For example, in Merton's analyses of possible responses to an anomic situation, mental disorder would belong to the type Merton calls *retreatism* (1967: 207-209). Retreatism as a form of behavior is characteristic of individuals who ignore both current social goals and culturally allowed means to achieve them. In addition to mental disorder, psychosis in particular, the types of behavior that Merton groups together under the name *retreatism* include the autistic persons, pariahs (outcasts), vagabonds, (chronic) alcoholics, and drug addicts. Merton's texts do not answer the question of whether and how mentally disordered people differ from other deviants whose deviation has the form of retreatism.

Symbolic interactionism is a sociological and sociopsychological theory that arose at the beginning of the twentieth century. It is linked to sociologists George H. Mead and Charles Cooley. The name of the theory itself comes from Herbert Blumer, one of Mead's students. The basic idea of symbolic interactionism is that people live in a world that is socially constructed. Objects, events and people have the meaning that we give them. We even see ourselves the way others see us, or rather how we believe that others see us.

The theory of symbolic interactionism was a rather important sociological theory until the 1970s when it was superseded by positivistic views in sociology. The most important representatives of symbolic interactionism are George H. Mead, Charles H. Cooley, John Dewey, Robert E. Park, Howard S. Becker, Edwin M. Lemert, Kai T. Erikson, and John Kitsuse.

I would note that labeling theory is usually equated with symbolic interactionism (the theory of social reactions). It is less often thought that labeling theory derives from symbolic interactionism or is some sort of "sub-theory" of symbolic interactionism.

Edwin M. Lemert and Thomas J. Scheff dealt with mental disorder more than the other symbolic interactionists or advocates of labeling theory. This is why I will devote some space to discussing their ideas on the nature and origin of mental disorder.

As symbolic interactionists focus their attention on deviant behavior, mental disorder interests them foremost as a form of deviant behavior. The symbolic interactionists consider behavior deviant if it deviates from socially expected forms of behavior and causes the organs of social control to react. The interactionists use the same interpretative principles when analyzing various forms of deviant behavior (criminals, bohemians, hippies, mentally ill, homosexuals /still in some environments/). Briefly put, in the explicative approach to every form of deviant behavior, the fact that the behavior deviates from the "average" is much more important for the symbolic interactionists than for each individual case to be a *specific* form of deviant behavior.

Since Scheff's concept of the sociogenesis of mental disorder has many elements of Lemert's teachings on primary and secondary deviation, I will first take a look at Lemert's views of what constitutes mental disorder in the social sense.

Primary and Secondary Deviation

Primary and secondary deviations are two key categories in Lemert's concept of deviant behavior, and of mental disorder as one form of deviant behavior.

Primary deviation is polygenetic: it is caused by numerous physiological, cultural and social deviations from the average, whether they appear individually or in constant or random combinations. Although primary deviation may sometimes be defined as undesirable from the individual's and society's viewpoint, it is of no great importance for the person who has committed the primary deviance. Should social-psychological problems arise as a result of primary deviation, they are normalized or ignored.

The concept of *secondary deviation* refers to a special type of socially-defined response that people use to deal with problems created by the community's reaction to their primary deviance. The community sometimes reacts negatively to primary deviance with stigmatization, repression and segregation. This "corrective reaction" of the community causes the person to feel resentment because the reaction does not suit the "cause," i.e., the primary deviance or deviances, and because the reaction takes the form of moral condemnation.

In some cases, an individual who feels unpleasant because the community has reacted to their primary deviance by stigmatizing, repressing and segregating them, takes on the social role of a deviant. Why? Because taking the role of a deviant in the given circumstances can help decrease or even remove the internal tenseness, resentment and even anger caused by the community's inappropriate reaction to the deviance. When the individual responds to stigmatization by taking the role of a deviant, their deviance takes the form of secondary deviation. Then the individual starts adjusting their behavior to the community's expectations. It could be said that they then meet society's expectations. This is the well-known social-psychological mechanism of a self-fulfilling prophecy.

Treating the phenomenon of mental disorder as a form of deviation, Lemert approached it the same way he did deviations, using the above framework defined by the concepts of primary and secondary deviation.

When defining the nature of mental disorder, Lemert (1951, 1972) started from the assertion that most symptoms that are denoted as neurotic or psychotic can be found in people who are not called mentally disordered and do not consider themselves as such. Here and there, mentally non-disordered individuals mention that they have hallucinations, express delusional-like ideas about their partner being unfaithful to them, about impending economic ruin, among other things.[17]

According to Lemert, the beginning of mental disorder coincides with the arising awareness that our behavior differs from the behavior of other people in the community where we live. This awareness results from the community's "symbolic responses" to primary deviant behavior or deviant opinion that every person shows or expresses more than once in their life-span. Awareness of the mentally disordered nature of these (primary deviance) manifestations results from their classification by the community as being mentally disordered.

According to Lemert's concept of mental disorder, societal reaction to activity that by no means expresses mental disorder is the fundamental event in the onset of mental disorder. In other words, the onset of mental disorder coincides in many respects with the process of secondary deviation or amplification, as secondary deviation is also denoted.

The difference between the mentally disordered and the mentally non-disordered lies in the fact that the former experience themselves as mentally disordered, i.e., they play the social role of being mentally disordered. Taking on this social role for them, as already mentioned, is a possible solution to all the problems, most often of a moral nature, created by the community's inappropriately harsh reaction to their primary deviance.

There are several questions Lemert needs to answer.

First, why, when and under which circumstances does the community respond with stigmatization, repression and segregation to just a small number of primary deviances that are almost everyday, ordinary and do not represent a significant deviation from the "average."

Second, why does the actor of primary deviances find some sort of solution to the tenseness inside them caused by the community's inappropriately harsh reaction by taking the social role of a mentally disordered person and not the role of another deviant? Does the community's reaction suggest to them or let them know that they are mentally disordered and therefore the most natural thing to do is take the role of a mentally disordered person and relieve the inner pressure caused by the fact that the community maintains that they are such and such, when they are not like that at all? Or perhaps the community's reaction to primary deviance does not contain any sign, suggestion or open message that the individual has lost their mind, but they themselves decide to start behaving like a mentally disordered person, taking on the role of a mentally disordered person? If this is the case, then the question arises as to why the actor of the primary deviance takes on the role of a mentally disordered person and not the social role of some other deviant. Does this mean that for some reason they feel closer to the role of a mentally disordered person than some other type of deviant? Or their behavior suggests that it could be related to burgeoning mental illness. Killian and Killian indicate that this could be the case: "Recent studies have found that behavior itself is of paramount importance in determining if an individual will be labeled mentally ill" (1990).

Lemert did not answer these questions because he did not pose them. Yet his writings did not allow us for inferring what his answers could be.

Residual Rule-breaking

Thomas J. Scheff, Professor of Sociology at the University of California, formulated a concept on the sociogenesis of mental disorder that is more interesting than Lemert's for those interested in defining mental disorder. Scheff tried to identify the specific features of mental disorder compared to other forms of deviation. Thus his concept of the nature and origin of mental disorder merits greater attention than Lemert's.

Scheff set out his concept in the book *Being Mentally Ill: A Sociological Theory* (1966) and in several texts published in journals (Scheff, 1963, 1968, 1974).

The author of *Being Mentally Ill* maintains that most offenses do not result in their actor being labeled as mentally disordered, rather as being uneducated, a criminal, a thug or debauched, depending on the type of norm that is broken.

Scheff asks us to look at the countless so-called unwritten rules that exist in every society. Respecting the unwritten norms is simply understood, it is taken for granted. Since these are general, unwritten rules, they have no special name. They are expected to be followed across the board.

For example, when we talk to someone, it goes without saying that we look them in the eyes and do not set our eyes on someone or something to the side. It is also understood that we stand at a suitable distance from our collocutor—not several meters away or right up close. Furthermore, it is also understood—even if we are politicians—that we follow the thread of the conversation, we answer questions and do not constantly talk about someone or something that has nothing to do with what was previously said.

Different cultures have different labels for those who break the unwritten rules, what Scheff calls *residual norms* because they are "remaining norms" that are left when the other ("named") norms are enumerated.

Those who more or less wantonly break the unwritten rules are usually called "eccentric," "foolish," "really odd," "peculiar," "lost a few marbles," etc. Why do people call them that? Because they find their behavior incomprehensible and inexplicable.

Scheff maintains that whoever breaks residual rules in our culture is labeled as being mentally disordered. Since this is residual rule-breaking, their deviant behavior is qualified as *residual deviance*.

Here is what Scheff says: "The diverse kinds of deviation for which our society provides no explicit label, and which, therefore, sometimes lead to the labeling of the violator as mentally ill, will be considered to be technically *residual deviance*" (1968: 10).

The reader should take note of the adverb of time "sometime" in the above sentence. Scheff wants to say that not every behavior that breaks the residual norms is labeled as mental disorder.

Scheff set out the basic points of his concept of the sociogenesis of mental disorder in nine propositions. In them he explains which kind of residual rule-breaking is called an expression of mental disorder, when and under which circumstances. Let us look at these nine propositions that Scheff set out in the text "The role of the mentally ill and the dynamics of mental disorder." It was first published in the journal *Sociometry* (1963) and then was reprinted in the collection *The Mental Patient: Studies in the Sociology of Deviance* (1968: 8-22). I will comment on each one of Scheff's propositions.

First proposition: *Residual rule-breaking arises from fundamentally diverse sources*. Here are the sources that Scheff feels lead to breaking unwritten rules.

A. Mental disorders resulting from an organic etiology.

B. Individual psychological peculiarities and differences in upbringing and training.

C. Different external stressors, for example fear of suffering that comes with conflicts of war, hunger, insomnia, etc.

D. Innovation or showing defiance.

Without going into an analysis of the above sources of residual deviance, I would draw the reader's attention to the first source—mental disorders resulting from an organic etiology.

If it is said that mental disorders resulting from an organic etiology are one of the sources of breaking residual rules, this implicitly states that such mental disorders do not have a social cause. They precede sociogenesis and are independent of it. This means that there are two types of disorder: those whose etiology is organic and those whose etiology is social. If Scheff considers that there are two large groups of disorders, which logically results from his stating the source of residual rule-breaking, then whenever he mentions mental disorder in the text, he must say which type of mental disorder he means: one with an organic cause or one with a social cause.

One must add also that since the etiology of the great majority of mental disorders is unknown, the obvious question that arises is what type of mental disorder Scheff meant when he writes "mental disorders resulting from organic etiology."

Psychiatrists are inclined to believe that organic factors play a greater role in the onset of psychosis than in the onset of other types of mental disorders. Does Scheff, who is a sociologist and not a psychiatrist, share this opinion? If he does, this means that he considers sociogenesis is involved solely in the case of non-psychotic disorders. As will be seen below, Sheff does not think that only or primarily non-psychotic disorders arise by social means. This is indicated by the following sentence, written at the end of the explanation of the first proposition on the sociogenesis of mental disorders. "The kinds of behavior deemed typical of mental illness, such as hallucinations, delusions, depression, and mania, can all arise from these diverse sources"(1968: 11).

I would note the following with regard to Scheff's last assertion. First, the enumerated symptoms are typical of psychotic and not non-psychotic disorders. Judging by this, Scheff is thinking of psychotic disorders when he speaks of mental disorders. If this is so, when Scheff speaks of mental disorders, he has an even greater obligation to say whether he is think-ing of (psychotic) mental disorders with an organic cause or (psychotic) mental disorders with a social cause. Scheff himself implicitly advocates this division when he says that the former (psychotic disorders with an organic cause) are one of the sources of breaking unwritten rules and that the latter (psychotic disorders without an organic cause) result from social reactions to breaking residual rules.

Second, it is hard to imagine how symptoms that are typical, not to say pathognomonic for psychotic disorders (hallucinations, delusional ideas, manias) can arise from "individual psychological peculiarities and from differences in upbringing and training."

Second proposition: *Relative to the rate of treated mental illness, the rate of unrecorded residual rule-breaking is extremely high.*

Scheff considers that not even very wanton residual rule-breaking are registered. They are considered an expression of capriciousness, eccentricity, bizarreness, etc. "Apparently, many persons who are extremely withdrawn or who 'fly off the handle' for extended periods of time, who imagine fantastic events, or who hear voices or see visions, are not labeled as insane either by themselves or others. Their deviance, rather, is unrecognized, ignored, or rationalized." This is actually denial.

It is rather logical that the number of people who break the residual rules without drawing the community's specific attention is far greater than the number of registered mentally disordered people. To give his assertions "scientific weight" Scheff cites the findings of epidemiological studies indicating that the number of mentally disordered people in a community is twenty (Pasamanick, 1961) or forty times (Hollingshead and Redlich, 1958) greater than the number being treated by psychiatrists. These data cover all types of mental disorders, including the "minor" or "mild" ones. When only psychotic illnesses are considered, it turns out that there are as many unregistered as there are registered psychotically ill.

In Scheff's desire to corroborate his assertion that the number of unregistered residual rule-breakers is far greater than the number being treated in mental hospitals, he makes a methodological mistake when he compares the unregistered mentally disordered people in a community to the number registered as mentally disordered. Why? Because not all unregistered residual rule-breaking expresses (untreated) mental disorder. Scheff actually states this earlier in the text when he says that mental disorders (with an organic etiology) are only one source of residual deviation, i.e., breaking unwritten rules. Innovative approaches or individual psychotic peculiarities, or differences in upbringing and training should not be considered untreated (unregistered) mental disorders. Thus there are no grounds to compare the number of unregistered residual (unwritten) rule-breakers and the number of registered (treated) mentally disordered people.

Third proposition: *Most residual rule-breaking is "denied" and is of transitory significance.*

If most of the residual rule-breaking is denied or transitory, then the question arises once again: why are only some forms of residual rule-breaking labeled as an expression of mental disorder? Scheff says that the person breaking the unwritten rules can "organize" their deviation so it is not labeled as mental disorder and passes almost unnoticed as eccentricity, bizarreness, being peculiar. Some residual rule-breaking stops as soon as the stressful situation stops that caused it. On the whole, deviation only stabilizes in a small number of cases.

When does deviant behavior stabilize? When the community labels it as mental disorder: "Residual deviance may be stabilized if it is defined to be evidence of mental illness, and/or the deviant is placed in a deviant status and begins to play the role of the mentally ill" (1968: 13).

In this phase of forming his views of the sociogenesis of mental disorders, Scheff cites the sociopsychological model of playing a social role. In a word, this model says that taking over a specific social role is completed when it becomes part of the individual's expectations and when those expectations are constantly reconfirmed in social interactions.

The next two propositions speak about how beliefs and acts are linked to mental disorder and the role they play in the development of mental disorder.

The fourth proposition: *Stereotyped imagery of mental disorder is learned in early childhood.*

There is no doubt—Scheff is right—that in the earliest years of their life, children acquire a notion, even though rather hazy, of what it means to be crazy, "have a screw loose," be idiotic, and so on.

Later in life this hazy notion about insanity takes on a clearer form and is reinforced. This is exactly what the fifth proposition says.

Fifth proposition: *The stereotypes of insanity are continually reaffirmed, inadvertently, in ordinary social interaction.*

Even though when people grow up they learn about medical views of mental disorder, the stereotypical picture of mentally disordered people determines their views about and attitude toward them. This is because the mass media and casual conversations expose them almost on a daily basis to the influence of stereotypes about mental disorder.

What happens in the smaller number of cases when residual rule-breaking is not denied, normalized or simply passes unregistered? In a smaller number of cases the reaction goes in the opposite direction: the scope and degree of the reaction to residual deviation is exaggerated and temporarily distorted. Scheff calls this pattern of exaggeration *labeling*.

The reader following the thread of Scheff's reasoning will now inevitably ask: why does the reaction go in the opposite direction in a smaller number of cases, i.e. why does the community recognize the residual rule-breakers as being mentally disordered in a smaller number of cases? The answer could lie in the fact that in our times, as Scheff asserts at the beginning of the text, someone who breaks the unwritten rules is considered to be mentally ill. But it is not enough for someone to break the residual rules to be labeled as mentally disordered. One more condition must be fulfilled: residual rule-breaking becomes a public issue. "In a crisis, when the deviance of an individual (residual deviation, D.K.) becomes a public issue, the traditional stereotype of insanity becomes the guiding imagery for action, both for those reacting to the deviant and, at times, for the deviant himself" (1968: 17).

How should we understand this sentence? Its author probably wanted to say that when residual rule-breaking becomes so obvious, not to say drastic, that it draws public attention, and in the newly arising situation when there are no conditions for the specific deviation to be "normalized" or ignored, then the stereotype about mental disorder is activated. The next sentence suggests that Scheff might be satisfied with such a reading of his text. "When societal agents and persons around the deviant react to him uniformly in terms of the traditional stereotypes of insanity, his amorphous and unstructured deviant behavior tends to crystallize in conformity to these expectations, thus becoming similar to the behavior of other deviants classified as mentally ill, and stable over time" (1968: 17).

Since the residual rule-breaker is labeled as mentally disordered in accordance with the stereotype about mental disorder, the manifestations of mental disorder arising by social means are uniform for the most part.

Two more phenomena help to reinforce or completely "coordinate" the role of a mentally disordered person. They are described in the sixth and seventh propositions.

Sixth proposition: *Labeled deviants may be rewarded for playing the stereotyped deviant role.*

Seventh proposition: *Labeled deviants are punished when they attempt to return to conventional roles.* It is well-known, for example, that doctors and particularly psychiatrists like patients who constantly provide new evidence that the diagnosis of their disorder made by the doctor (psychiatrist) is accurate. It is also well-known that the public is not inclined to treat an ex-psychiatric patient the same way they would someone who has never received psychiatric treatment. The stigma of mental disorder with all its implications and repercussions clearly indicates that the mentally disordered are not expected to take back their earlier (pre-illness) social roles.

Eighth proposition: *In a crisis occurring when a residual rule-breaker is publicly labeled, the deviant is highly suggestible and may accept the proffered* (more exactly: imposed, D.K.) *role of the insane as the only alternative.*

Allegedly, when an unwritten rule is wantonly and publicly broken, the person doing it is very confused, anxious, embarrassed. In such a state they are sensitive to messages they receive as part of the community's reaction to their act. But people around the actor are confused too. Confronted with an act they do not understand (why, how) and the need to do something, they resort to the stereotype of insanity that is almost always close at hand. So they start to label the actor as being mentally disordered. The actor, confused, embarrassed and tense, experiences the label almost like some sort of solution (now I know why I do such idiotic things, why I act so weird), and they start acting according to the stereotype of a mentally disordered person, a stereotype they know all about because they have come across it in other people and have been fostering it their whole life. Thus the person breaking the unwritten rules starts their career of being mentally ill.

Ninth proposition: *Among residual rule-breakers, labeling is the single most important cause of careers of residual deviance.*

Scheff wants to say that if there are no grounds for taking on the role of insanity, primary deviation will not lead to the career of a deviant. In other words, the career of a deviant, i.e., someone who is mentally ill or permanently playing the role of someone who is mentally ill, is not directly linked to the nature and origin of the primary deviation. Secondary deviation, which is when someone takes the role of being insane after the community has labeled them as insane, results from contingencies.

There are a great many contingencies that lead to labeling and not to normalization or ignoring the primary or residual deviation. It seems, writes Scheff, that labeling as mentally ill resulting from the secondary deviation is a function of: (1) the degree, scope and social visibility of the deviance, the residual rule-breaking; (2) the social power of the deviant and the social distance between them and the organs responsible for keeping law and order; (3) the community's tolerance of deviance; and (4) the accessibility (in the community's culture) of alternative non-deviant roles.

Let me summarize my remarks about Scheff's concept of the socio-genesis of mental disorder.

1. Scheff asserts that there are mental disorders with an organic etiology. Since the goal of his concept of the onset of mental disorders is to show that social causes lead to mental disorders, whenever he mentions mental disorders, he must clearly denote whether he is thinking of mental disorders with an organic etiology or a social etiology. Scheff did not do this, thereby making parts of his concept confusing, to say the very least.

    Although he says that the origin of primary deviation, i.e., breaking unwritten rules, has no direct link to the situation in which the actor is labeled as mentally disordered (wanton and public breaking of the norms), in a number of cases the possibility remains that mental disorders with an organic etiology are the source of primary deviation. It is hard to explain how a psychotic disorder with an organic etiology as the source of primary deviation (breaking unwritten rules) becomes a psychotic disorder with a social etiology by the process of labeling. It turns out that a person's psychosis is first exclusively organic and then exclusively social!

2. Scheff makes a methodological mistake when he compares the number of cases of unregistered residual deviations (breaking unwritten rules) with the number of mentally disordered people receiving some sort of psychiatric help. To this effect, he can only compare the number of psychiatrically untreated and the number of psychiatrically treated mentally disordered people. Unregistered cases of residual deviation cannot be considered as psychiatrically untreated mentally disordered people. This is counter to Scheff's very concept of the sociogenesis of mental disorders. According to Scheff, mental disorder becomes structured only with secondary deviation when, under specific circumstances, only a small number of those breaking unwritten rules are labeled as mentally disordered.

3. Scheff's entire construction of the concept of the onset of mental disorder is based on several elements. Unwritten rules of behavior exist in every community. Since they are unnamed, such rules are residual. They are what is left when the other rules are named. Obeying residual rules is something that goes without saying (which is why residual rules have no names), so much so that breaking them is considered unreasonable and incomprehensible. It cannot be imagined that someone "in their right mind" would break residual rules of behavior (residual norms). Most residual rule-breaking passes unnoticed because it is transitory, insignificant, becomes normalized or is ignored. But when residual norms are broken wantonly and in public, the community has no other choice but to label the deviant as mentally disordered, pursuant to the stereotyped picture of someone who is mentally disordered. Since the deviant is confused and embarrassed about their wanton and public breaking of the unwritten rules and thereby suggestible, they accept the role of being mentally ill, which is offered to them or imposed on them by the community. Once the person starts to play this role, it is hard to abandon it.

As much as I consider that there are unwritten rules in every community, I do not agree that breaking only these rules is perceived as unreasonable or incomprehensible. Thus, remaining within the framework of the sociogenesis of mental disorder, I do not see why breaking only unwritten rules (residual deviation) would be the initial phase in the onset of someone's mental disorder. I feel, as stated at the beginning of this text, that behavioral-functional deviation from the behavior and belief standard of a given community is one of the characteristics of mental disorder irrespective of which factors played a more important role in its genesis.

4. If "being mentally disordered" is nothing more than playing the social role of being mentally ill, i.e., behaving in accordance with the stereotype of mental disorder, which stems from Scheff's propositions, the following question arises: what about the *experienced* aspects of mental disorder? Does playing the role of being mentally disordered, which is what Scheff considers mental disorder to be, mean that the person experiences hallucinations and has delusional ideas, that their mood is very low, that their awareness has altered, which are all *experienced* phenomena characteristic of the mentally disordered? It is hard to believe that playing the social role of a mentally disordered person could include the above-mentioned and many other dimensions as well as specific experience of *being mentally disordered*, regardless of how strongly someone identifies with the "spitting image" of the mentally disordered. Particularly since the stereotype of mental disorder determines the content of the social role of being mentally disordered and the stereotype of mental disorder is an extremely simplified picture of mental disorder that does not include different expressions of some forms of mental disorder.

5. Scheff's concept of the sociogenesis of mental disorder, as already mentioned, is an example of the sociological approach to mental disorder. It therefore has all the deficiencies of the other concepts of mental disorder that belong to the sociological model of mental disorder.

Roger Bastide (1965: 43-44), a French anthropologist who was dealing with social aspects of mental disorders, criticizes the sociological approach for being too general and too specific.

First about the specific quality of the sociological approach to mental disorder. Basic sociological concepts of mental disorder interpret it in the context of either an adaptive response to an anomic situation (Merton) or deviant behavior (Lemert, Scheff). Both the adaptive response to an anomic situation and deviant behavior are treated as exclusively social phenomena. Mental disorder is interpreted in the same way. Only one dimension of a mentally disordered person: their deviation from the average of normative expectations, is considered to be the constitutive feature of a mentally disordered form of existence.

This equating the sociology of mental disorder with the sociology of deviant behavior or the sociology of social deviations has two obvious deficiencies. First, it leads to the wrong conclusion that behavior that is not outside the given normative framework is an expression and indicator of mental health or mental non-disorder (mental health, as I will show in the next chapter, may not be reduced to normalcy), and second, it neglects the organic-biological and psychological dimensions of mental disorder.

With regard to its being too general as the second basic limitation of the sociological approach to mental disorder, this is shown by its making no distinction between individual types of mental disorder. For example, Scheff, the creator of the most well-rounded social concept of mental disorder, feels that the clinical pictures of mental disorder are very similar.

6. When Scheff speaks of breaking residual norms, he is clearly thinking of the public breaking of unwritten rules. What about secret, hidden unwritten rule-breaking? Is it, as Len Bowers (1998: 15) notes, excluded as a possible reason for secondary deviation, i.e., taking over the role of a mentally disordered person?

7. In order for someone to take the social role of being mentally disordered, is it enough for the community to label them as mentally disordered? Or do psychiatrists, who are professionally trained and socially responsible for this job, need to make a diagnosis of mental disorder? In other words, could someone start to play the role of a mentally disordered person even before being labeled or diagnosed by a psychiatrist as mentally disordered, while being sound of mind? Are psychiatrists, as professionals, included in this last phase of the sociogenesis of mental disorder when the primary deviant is labeled as socially disordered and when they accept the role of being mentally disordered? If this is true, if their word is needed, then the sociogenesis of mental disorder could be largely reduced to psychiatrists' wrong diagnosis or labeling, which is the same thing in the given context.

8. Scheff does not make a clear distinction between "diagnosing" a specific behavior (residual deviation) as being mental disorder by laymen and the diagnosis of mental disorder made by psychiatrists. According to Scheff, a person is mentally disordered because the community has recognized their breaking the (social) residual rules as an expression of mental disorder and not because a psychiatrist, using criteria of mental disorder which are not the same as those of laymen, has diagnosed (recognized) someone's behavior, way of feeling and thinking, relationship towards themselves and others, in the specific features of their experiences, as being mentally disordered. Thus Scheff's explanation of the difference between mental disorder and non-disorder corresponds to that of a layman.

The sociological definition of mental disorder, both the theory of anomie and social interactionism (labeling theory), has not helped make a clearer distinction between mental disorder and non-disorder primarily because mental disorder is reduced to exclusively social phenomena: deviant behavior, society's reaction to deviant behavior, playing the social role of being mentally disordered, the stereotype about mental disorder and breaking residual norms.

Mental disorders are primarily personal and only then social problems. For sociologists, studying personal problems is studying social problems. This is what C. Wright Mills wrote in the book *The Sociological Imagination* (1959) that was used by generations of sociologists as some sort of guidebook to sociological research. This is why the sociological study of mental disorders "can truly serve as a social mirror" (Pearlin, Avison, Fazio, 2008: 36), that is, help to better understand different aspects of a given community, but not to better understand mental disorder. It cannot help to better define mental disorder, i.e., to accurately distinguish mental disorder from non-disorder.

Consequences of Unclear Border between Mental Disorder and Non-Disorder: Confusing Results of Epidemiological Studies

If there was an agreed-upon operational definition of mental disorder, there would be a clear border between mental disorder and non-disorder. This does not mean that that border would correspond to the border, if any, in *rerum natura* because, as stated, at this stage, validity of generic mental disorder, and the majority of individual mental disorders, for that matter, cannot be assessed. If there was an agreed-upon definition of mental disorder, we would only agree on where a border between mental disorder and non-disorder is.

Psychiatric epidemiologists cannot do without a clear-cut definition of mental disorder. That is why two main concepts of psychiatric illness epidemiologists operate with are based on clear definitions of mental disorders. As noted by Sandanger, Nygard, and Sorensen (2002), particular symptoms will be called illness when they exceed a certain level: *How much of it has s/he got?* "The second alternative concept is the criteriological, essentialist view that people either have or do not have disorders: *Has s/he got it?*"

The results of epidemiological research of the prevalence of mental disorders carried out in the last twenty years, or so, demonstrate the consequences of a lack of valid diagnosis of mental disorders.

The work of the epidemiologist on establishing the number of mentally disordered in a community, the prevalence of different types of mental disorder and the links between biological, psychological and social factors, and the onset and duration of mental disorders, is no less important than the work of psychiatrists who on clinical level evaluate who is disordered and what they are suffering from. The findings of epidemiological research are extremely important for public health in particular. They indicate the number of sick or mentally disordered in a specific population. These findings determine the amount of funds that should be invested to protect the population's mental health, and particularly which mental health protection programs should have priority. They speak of the amount of funds needed for psychiatric services, the number of mental health workers that are needed, among other things. In a word, it is extremely important for epidemiological research to provide an *accurate* picture of how many mentally disordered people there are in a community at a specific point in time or over a specific period of time, and the frequency of newly arising cases in that specific period of time.

It is particularly important for epidemiological research to show the *real prevalence* of mentally disordered people. Unlike *clinical prevalence* that shows how many mentally disordered people are receiving psychiatric help, *real prevalence* shows the total number of mentally disordered in a community. It consist of the sum of the number of disordered people registered by psychiatric services and the number of untreated mentally disordered people, i.e., those people who are first identified by psychiatric epidemiological research as being disordered.

From the public health viewpoint, *real prevalence* is a more important figure than *clinical prevalence*. A large number of factors influence the size of *clinical prevalence* that have nothing to do with the real number of mentally disordered, such as the accessibility of psychiatric services, the tolerance of the environment to manifestations of mental disorder, the bias of the environment towards the mentally disordered and psychiatry, whether outpatient forms of providing psychiatric care are developed, whether the state covers the cost of psychiatric services or the patient pays partially or in full.

The basic diagnostic instrument used by psychiatrists is the psychiatric interview. It cannot be used as a basic diagnostic instrument in epidemiological research not only because of the problem of the low (inter-psychiatrist) inter-rate reliability of the diagnosis of mental disorder, particularly mild forms of mental disorder, but the very long time that would be needed to conduct epidemiological research in which the psychiatric interview was the basic diagnostic instrument, along with the enormous amount of funds that would be needed for such research. This is why structured interviews or structured questionnaires are used for diagnostic purposes in epidemiological research. In the first case, laymen who have been trained at a short course ask the subjects questions that are clearly defined in the questionnaire. The number of positive answers above a specific cutoff indicates the probability that the individual is mentally disordered. In the second case, the subjects themselves fill out a questionnaire that contains all the questions needed to make a diagnosis. The data is then fed into a computer and an algorithm calculates the number of mentally disordered people in the given population based on this information.

In the past twenty years several large epidemiological studies have been made in the United States, *inter alia* on the incidence and prevalence of mental disorders. A number of results from these studies indicate that psychiatric epidemiologists do not have a valid definition of mental disorder. In the text that follows I will discuss these results as empirical proof of psychiatric epidemiologists' unsatisfactory success in distinguishing mental order from non-disorder.

All except one of these epidemiological studies—Regier, Myers, Kramer et al., 1984; Kessler, McGonagle, Zhao et al., 1994; Kessler, Berglund, Demler et al., 2005; Kessler, Chin, Demler et al., 2005—used the operational definitions of mental disorders set out in DSM-III and DSM-IV that "rely" on the definition of generic mental disorder found in these classifications. DIS (*Diagnostic Interview Schedule*) and CICS (*Composite International Comorbidity Survey*) were used as research instruments. Since DSMs are based on symptoms, epidemiologists had a rather easy time turning the criteria to diagnose patients in clinical conditions into questions for epidemiological research of the entire population. The authors of the above study started from the assumption that a structured diagnostic interview, such as DIS, would allow researchers to diagnose mental disorder in the population almost the same way that a psychiatric would in clinical conditions.

What did the results of this epidemiological research show? How high is the prevalence of mental disorder in the United States? It established that the *twelve-month prevalence of mental disorder ranged from 26.2 to 30.2 percent*[18] (ECA, Epidemiological Catchment Area, Robins and Regier, 1991; NCS, National Comorbidity Survey, Kessler, McGonagle, Zhao et al., 1994).

As to how many Americans will suffer from mental disorder during their lifetime, it turned out (Kessler, Berglund, Demiler et al., 2005) that almost half of the population of the United States will have some form of mental disorder during their lifetime.

It has been estimated (Wakefield and Spitzer, 2002: 31-32) that the finding that around one-third of Americans satisfy the criteria of at least one mental disorder—which is a truly high percentage—stems from the fact that the DSM system is overly inclusive. This is why the DSM-IV Task Force added the clinical significance criterion to the definition of many disorders in DSM-IV. When these criteria were added *post hoc* to the ECA and NCS data, the prevalence rate of overall mental disorders decreased 30 percent compared to the initial finding.

Both the initial findings of the ECA and NCS on the prevalence of mental disorders in the United States and their one-third decrease after adding the significance criterion to many of the mental disorder definitions in DSM-IV were considered much too high. Questions were raised in the psychiatric community and beyond as to whether psychiatric epidemiological research was able to provide accurate information on the prevalence of mentally disordered people in a community, in other words whether psychiatric epidemiological research clearly distinguished mental disorder from non-disorder. Such questions were all the more justified since some scholars (e. g., Kendell, 2002: 5) considered that the *post hoc* addition of the clinical significance criterion did not completely eliminate the false positive cases, and other scholars (e. g., Wakefield and Spitzer, 2002: 37) wrote that adding this criterion resulted in identifying people who were mentally disordered as non-disordered (false negatives).

It is quite probable that using some other definition of generic mental disorder and other diagnostic criteria than that found in DSMs would produce different results as to how many people are mentally disordered in a given population.

The data that around one-third of Americans have at least one mental disorder, then reducing that number by one-third after the *post hoc* addition of the clinical significance criterion, and finally doubts whether the addition of this criterion successfully eliminated false positive or false negative cases indicates that psychiatric epidemiological research *does not use conceptually valid criteria to distinguish mental disorder from non-disorder*. They are not used because they do not exist.

The problem lies *inter alia* in the imprecise and unclear criteria to identify mental disorder, i.e., insufficiently *specific* criteria. I would remind the reader that the specific features of diagnostic criteria denote the degree to which they can be used to identify *only* that disorder.

Even the slightest problem with the specific features of diagnostic criteria can greatly influence the validity of the results of epidemiological research on the prevalence of mental disorder in a population. One of the basic reasons is that the general population sample used for epidemiological research has far more people who are not mentally disordered than disordered.

Let me cite the example given by Jerome C. Wakefield (1999b: 41) of the enormous influence that insufficiently specific diagnostic criteria can have on the results of the prevalence of mental disorder in a population.

Let us assume that the real prevalence of a certain disorder is one percent of the total population. Let us also assume that diagnostic criteria to identify mental disorder have a 10 percent degree of error for false positive and false negative. In other words, the diagnostic criteria can establish 90 percent of all those who are really mentally disordered as being disordered, with 10 percent of the subjects being incorrectly classified as non-disordered. At the same time, the diagnostic criteria will accurately identify 90 percent of those who are not disordered as being non-disordered and will incorrectly identify 10 percent of them as disordered. Although it is the same degree of error for false positive and false negative, both degrees of error have very different effects on evaluating the prevalence of mental disorder because the two populations, the population of non-disordered and disordered, are of very different sizes.

The degree of false negative means that 10 percent of the one percent of the disordered population, or 0.1 percent are wrongly diagnosed as non-disordered. On the other hand, the degree of false positive means that 10 percent of the 99 percent non-disordered population or 9.9 percent of the population is incorrectly diagnosed as disordered.

This indicates that the 10 percent false positive has a *99 times greater impact* than the 10 percent false negative on the estimated degree of prevalence of mentally disordered in a given population.

This example convincingly shows that a *small* error in establishing the specific features of diagnostic criteria for mental disorder causes a *large* error in establishing the prevalence of mental disorders.

We have now returned to the beginning of this part of the text, to the title that asks whether epidemiologists know what constitutes mental disorder. They do know—would be the answer—as much as other psychiatrists, which means not enough. Psychiatric epidemiologists, who include many sociologists and psychologists, do not have valid diagnostic criteria for mental disorder, and neither do clinical psychiatrists and psychologists who endeavor on a daily basis to establish whether the people they interview in psychiatric outpatient clinics are mentally disordered. The lack of such criteria is the basic reason why it is hard to have faith in psychiatric epidemiological estimates of the prevalence of mental disorder in a specific community.

What Makes It Difficult to Define Mental Disorder: The Nature of Mental Disorder or Imperfect Psychiatric Diagnostic Instruments?

The numerous difficulties that stand in the way of successfully distinguishing mentally disordered people from those who are non-disordered spurred Deborah A. Zarin and Felton Earls from the Developmental Epidemiological Research Unit, Judge Baker Children's Center in Boston, to put forward their observations in the introduction to the work "Diagnostic decision making in psychiatry" (1993). These deserve mention in the context of defining mental disorder, particularly since the authors quite correctly link the definition of mental disorder with the diagnosis and classification of mental disorders.

Zarin and Earls noted that a large number of relevant works point to deficiencies in the classifications of mental disorders, diagnostic criteria and diagnostic tests used in psychiatry.

The following question is therefore fitting: why does psychiatry face up to so many problems regarding the definition of mental disorder, diagnosing and the classification of individual forms of mental disorders? Opinions range from blaming the nature of mental disorders for this unenviable state in psychiatry, which virtually means that no improvement can be expected, to those that psychiatrists are where they are with regard to diagnosing mental disorders because they have been unable to find better instruments to detect mental disorders. Thus, work is needed to improve psychiatric diagnoses.

Regardless of which of these opinions enjoys our (greater) trust, conclude Zarin and Earls, even when psychiatrists use the best diagnostic instruments, there is considerable overlap between the mentally disordered and non-disordered.

With regard to conceptualizing generic mental disorder, I feel that a consensus could probably be reached for its definition, but not in the same way as the consensus concerning the operational definitions of individual types of mental disorder set out in DSMs. This was preceded by empirical studies intended to establish how much a set of specific symptoms could be considered a separate pathological entity. The conclusion in this regard was reached after studying whether, over a long period, the same symptoms appeared together in the same patient; what was the course and outcome of the specific clinical syndrome; how did it respond to this or that type of treatment; how frequent it was among the patient's relatives; whether it had biomarkers and what they were.

Such studies *cannot* provide data that would help to reach consensus about one single definition of generic mental disorder: which set of symptoms should be singled out and monitored for generic mental disorder in order to see whether they appear together over a longer period; what is their outcome; whether they appear and how frequently among the person's relatives, whether they react to the same therapy the same way. In other words, it cannot be said which set of symptoms is characteristic of generic mental disorder.

By definition, generic mental disorder includes what is essential for all individual forms of mental disorder, what they all have in common. But the definition of generic mental disorder cannot contain several hundred symptoms of individual mental disorders or even a special selection of symptoms that would be representative of the symptoms of all types of mental disorder. The definition of generic mental disorder contains a description of the *nature* of mental disorder that is valid for mental disorder *as such* and for all types of mental disorder.

With regard to individual types of mental disorder, the biological structural-functional basis of each one must be determined to establish its validity. Only an appropriately high degree of validity of a specific diagnostic definition is proof that this definition is correct, that it corresponds to the reality of what it defines and what it defines exists as a separate entity.

Now comes the question that is as logical and inevitable as it is rarely discussed in texts on the diagnosis and classification of different forms of mental disorder.

How is it possible to establish the cause of a specific mental disorder if, on the level of its symptoms, its clinical picture, a clear boundary cannot be drawn between this mental disorder and another mental disorder, or between this mental disorder and a mentally non-disordered state? How can we look for one single or many causes of a phenomenon, if prior to our research features that distinguish this phenomenon from other phenomena have not been identified?

This was written about in detail in the "Distinguishing between the validity and utility of psychiatric diagnoses" (2003) by Robert E. Kendell and Assen Jablensky. I will return to this critical work in the chapter "Physical Diseases and Mental Disorders: Should They be Differentiated?"

This same question can be raised when determining the validity of generic mental disorder. How can we determine the validity of generic mental disorder, when we do not know which symptoms comprise generic mental disorder? Which symptoms of generic mental disorder would have a biological basis when we do not know which symptoms comprise generic mental disorder?

Dimensional Definition of Mental Disorder and Defining Mental Disorder Using Prototypes

The difficulty in determining the characteristics that are specific to mental disorder (alone) is shown by attempts to use two other approaches instead of the categorial approach ("sick" and "healthy" are two completely separate and independent categories) when defining mental disorder. These approaches are the *dimensional* approach and determining a *prototype* of mental disorder. As shown below, these two attempts were unable to rectify the defects in the categorial definition of mental disorder.

The concept of a *dimensional* definition[19] of mental disorder is based on the assumption that there is no clear boundary between a disordered and non-disordered state, that one state shifts almost imperceptibly into the other. The state of complete mental health or non-disorder would be on one end and the state of complete mental disorder on the other end of the imagined dimension of "mental health-mental disorder."[20] Between these two extreme points would be states of greater or lesser mental disorder and more or less non-disordered states, and which of these states was (momentarily) dominant would be determined for each individual case.

The difficulty, however, is that for the needs of psychiatric-epidemiological research a point on the imagined dimension "mental health-mental disorder" *must* be defined as the watershed between mental disorder and non-disorder. In order to be able to compare the results of different psychiatric-epidemiological studies, the same dimensional definition of a specific disorder must be used in all psychiatric-epidemiological studies on some aspect of that mental disorder (e.g. incidence, prevalence, association of the disorder with some biological, social or other factor or factors). Furthermore, the same number of dimensions would have to be used to define the disorder, and finally, the point on the dimension for a specific quality would have to be defined in the same manner up to which that quality is *normal* and after which it is *pathological*.

Such kind of methodological uniformity of epidemiological studies is not easy to procure. This is only one of the reasons why the dimensional approach might be less suitable for epidemiological studies. In any case, it is easier to compare the results of studies performed by using the categorial rather than dimensional concept of mental disorder.

What would be the definition of mental disorder using a *prototype*? The prototype of something includes the most frequent characteristics of the members of a specific category, the characteristics that we are more likely to find among members of that category than among members of other categories.

Juan E. Mezzich (1989) compared the categorial definition of mental disorder, which he called classical, and the definition of mental disorder using its prototype. He states that in the categorial model the members have homogenous characteristics and in the model based on stereotypes they are heterogeneous to a certain degree. The boundaries between entities in the categorial model are clear and in the model based on stereotypes they are unclear. While every defining characteristic of the mental disorder is needed in the categorial model, and all together they are sufficient to define the mental disorder, in the model based on stereotypes the characteristics that are chosen as defining the mental disorder are only in correlation with membership to the group of mentally disordered. Finally, it can be said that the categorial approach to mental disorder is deterministic, while the approach based on stereotypes is probabilistic.

In conclusion, neither the dimensional approach nor the approach to defining mental disorder based on prototypes overcame the numerous difficulties that appear when trying to define mental disorder. The number of questions and dilemmas only increased.

Conclusion

Robert E. Kendell (1975a: 9) wrote that "that there is no concept in medicine more fundamental than that of disease and illness." He was also thinking about psychiatry, of course, as a branch of medicine.

Many authors—interestingly enough more philosophers, psychologists and anthropologists than psychiatrists—have tried to define mental disorder. The definitions are quite different, although a relatively small number of characteristics of mental disorder appear in them (e.g., deviancy, dysfunction, impairment, incapacity, distress, harmful dysfunction), thought by the authors of the definitions to be characteristic of mentally disordered people.

I have set out and stated the reasons for my definition of mental disorder. Mental disorder is characterized by deviation from the behavior and belief standard of a given community, damage to one or more mental functions, psychological dysfunction, these events happen against the individual's will, and cause suffering (distress).

With regard to dysfunctional deviation of the mentally disordered from the prevailing behavior and belief pattern of a given community, this is always behavioral-functional *deviation* regardless of the specific sociocultural community. It is at the same time always deviation from the specific behavior and belief pattern that prevails in the community.

In addition, I have critically analyzed two of the most important and most discussed definitions of mental disorder in the past thirty years (the definition of mental disorder in DSMs, and Wakefield's definition).

I have shown why psychosis-like experiences do not, in fact, substantiate the allegations that there is no such a thing as psychosis—and mental disorder, for that matter—as in psychopathological terms a qualitatively distinct phenomenon.

Also it has been indicated that attempts to deceive psychiatrists performed by Rosenhan and Slater left unanswered the question of whether "sanity and insanity exist," and "how we shall know them."

The sociological definition of mental disorder—as I have shown— cannot be used by those who want to establish the specific features of mental disorder: whether and how a mental disorder differs from a state with which it shares certain common characteristics.

Numerous are the consequences of difficulties to draw a clear-cut border between mental disorder and non-disorder. One of the consequences is the considerable difference in the prevalence and incidence of mental disorders in the same community from one epidemiological study to another.

There must be a correspondence between the characteristics (of the definition) of generic mental disorder and the characteristics (of the definition) of each individual mental disorder. Defining the basic characteristics of generic mental disorder should precede the definition of the individual types of mental disorder. Any type of mental disorder that does not contain the characteristics of generic mental disorder should not be diagnosed as mental disorder.

A good definition of generic mental disorder is one that contains the *specificity of the characteristics* of mental disorder compared to other states that are more or less similar to mental disorder ("closest neighbors").

A good definition of generic mental disorder is one that does not depend on changes in the classification of mental disorders, changes in diagnostic criteria for individual disorders, changes in the boundary between different types of mental disorder, changes in the names of mental disorders, introducing new mental disorders to the classification and removing others.

The validity (of the definition) of generic mental disorder cannot be determined on a biological structural-functional basis because there is not a clinically defined, widely agreed upon definition of mental disorder. We could—purely hypothetically—talk about establishing the structural validity of a definition of generic mental disorder only if the structural-function basis of almost all types of mental disorders were determined, so that the *common denominator* of biological structural-functional changes of all individual types of mental disorder would be taken as the biological basis of generic mental disorder. This common denominator of the biological basis of different types of mental disorder would be the *biological specificity* of mental disorder as such.

In addition to the difficulty in identifying the specific characteristics of mental disorder *per se*, the *degree of intensity* of these characteristics appears as a considerable obstacle on the path to finding a better definition of generic mental disorder, and this means a definition of generic mental disorder that can be used with a high degree of certainty in distinguishing mental disorder from non-disorder. Denoting the degree of intensity as *significant* did not prove to be a good solution.

Definitions of generic mental disorder to date, including mine, should be understood as attempts to come closer to a definition of mental disorder that would include characteristics that are specific only and exclusively to mental disorder. Such a definition would certainly be widely accepted. To date there is no generally accepted definition of generic mental disorder that would satisfy all psychiatrists and clinical psychologists, regardless of their theoretical orientation and the nature of their daily practice.

Notes

1. Alluding to doctors' unwillingness to address the issue of defining illness/disorder, Peter Sedgwick writes in his text "Anti-psychiatry, Disorder and the Mentally Ill","

published as an introduction to *PsychoPolitics*, edited by Sedgwick, as follows: "Any inspection of the current state of discussion in medical press about the real nature of illness and disease will undermine any confidence the reader may have that our doctors have the faintest idea of what is, in the most general sense, that they are trying to cure, treat or palliate" (1982: 11).

2.   It is important to note the difference between viewing as normal and thereby desirable a behavior and belief pattern that is most frequent in a society and viewing it as valid. The following Fromm's comment may help us to make this distinction. Erich Fromm writes: "It is naively assumed that the fact that the majority of people share certain ideas or feelings proves the validity of these ideas and feelings. Nothing is further from the truth. Consensual validation as such has no bearing whatsoever on reason or mental health. Just as there is a *folie à deux* there is a *folie à millions*. The fact that millions of people share the same vices does not make them virtuous, the fact that they share so many errors does not make the errors to be truths, and the fact that millions of people share the same forms of mental pathology does not make them sane" (1954).

3.   The notion of "abnormal" is used in psychopathology and psychiatry to denote a degree of pronouncement of some characteristic. What is *quantitatively* below or above the defined limit of "normal" for a specific trait or amount is abnormal. The concept of "abnormal" should not be confused with the concept "pathological" that denotes primarily a *qualitative* deviation from the behavior and belief standard of a given environment. In the same manner, psychoanalyst Heinz Hartmann distinguishes "abnormal" from "pathological": "abnormal" in the sense of deviation from the average is not synonymous with "pathological" (1939).

4.   It is true that a certain number of mentally ill people are found among those who foster an alternative lifestyle. It happens that mentally disordered individuals who cannot properly play most of social roles that they carried out successfully before their mental disorder choose an alternative lifestyle that does not include the regular execution of the social roles that are carried out by the majority in a given community. Thus, it sometimes happens that an alternative lifestyle hides the disorders of its members.

5 .   This does not mean that psychiatrists in one and the same society are not members of psychiatric schools and orientations that are so different that one might almost speak of different types of psychiatry. This was the case in Argentina until recently where two quite different types of psychiatry existed; their supporters held to the principles of two completely different models. One group followed the theory and practice of the French psychoanalyst Jacques Lacan, and the other group advocated the biomedical model. This division lasted for decades. Recently, after a merciless offensive by pharmaceutical companies, the biomedical model supplanted Lacans' supporters (See Lakoff, 2005).

6.   We can only guess how Aubrey Lewis would comment on attention that has been paid lately to findings about mentally sound people having auditory hallucinations or delusions, and in particular on conclusions drawn from these findings.

7.   Julka Varelius (2009) believes that psychiatric patients lack control over their behavior because it is not based on autonomous choices and decisions. According to this scholar, a diminished psychological capacity for autonomy is the fundamental characteristic of mental illness.

8.   Even though it does not refer to primary but rather secondary prevention, it is worth mentioning, in this context, early intervention in psychosis. Over the last ten years, the issue of early intervention in psychosis has attracted psychiatrists' attention across the board. In the early nineties, Patrick D. McGorry, Professor at Orygen Research Centre in Melbourne, initiated a systematic research on how it would be

possible to perform secondary prevention of psychoses, primarily of schizophrenia. McGorry and other psychiatrists and psychologists dealing with early intervention in psychosis have extensively reported on their research and practical activities, as well as on the challenges they have faced (for example, McGorry, Killackey, Yung, 2008; Yung and McGorry, 2007; McGorry, Hickie, Yung, *et al.*, 2006; McGorry, Nordentoft, Simonssen, 2005).

There are two major goals of early interventions in psychosis. First, to detect those at risk of onset of psychosis, and then to treat them by CBT, atypical antipsychotics, omega-3 fatty, glycine, skills training, psychoeducation and family interventions so as to prevent or delay a full-blown psychosis (pre-onset intervention). Second, to start treating those with psychosis in the earliest possible stage of disorder in order to minimize duration of untreated psychosis (DUP) (post-onset intervention). The earlier the treatment the better outcome is the idea underlying such a strategy.

As my book deals with controversies and dilemmas in contemporary psychiatry I will point at some major questions that arise in regard to early intervention in psychosis.

Prodromal symptoms for psychosis are heterogeneous, i.e., non-specific. That is why criteria had to be defined for the selection of those who are at highest risk of psychosis: a group of ultra-high risk (UHR) of psychosis. In addition to age (between 12 and 25), three criteria are used: (1) Attenuated Psychotic Symptoms Group: have experienced subtreshold, attenuated positive psychotic symptoms during the past year; (2) Brief Limited Intermittent Psychotic Symptoms Group: have experienced episodes of frank psychotic symptoms that have not lasted longer than a week and have spontaneously abated; (3) Trait Plus Risk Factor Group: have a first-degree relative with a psychotic disorder or the identified client has a schizotypal personality disorder and they have experienced a significant decrease in functioning during the previous year (Yung, Yuen, Berger *et al.*, 2007).

A key issue has continued to be the predictive validity of the prodromal or UHR selection criteria (Cannon, Cornblatt, McGorry, 2007). Studies report a transition rate to a full psychotic disorder of, on average, about 30 percent. In other words, about two thirds of those who meet criteria for ultra high risk of psychosis do not develop psychosis.

Many questions arise in regard to such a high number of false positive. Do characteristics of those with UHR of psychosis constitute a prodrom or a risk syndrome? As noted by Stephan Heckers (2009), the prodrom is, by definition, the nascent stage of a disorder. "In contrast, a risk syndrome is not necessarily linked to a disorder. The value of a risk syndrome increases with the accuracy in predicting future outcomes." Given such a high percentage of those with UHR of psychosis who do not transit to psychosis, it seems that UHR is more a risk syndrome than a prodrom. And "a risk syndrome is not part and parcel of the disorder."

Further on, "it has been estimated that the false positive rate would jump from about 70 percent in specialty clinics to about 90 percent in general practice. This means that as many as astounding nine in ten individuals identified as "risk syndrome" "would not really be at risk of developing psychosis" (Frances, 2010). And still they will be given antipsychotics that have unpleasant side-effects such as weight-gain and the risk for metabolic syndrome. And they will be stigmatized as mentally disordered, as well.

The term "pre-onset" intervention is justified if pre-psychotic and psychotic— and non-disorder and disorder, for that matter—can be differentiated. And that is not always the case. Thus, Alison R. Yung and Patrick D. McGorry (2007), the most enthusiastic advocates of early intervention in psychosis, write that "the onset of psychosis is arbitrarily defined and does not differ qualitatively from subtreshold psychosis." Parnas on his part draws our attention to the difficulties in dating the illness onset. "In a polydiagnostic scenario, a patient diagnosed as being 'pre-onset' by one diagnostic system may be already considered as 'post-onset' by another system. The notorious 'fuzziness' of the schizophrenia concept makes dating the illness onset not only a psychometric problem, but a theoretical issue intimately associated with the conceptual validity of schizophrenia, that is what we take schizophrenia to be in the very first place" (Parnas, 2005).

The efficacy of clinical interventions in preventing or delaying the transition into psychosis is what clinicians are most interested in. William T. Carpenter (2009) writes that data from "clinical studies suggest that clinical intervention may be effective in delaying or preventing exacerbation into psychosis, but evidence to date is very weak." This view is shared by Thomas H. McGlashan (2005). He maintains that "the data informing the benefit: risk ratio are insufficient to justify prodromal intervention research." De Koning, Bloemen, van Amelsvoort *et al.* (2009) too maintain that a definitive conclusion about the efficacy and safety of the interventions aimed at delaying or preventing the transition into psychosis "cannot be drawn at this moment."

Also, there is no consensus as to whether the earliest possible treatment yields the best outcome. While fervent advocates of the idea of early intervention in psychosis have no doubt that the shorter DUP the better outcome, other authors are cautious about such type of correlation. Thus, for example, Larsen, Friis, Haahr *et al.* (2001) write: "Regarding secondary prevention we conclude that it is still an open question if a reduction in DUP leads to better outcome for first-episodes patients." Yet Warner (2005) is unequivocal: "The belief that early intervention in psychosis leads to better outcome is based on a misinterpretation of the available data."

Two meta-analyses (Marshall, Lewis, Lockwood *et al.* 2005; Perkins, Gu, Boteva *et al.* 2005) have shown that longer DUP is associated with poorer outcome. Yet the key question, as rightly noted by Svein Friis (2010), is how lasting are the effects of early specialized or integrated treatment, which encompasses assertive community treatment, family involvement, social skills training, regular contact with a team member responsible for treatment coordination, etc. The results of the part of the Lambeth Early Onset (LEO) study that deals with long-term effects of the 18-month specialized early intervention (Gafoor, Nitsch, McCrone, *et al.* 2010) have demonstrated that the members of the specialized care group as compared to the members of standard group did worse in the long run. They had more hospital admissions and total duration of admissions. And the results of the part of the Danish National Schizophrenia Project (OPUS) that deals with long-term effects of integrated treatment versus standard treatment (Bertelsen, Jeppesen, Petersen *at al.* 2008) have shown that the difference between the integrated and the standard group were no significant after five years. The intervention, that is, the integrated treatment lasted for two years.

Indeed, the idea of early intervention in psychosis, and its feasibility in particular, has been welcomed by many mental health workers all over the world. Hundreds of centers dealing with early intervention in psychosis have been set up over the last ten years or so. Moreover, the introduction of Psychosis Risk Syndrome as a diagnostic entity into DSM-V has been hotly debated (e.g., Frances, 2010).

In discussing the pros and cons of early intervention in psychosis due attention should be assigned to the most recent assessment made by Max Marshall and John Rathbone (2010). They write: "We sought to review all trials that involved early intervention for people with prodromal symptoms, or a first episode of psychosis. We identified seven studies, most were underpowered and at present we have insufficient data to draw any definitive conclusion, although further trials are expected."

Knowing the poor prognosis of a good number of psychotic and especially schizophrenic disorders psychiatrists could not help but greet the possibility of preventing this kind of mental disorders and/or making the life of those affected easier. Yet the following warning is more than well placed. "There is a danger that our lack of effective treatment strategies for psychoses may weaken our critical attitude towards new ideas that are marketed strongly" (Larsen, Friis, Haahr, *et al.* 2001).

9.   Allen J. Frances adds (2009a) that "having in mind the unfortunate experience of the past," there is a looming danger that marketing strategists would greatly enlarge the ranks of the false positives.

10. After reviewing how "distress" has been used in DSM-IV and ICD-10, Michael R. Phillips concludes that "both diagnostic systems use distress as a stand-alone symptom, as a qualifier of other symptoms and as a general measure of severity; but neither the DSM-IV nor the ICS-10 provides a definition of the term, so there can be a wide range of interpretations of the corresponding diagnostic criteria" (2009). Phillips stresses out that the frequent use of various qualifiers for distress in the diagnostic criteria, like "clinically significant," "marked," "excessive," indicate that distress is conceived of as a dimension. "But the diagnostic systems do not assess the degree of distress and do not provide further clarification about the cut-off between distress that is and is not diagnostically important."

In other words "distress" has not been operationalized, the same as "disability (i.e., impairment in one or more important areas of functioning) has not been operationalized in DSMs.

Phillips maintains that "if it is not possible to develop a unique, non-overlapping operational definition of distress" "distress" should be dropped from the diagnostic criteria.

The truth is that a very small number of diagnostic criteria for a generic mental disorder can be operationalized. However, this does not mean that they should not be used in differentiating mental disorder from non-disorder. If all diagnostic criteria for the generic mental disorder were operationalized this would significantly reduce psychiatrists' dilemmas about whether a bunch of particular symptoms are to be considered as a mental disorder. However, this does not mean that by using the operationalized diagnostic criteria for the generic mental disorder psychiatrists will *more accurately* differentiate mental disorder from non-disorder. Nor does it mean that psychiatrists will be more willing to use such criteria than they are (un)willing to use the existent diagnostic criteria, defined in DSMs and the ICD-10, for the generic mental disorder.

11. Dan J. Stein, Katharine A. Phillips, Derek Bolton *et al.* (2010) proposed a revision of the definition of a mental disorder as part of the process of developing DSM-V. They, in fact, suggested very slight changes in the DSM-IV definition of mental disorder. They maintain that "clinical significant" should be used when mentioning distress and disability as the consequences of a behavioural or psychological syndrome or pattern that occurs in the individual rather than as a characterization of a behavioural or psychological syndrome. Also, they suggest that the DSM-IV "E" criterion that runs "A manifestation of a behavioural, psychological or biological dysfunction in he individual" should be rephrased and run (a behavioural or psychological syndrome or pattern) "that reflects an underlying psychobiological dysfunction."

The cited authors add two more criteria to characterize an individual mental disorder. "First, any disorder in DSM should have diagnostic validity, on the basis of a number of key validators (e. g., prognostic significance, evidence of psycho-biological disruption, or prediction of response to treatment)."

Such a criterion is, at this stage, unrealistic, to say the very least. If we were able to establish diagnostic validity of any disorder in DSMs, or in any other classificatory system, the majority of problems associated with the diagnostics of mental disorders would be solved.

"Second, any disorder in DSM should have clinical utility...That is, we suggest that receipt of a DSM-V diagnosis needs to convey something important about that individual that is relevant in a treatment setting."

My only comment is that depending on the psychiatric model one signs up to—and many other factors, as well—a (new) diagnosis "conveys something important about that individual that is relevant in a treatment setting." In other words, this criterion is rather loose.

12. Ronald C. Kessler, Kathleen R. Merikangas, Patricia Berglund *et al.* (2003), feel that mild disorders, with all the ambiguities linked to their definition, should not be excluded from the fifth revision of the American classification of mental disorders because the proper treatment of milder cases prevents a considerable number of future serious cases. Gordon Parker, one of the greatest experts in the field of depression, does not agree with this opinion. He feels that there is not enough data to show the purposefulness of treating "mild depression." "Those who advance this component of the unidirectional model (i.e. subsyndromal depression is a driver of substantive morbidity and disability) often then argue that findings establish the need for assertive treatment of the 'depression'. In reality, the evidence base supporting such advocacy is quite limited, and even more desultory than evidence in regard to major depression. By itself, it does not validate the extreme consequences of the dimensional approach: that expanding the boundary of 'depression' is necessarily associated with successful intervention across the spectrum" (2008).

13. The most comprehensive analysis to date of Wakefield's definition of disease (disorder) as "harmful dysfunction" was carried out by Derek Bolton in his book *What is Mental Disorder?*, 2008, pp. 116-162.

14. For instance, Feelgood, S. R., Rantzen, A. J., 1994; Chedru, F., Feldman, F., Ameri, A. *et al.*, 1996; Olfson, M., Lewis-Fernandez, R., Weissman M. *et al.*, 2002; Schreier, H. A., 1999; Verdoux, H., van Os, J., 2002; Eaton, W. W., Romanosky, A., Anthony, J. C. *et al.*, 1991; Johns, L. C., Canon, M., Singleton, N. *et al.*, 2004; Dhossche, D., Ferdinand, R., van der Ende, J. *et al.*, 2002.

15. For instance, Freeman, D., Garety, P. A., Bebbington, P. E. *et al.*, 2005; Johns, L. C. Canon, M., Singleton, C. *et al.*, 2004; Verdoux, H., Maurice-Tison, S., Gay, B. *et al.*, 1998; Poulton, R., Caspi, A., Moffitt, T.E. *et al.*, 2000.

16. It is of note that Louis A. Sass, Professor of Clinical Psychology at Rutgers University, in the United States, also opines that schizophrenia and modern times are closely connected. Thus, he writes that "schizophrenia's emergence coincided with the birth of modern episteme" (1996: 365-366), and, further on, that "whether considered from a historical or a cross-cultural standpoint, modern Western civilization does seem to have a statistical association with schizophrenia, or at least with its severely chronic or autistic forms" (1996: 366). Sass considers the following characteristics of modern human beings' psyche as, to say the very least, similar to the way people with schizophrenia relate to themselves and other people: a pervasive detachment, a "disengagement," a sense of inwardness, a state of permanent reflectiveness and subjectivization, intellectuality and cautious deliberation. "If schizoids and schizophrenics, like other human beings, are subject to the influences of their social milieu, it is not hard to see how a number of their core traits (the asocial turning inward, the lack of spontaneity, the detachment from emotion, the hyperabstractness, the

anxious deliberation and cognitive slippage, and the exquisitely vulnerable sense of self-esteem, for example) might be exaggeration of tendencies fostered by this civilization" (1996: 370).

Thus, Sass, like Devereux, regards the symptoms of people with schizophrenia an exaggeration of tendencies fostered by modern civilization. There is no mention—at least not in this passage—of specific experiential dimensions of a schizophrenic patient. It turns out that the difference, if any, between those who suffer from schizophrenia, on the one hand, and mentally sound people, on the other, is quantitative ("exaggeration") rather than qualitative. Modern times engender specific imperfections of people living in those times. When exaggerated, those imperfections become the characteristics of schizophrenic patients.

It is of note that there are other scholars who also claim that there is an association of modern times and schizophrenia. Thus, Liah Greenfeld, University Professor and Professor of Political Science and Sociology, Boston University, maintains (2005) that modern culture "at the core of which lies the vision of nationalism," and which is "inherently and pervasively *anomic* culture," increases the rate of the most serious mental disorders such as schizophrenia.

She stresses more than Sass the etiological link between modern culture and schizophrenia. In other words, she does not claim that there is a similarity between modern human beings' psyche and the symptoms of those who are diagnosed with schizophrenia. Rather, she claims that modern culture is responsible for the increased rate of schizophrenia in modern times. However, there is no conclusive evidence that the incidence of schizophrenic patients has increased over the last few centuries. Nor there is evidence that anomie, i.e., anomia, which is a subjective equivalent of anomie, can engender serious mental disorders, such as schizophrenia (Kecmanovic, 2007).

17. By asserting that many mentally healthy people experience phenomena that are usually identified with mental disorder, Edwin Lemert can be considered the precursor of the psychosis-like experiences movement.

18. The subject of this research was not only the prevalence of all mental disorders but the frequency of individual types of mental disorder and many other epidemiological aspects of mental disorder.

19. The difference between the categorial and the dimensional model of mental disorders is well elaborated in the paper "Plato versus Aristotle: Categorial and dimensional models for common mental disorders" (2000) by David Goldberg. I thank Professor Vladan Starcevic for drawing my attention to this article

20. Corey L.M. Keyes by using self-report measures of mental health has confirmed empirically "that mental health and mental illness are not opposite ends of a single continuum: rather, they constitute distinct but correlated axes that suggest that mental health should be considered as a complete state" (2005).

2

From Normality to Mental Health

There is hardly a term in current psychological thought as vague, elusive, and ambiguous as the term "mental health."

Marie Jahoda, 1958

Mental health is sought after. It is highly valued. It is good to have, and bad not to have in good shape.

When young people compete, apart from physical stamina, they boast of how smart they are. When toying with the idea of getting married, their parents make inquiries regarding the physical and mental health of the would-be son-in-law, or daughter-in-law as well as of their close relatives. When they reach old age people are concerned above all about their mind: when and how much it is going to decline.

A sane society is said to consist of sane individuals. According to the well-known saying, "the world belongs to the young." It is why the leaders in a society frequently stress how much pride they take in the health of their youths. Although the hidden message is that young people are healthy because they are not in opposition to the regime, by stressing how much they are healthy the leaders wish to underscore at the same time that social conditions in that particular society are so favorable that nobody should be mentally deranged.

There are other indicators of how much people appreciate mental health. People are voicing the view in an increasing number of countries that the mental health of the candidates for the position of prime minister and/or the head of the state should be assessed. Certainly not because those whose mental health is not the best run for top jobs but rather because people are adamant that the holders of such high positions should be mentally healthy. And if the assessment of the mental health of the runners was not carried out on time, it should be performed when those who have been elected are due to assume job. The reassessment of the status of mental health of prime ministers and/or presidents in the course of their mandate is also highly recommendable, in particular if they start to make decisions that go against the interests of those who have elected them, and even, directly or indirectly, harm them (Post, 1995).

Without exaggerating the role played by the personality in shaping history, it is sensible to say that history would be different if leaders were toppled whenever they showed signs of disturbed mental health, let alone mental illness. This holds in particular for the leaders of big nations and empires.

Moreover, good mental health is prerequisite for doing many jobs. Piloting a plane, working in submarines and/or intelligence requires, among other things, excellent mental health.

Interestingly enough, people's awareness of the importance of mental health does not correspond to the knowledge they have about mental health. Mental health matters, people have a high opinion of mental health, but as a rule they are not able to tell what mental health is. It is true, however strange it might sound.

For example, if you ask people with no psychological or psychiatric training: what is mental health, they will give spare responses, if any responses at all, and their description of mental health will be quite different from one individual to another.

If you pose the same question to those who have psychological or psychiatric training, the answers will be less deficient, but most likely as different from one individual to another as the responses of those who have not graduated in psychology or psychiatry.

In this chapter, I will first deliberate about why mental health is not in the psychiatrists' focus of interest, and why they should deal much more with this topic, in particular with the definition of mental health.

Then I will analyze three concepts of mental health: the clinical-pragmatic concept, the positive psychology view of mental health, and the concept of mental health as a critical attitude towards the given society. There are reasons for the choice of each of these concepts of mental health. The first is most frequently used in psychiatrists' everyday practice. The second is today most talked about concept of mental health. The third introduces to the definition of mental health a crucial element which is lacking in the first and the second definition of mental health, and that is people's attitude towards the given society.

Also, I will provide my definition of mental health.

Finally I will sketch a possible classification of mental health states, and explain why this classification would benefit psychiatrists, psychologists, as well as those mentally health people who need psychological-psychiatric assistance.

Why are Psychiatrists Not Interested in Mental Health?

Psychiatrists deal with mental disorders. One might say that mental disorder is a *terminus technicus* in psychiatry. And what about mental health?

According to the WHO (1948), health is defined as a state of complete physical, mental, and social well-being and not merely the absence of disease or infirmity. This definition is of no much help in indicating which profession or discipline should deal with mental health.

Psychiatry textbooks devote very limited space to mental health, its dimensions and its definition. With the exception of very few textbooks—for example, Jesse O. Cavenar and H. Keith H. Brodie (eds.) *Signs and Symptoms in Psychiatry*, 1983; *Kaplan and Sadock's Comprehensive Textbook of Psychiatry*, 2005—there is no psychiatric textbook in which a chapter deals with mental health and the numerous questions that arise when trying to define it.

I will cite several possible reasons for psychiatrists' negligence of the issue of mental health, for rarely discussing this topic at psychiatric conferences and in psychiatric journals.

First, the majority of psychiatrists are more interested in practical aspects of their job than they are keen on pondering issues related to the basic notions of psychiatry, such as mental disorder and mental health. Psychiatrists leave the deliberation about these topics to those among them whom they consider as theoretically-minded. And they are certain these people deal with less important issues than they do. They themselves care for those in need, as they put it, all day long, without asking themselves and others how to tell the difference between mentally sound and mentally deranged people, what kind of general concepts underpin this or that definition of mental disorder and/or mental health, and what are conceptual grounds of psychiatry. Question as "what is mental disorder" are considered purely theoretical and as such have nothing to do with their day-to-day practice.

Second, any deliberation about the cited questions cannot help but imply a critical view of psychiatry because psychiatrists have not provided satisfactory answers to those questions. The key psychiatric concepts are in question. "The paired concept 'normal' and 'abnormal' are the key concepts of psychiatry, and the determination of the exact locus of the boundary between them is the crucial problem of psychiatry," as George Devereux put it (1980: 3). (Devereux means "pathological" by "abnormal.")

Since these questions are related to the basics of psychiatry, the majority of psychiatrists believe that considering such questions is, in fact, criticism of psychiatry. And no one likes to have the fundamentals of the job they do disputed. Therefore, psychiatrists prefer to keep away from discussing the key concepts of psychiatry including mental health.

Third, psychiatrists often mention that mental health is the topic of psychology rather than that of psychiatry. The wide-spread belief is that psychologists, with the exception of clinical psychologists, deal with undisturbed, and psychiatrists with disturbed psyche. Though there is a ring of truth in such a belief, the question might be raised why *clinical* psychologists treat issues related to mental health more frequently and more studiously than psychiatrists do.

The possible answer is that psychology students are thought more subjects related to the mental sides of human beings than psychiatrists are, and thereby psychologists are more familiar with mental health issues, more qualified to discuss them, and more interested in them. When these circumstances are taken into consideration, it becomes clear why psychologists more than psychiatrists deal with mental health, and why psychiatrists are not intent on changing anything in such a division of labor regarding deliberations about mental health.

Fourth, mental health has more numerous and more various meanings than mental disorder. And what is particularly important, the category of mental health is used in more areas of social life than the category of mental disorder.

Here are some meanings of mental health.

Mental health is a norm; a form of behaving, feeling, relating to one-self and others that is most widespread in a given society; an ideal belief and behavior pattern; one of the key dimensions or manifestations of a human being; it is built into the foundations of the social life insofar as a mentally healthy individual is the individual who is able to love and work (S. Freud), and there can be no community where people are not able to love and work. Also, mental health is a state of mental homeostasis, as well as resistance to stress, and the capability of living with one's own contradictions and frailties. Those who are in power in a given society rely on mentally healthy, as in the sense of mentally normal, individuals. They cannot stay in power without mentally normal people who are crucial to keeping the social *status quo* alive and well.

Psychologists, philosophers, sociologists, and anthropologists are much more interested than psychiatrists in these trans-psychiatric dimensions of mental health. In other words, psychiatrists are mostly interested in disease or medical definition of mental health, which is—as the reader will see—a negative definition.

Fifth, psychiatrists cannot charge the services they provide to mentally healthy people. Insurance companies are reluctant to cover the bill for services provided to mentally healthy people. Insurance companies merely disregard the fact that a good number of the mentally healthy people have mental problems, and that they need assistance of general practitioner, clinical psychologist, or psychiatrist.

Since they cannot have the bill covered for the services provided to mentally healthy people who are in need of psychological-psychiatric help, psychiatrists pathologize the mental difficulties of healthy people, their problems in living: they diagnose them as mental disorders. Over time, they forget that they have pathologized problems in living, and start believing that they actually represent those same mental disorders. Thus even when they treat mentally healthy people, they do not think they should deal with mental health, study it, and analyze its various manifestations or states.

Sixth, psychiatrists tend to misidentify mental health states as pathological states. A good example is conflating sadness "with cause," or normal sadness, and depressive disorder which develops for no apparent reason. Allan V. Horwitz and Jerome C. Wakefield (2007) have shown that the recent epidemic of depressive disorder results from covering quite normal states of sadness which develop secondary to some loss with the notion of depressive disorder. The guess is that if psychiatrists were more cognizant of mental health and its various manifestations, they would not confuse sadness (mental health) with depression (mental disorder).

Seventh, questioning the very existence of mental disorder has a long history, as long as the history of psychiatry is. It goes without saying that those who question mental disorder are actually questioning psychiatry. A number of psychiatrists reacted angrily to this questioning and published papers and books, showing that claims about the dubious existence of mental disorder are unsubstantiated. Thus psychiatrists, or at least a number of them, were forced into thinking and re-thinking about mental disorder, analyzing its definition, trying to figure out what mental disorder is all about. Antipsychiatrists were the leading figures of such attacks on psychiatry in the 1960s and 1970s.

Yet the existence of mental health has rarely been questioned; in any case much less frequently than the existence of mental disorder. So the psychiatrists did not feel prompted to explain mental health, what it consists of, how it is defined.

When someone challenges mental disorder, psychiatrists as professionals feel threatened. Questioning the existence of mental health does not cause the same feeling among psychiatrists.

Eight, the costs of mental health services are mounting. So are the costs incurred by work absenteeism, diminished productivity, and invalidity of mentally ill people (Murray and Lopez, 1996). As a result, the significance of mental illnesses for public health is enormous. Since mental disorders are in the focus of public attention, mental health is given second-rate importance.

Why Should Psychiatrists be More Interested in Mental Health?

Is there any need for a definition of mental health, be it scientific or non-scientific? Furthermore, is it better to have one universally agreed-upon definition of mental health, or is it more appropriate to have many different definitions?

John K. Wing wrote that he is not sure that a scientific definition of mental health should be sought. "Virtually all that is scientifically useful seems to be better dealt with by discussing the prevention of disease, and here various concepts of fitness may be useful. The remaining component is the definition of mental health can then be seen for what it is—pertaining to art, myth, and social tradition, rather than to science" (1978: 33).

This is the view of a renowned English psychiatric epidemiologist (his mentioning of prevention has to do with his work with epidemiology) who seemed unsympathetic towards explanations that did not look (sufficiently) scientific. Since—as will be shown further on in the text—the notion of mental health is value-laden, just as the notion of mental disorder, there is no doubt that mental health cannot be scientifically defined, if what is meant by *scientific* is value-neutral.

Indeed, opinions are split as to whether there should by a definition of mental health. Some authors (for example, David Freides, 1960) are of the view that the notion of *mental health* should be eliminated.[1] They cite the multitude of the definitions of mental health as corroborating their position. Others (for example, Maurice Korman, 1961) are of the opinion that the notion of *mental health* should be kept, and that an operational definition should be formulated.

I am of the opinion that mental health workers need to know what mental health is all about. They should deliberate about the nature of mental health, about its dimensions and manifestations as well as about its definition. Mental health should be high on the agenda of those who provide care to the mentally healthy and mentally ill people alike.[2] I will substantiate my claim as follows.

First, there is belief that no one is totally mentally healthy or mentally disturbed, but rather both at the same time, only to various extents.[3] Thus the relationship between mental disorder and mental health should be inspected. Can they be presented dimensionally, or are mental health and mental illness qualitatively different, and cannot be presented on one dimension?

When they treat people with mental illness psychiatrists try to boost health potential in patients, to make it stronger. The idea is that it will develop and eventually prevail. In order to know what the health potential is like psychiatrists should get acquainted with the concept of mental health, with mental health dimensions; briefly, they should know what mental health is all about.

Marie Jahoda rightly noted that "it will take special efforts to introduce concern with health into clinical work with the sick." And she added: "But such efforts may well be worth while" (1958: 75).

Second, in psychiatric research the notion of mental health cannot be avoided, at least not in any research in which control group is used as a methodological device. A control group consists of mentally healthy subjects. Since in terms of methodology the control group is as important as the experimental group, one could expect researchers to pay as much attention to mental health as they do to mental disorder. Members of experimental groups are required to be the same in regard to as many variables as possible, first of all in regard to diagnosis. They have to suffer from the same mental disorder. It is extremely rare for the question to be raised whether the members of the control group are the same as far as their mental health is concerned. It is taken for granted that they are the same due to the mere fact that they are mentally healthy, that is, that they do not display the symptoms of any mental disorder. However, that is not the case. The manifestations of mental health are numerous and various. If mentally healthy people are the same, they are not the same in the same way.

To date, psychiatric researchers have been focused on mental disorder, on diagnostics and the classification of mental disorders. It is high time they paid more attention to mental health, if for no other reason than to make the members of the control group as similar to one another as possible. And this cannot be done without knowing what mental health is, and who mentally healthy subjects are.

Third, as demonstrated by Corey L.M. Keyes (2002), a great many individuals who are not mentally disordered do not feel healthy and do not function well. Nearly half of adults receive mental health services annually because a mental health problem is inferred, meaning that there was no diagnosable disorder.[4] Since they so often treat mental health problems in people who have no diagnosable disorder psychiatrists should learn more about mental health, its manifestations, its deficiencies and imperfections.

Fourth, mental health is the key category of any kind of psychiatric treatment. The same question re-emerges all the time: what is the goal of the treatment? To reduce the number and intensity of symptoms, or to make the patient as healthy as they were before they fell ill, or to make them healthier than they were before they fell ill, or to make them as healthy as the "normal mean" (This last goal is quite often mentioned in the context of psychodynamic psychotherapy).

Ernest Jones, the most renowned biographer of Sigmund Freud, also thinks that the definition of mental health will be helpful in the assessment of the result of the therapeutic intervention. "What constitutes a normal mind, and whether such a thing can actually exist, are questions of considerable technical, and sometimes of practical, interest. Even if we conclude that in an absolute sense no mind can be entirely and completely normal, it is nevertheless worth asking what would be the attributes of such a mind. For, with such a standard before us, it would be easier to determine how far a given mind under treatment had progressed in the direction of normality" (1942).

Obviously the notion of mental health is unavoidable whenever the goal of the treatment is discussed, whenever the question is raised: what do we want to achieve by the use of a particular treatment. In this sense Aubrey Lewis rightly remarked that if psychiatrists could agree on the concept of mental health, there would be more accordance in regard to therapeutic efficacy and treatment goals (1953).

Fifth, a definition of mental health has to underpin programs aimed at improving the mental health of the population. How can mental health be improved if there is no knowledge of what mental health is, if we do not know what we would like to improve.

As stated, the notion of mental health has been interpreted in various ways. In my view, today, there are three basic approaches to mental health: *the clinical-pragmatic view of mental health, the positive psychology view of mental health, and the humanistic-philosophical approach to mental health.*

Clinical-Pragmatic View of Mental Health

Clinical-pragmatic view of mental health is also called the medical or disease model of health. There is a *pragmatist* and a *pragmatic* definition of mental health. According to the first, individuals who do not seek psychological and/or psychiatric assistance are mentally healthy.

It goes without saying that this definition is flawed. There are a great many reasons why someone who needs psychiatric help does not seek it: lack of knowledge about those who provide psychiatric help; fear of stigmatization; unavailability of mental health services; lack of insight into one's own mental condition, and so on. None of these circumstances is an indication of someone's real need for psychiatric assistance. Therefore, those who do not seek psychiatric help include the very seriously mentally deranged, and the mentally sound as well.

Psychiatrists do not use this pragmatist definition of mental health. They find the pragmatic definition more useful and closest to the mark. This definition is as follows: *mental health is the absence of mental disorder.* Being not ready or unwilling to deal with the definition of mental health, to discuss it or to bother about it, they use a shortcut: if someone is not mentally disordered they cannot be anything else but mental healthy.

When psychiatrists describe the current mental condition of a client based on an interview which is the key diagnostic instrument in psychiatry, they note, among other things, the status of the client's mental functions. If none of mental functions shows deviation, any kind of distortion or deficiency, psychiatrists tend to conclude that the individual is not mentally ill, which, in fact, means that they are mentally sound.

Psychiatrists usually do not bother about the notions of mental health and mental disorder. "It seems crucial that psychiatrists have workable schemata to use clinically when faced with a patient who comes either voluntarily or is forced to come by some outside agency for evaluation" (Cavenar and Walker, 1983: 33).

Here is a simplified description of a healthy person's mental status. The individual is well oriented in time, space and towards other persons. Verbal contact with them can easily be established. Their memory of recent and remote events is well preserved. Their basic mood is euthymic.

Affect corresponds to the topic of conversation and to the ambience. The affect expression is appropriate. They have a projection of themselves onto the future, and realistically assess the relation between what they would like to have or to achieve, and how much it is likely that their desires and dreams will come true. They are interested in other people and matters. Thinking does now show pathological distortion in terms of content and form. They deny perceptual disturbance. Cognition is intact. There is no suicidal ideation.

The truth is that, apart from assessing the state of the client's mental functions, in the diagnostic procedure psychiatrists and clinical psychologists rely on how they experience the client, on how they feel the client as a whole. Thus when they explain the diagnosis of the client's disorder, in addition to citing the kind of disturbance of the client's mental function(s), they usually cite their overall impression about the client's mental condition.

The important thing, in this context, however, is that those who are not mentally ill are considered to be mentally healthy in the eyes of psychiatrists. Most often this is an implicit rather than explicit statement, for psychiatrists usually are not keen on declaring anyone as ('totally') mentally sound.

However practical this view of mental health might be—you are mentally sound if you are not mentally disordered—it represents a more negative than positive definition of mental health.[5] It does not substantiate mental health. It does not say what is there in mental health that makes it desirable, attractive, positive. Why is it good to have it except for sheer fact that if you are mentally healthy you are not mentally disordered.

Hence, it is not surprising that this negative definition of mental health has been criticized. For example, Corey L.M. Keyes writes: "This is an unfortunate bias in the scientific and policy community, which is the assumption that individuals who are not ill are therefore healthy" (2006). In another paper he says: "Science, by default, portrays mental health as the absence of psychopathology" (2005).

According to WHO: "It is generally agreed that mental health is broader than a lack of mental disorders" (2001).

Finally, as mental disorder is not well defined it may be unhelpful to define mental health by the absence of mental disorder. "The apparent difficulty in clearly circumscribing the notion of mental disorder makes it unlikely that the concept of mental health can be usefully defined by identifying it with the absence of disease" (Jahoda, 1958: 14).

And, if mental health is not the absence of mental disorder, what is it? It is well-being. That is what positive psychologists say. They have been striving to define mental health in terms of subjective well-being (henceforth: SWB) for the last few decades.

Positive Psychology View of Mental Health

Well-being has been considered as an indicator and reflection of a good life from time immemorial. Psychologists and sociologists began paying more attention to it in the 1950s. This resurgence of interest in well-being was the result of the social climate after the Second World War. Along with the reconstruction of devastated countries and the comparatively fast increase in the living standard in most west European countries and North America, well-being came high on the agenda. How people feel about themselves became important. The questions raised were: has economic development been accompanied by an increase in happiness? Does economic development encourage human development? What should be done to make people happier? What does contentment and life satisfaction depend on? Are we and people around us mentally healthy?

All these questions required answers. Psychologists Abraham Maslow and Carl Rogers, and philosophers Erich Fromm and Herbert Marcuse, among others, provided answers by developing concepts that involved human happiness, but also questioned assumptions about an increase in happiness as the result of material progress.

In the mental health field, the monograph *Current Conceptions of Mental Health* (1958) was the first comprehensive undertaking aimed at answering those questions. This monograph opened a series of monographs published by "The Joint Commission on Mental Illness and Health." Other monographs, published by the Commission deal with topics such as economics and mental illness, mental health manpower, research resources in mental health, the epidemiology and etiology of mental disorders, and others.

Marie Jahoda, who at the time was Professor of Social Psychology, New York University, and director of the N.Y.U. Research Center for Human Relations, selected and systematized the opinions about mental health of various authors who directly or indirectly dealt with mental health.

Even though she did not mention well-being among the six features (attitude of an individual towards their own self, growth, development, or self-actualization, integration, autonomy, perception of reality, environmental mastery) which she identified as defining mental health,

Jahoda devoted a few pages to well-being. She writes that "in an informal inquiry conducted by the director of the Joint Commission on Mental Illness and Health to ascertain the meaning attached to mental health by a group of experts, a fair number described their ideas in terms of happiness, well-being, and contentment" (1958: 19).

In 1984, Ed Diener published his now classical text "Subjective well-being" in the *Psychological Bulletin*, which gave a new impetus to the study of well-being. Huge interest in SWB has virtually not subsided since then. It was said that psychologists have dealt with unhappiness for long time, and that the time had come to turn to happiness, to the "sunny sides of humans."

Then in the 1990s positive psychology[6] took shape. Happiness and life satisfaction, how to increase or acquire them are common topics of research on SWB and positive psychology. Since they shared the same interest, these two fields coalesced into one single discipline. Many scholars have contributed to the field. I will mention just a few of them: Carol D. Ryff, Corey L.M. Keyes, Richard M. Ryan, Edward L. Deci, David G. Myers, K.M. Sheldon, Martin E.P. Seligman, Mihaly Scikszentmihalyi, Sonja Lyubomirsky, among others.

What is Subjective Well-being?

SWB comprises a high level of positive affect, a low level of negative affect, and a high degree of satisfaction with one's life. The dominance of positive affect is usually called happiness, and it constitutes the core of the *hedonic* stream of well-being, or the *hedonic well-being*. Life satisfaction involves a cognitive element, and therefore it is not a strictly hedonic concept. "Viewed as a cognitive component, life satisfaction was seen to complement happiness, the more affective dimension of positive functioning" (Ryff and Keyes, 1995).[7]

The *eudaimonic*[8] stream of well-being, or the *eudaimonic well-being* refers to living well and actualizing one's human potentials (Deci and Ryan, 2008).

As it is often the case when the ancient Greek words are used, there are arguments about the original meaning of the notion *eudaimonia*, about what the right translation of the word is.

I will cite the meaning given to eudaimonia by various researchers in the field of SWB.

"Eudaimonia is concerned with living well and actualizing one's human potentials.... It is a process of fulfilling or realizing one's virtuous potentials and living as one was inherently intended to live" (Deci and Ryan, 2008).

"The term eudaimonia is valuable because it refers to well-being as distinct from happiness per se. Eudaimonic theories maintain that not all desires—not all outcomes that a person might value—would yield well-being when achieved. Even though they are pleasure producing, some outcomes are not good for people and would not promote wellness. Thus, from the eudaimonic perspective, subjective happiness cannot be equated with well-being" (Ryan and Deci, 2001).

"Had Aristotle's view of eudaimonia as the highest of all good been translated as realization of one's true potential rather than happiness, the past 20 years of research on psychological well-being might well have taken different directions" (Ryff, 1989).

"The affective dimension of subjective well-being when the concept of eudaimonia is acknowledged ... is strictly related to personal goals and prospects, the destination of which is growth, meaning and self-realization in a purely personal phenomenal sense" (Simsek, 2009).

"Eudaimonia as a subjective state refers to the feelings present when one is moving toward self-realization in terms of the developing one's unique individual potentials and furthering one's purposes in life" (Waterman, Schwartz, Conti, 2008).

"The essence of eudaimonia is the idea of striving toward excellence based on one's unique potential" (Ryff and Singer, 2008).

The notion of eudaimonia covers so many constructs that it is difficult to say what it really means. The term has entered the lexicon of psychology with minimal scientific scrutiny (Biswas-Diener, Kashdan, King, 2009).

The realization of one's true potentials—the notion that SWB theorizers took from humanistic psychologists—seems to be the common point in the cited interpretations of eudaimonia. Yet even this seemingly common point is not conceived of in the same way by various interpreters of eudaimonia. Does eudaimonia refer to the realization of one's true potentials, or to strivings to realize one's true potentials; in a word, does it refer to a state or to a process? Given that self-actualization is a never-ending course, the making of efforts to realize one's true potentials would be closer to the mark. In that sense the interpretation of eudaimonia as the realization of one's true potentials (Ryff, 1989) does not accurately translate the meaning of this notion.

Furthermore, the notion of *one's true potentials* is rather moot. How can we detect what are the true potentials of a particular person? Would a person themselves be able to say what their true potentials are, or someone else should do this job? And how, on the basis of which data, someone other that the person in question would be able to find out what the true potentials of that particular person are? It turns out that the presumptions of the process of the realization of one's true potentials, which is one of the key elements of the eudaimonic well-being, are fraught with difficult-to-answer questions.

There are some other contentious issues. Edward L. Deci and Richard M. Ryan (2008) mention "fulfilling and realizing one's *virtuous* potentials" (my emphasis) as the basic characteristic of eudaimonia. The adjective *virtuous* indicates something that has moral virtue. If eudaimonia is confined to fulfilling and realizing of only virtuous potentials—probably in an attempt to confine varying sorts of potentials to the noble ones—we open a can of worms, and have low or nil chances of closing it. Briefly, the introduction of virtuousness criterion would make the notion of potentials even more clouded.

Given the number of moot points and hard-to-resolve issues relating to eudaimonia, it is questionable whether it is opportune to keep on insisting on the existence of two streams of SWB. In that sense Robert Biswas-Diener, Todd B. Kashdan and Laura A. King are right, when, replying to the comments on their critique of the distinction between eudaimonic and hedonic forms of happiness, they say: "We remain steadfast in our original assertion that existing evidence does not support a conceptualization of two *qualitatively distinct* forms of happiness" (2009, emphasis in original).

The hedonic and eudaimonic components of SWB reflect the two traditions in the conceptualization of SWB. The hedonic view of SWB is older, and it has been complemented by the eudaimonic one. Both those who overemphasize the importance of happiness as a component part of SWB, and those who believe that SWB should be viewed more in terms of *eudaimonia*, or more accurately, in terms of *eudaimonia* as well, agree that there is no SWB without happiness.

However different the concept of hedonic and eudaimonic well-being are, "they are not, however, independent constructs" (Waterman, Schwartz and Conti, 2008). They considerably overlap (Bauer, McAdams, Pals, 2008; Ryan and Deci, 2001).

Summarizing the relationship between hedonic and eudaimonic well-being Alan S. Waterman, Seth J. Schwartz and Regina Conti say that there are three conceivable categories of activities: "(a) those for which both hedonic enjoyment and eudaimonia are experienced; (b) those for which hedonic enjoyment, but not eudaimonia, is experienced; and (c) giving rise to neither hedonic enjoyment nor eudaimonia." Then the cited authors add: "From a eudaimonistic philosophical perspective, the category of activities giving rise to eudaimonia but not hedonic enjoyment is a theoretical null" (2006).

It turns out that there is no eudaimonia without hedonic enjoyment. In that sense Elizabeth Telfer (1990) was right when she wrote that hedonic pleasure sometimes occurs in the absence of eudaimonia, but eudaimonia never occurs in the absence of hedonic pleasure.

Carol D. Ryff, director of the Institute of Aging at University of Wisconsin, and Corey L.M. Keyes, Professor at Emory University, GA, among others, tried to correct the confinement of SWB to only the affective category. In their interpretation SWB covers not only one but many mental functions or aspects of a person.

Thus Ryff and Keys (1995) define six dimensions of well-being.

Table 2.1
Definitions of Theory-Guided Dimensions of Well-Being
(Ryff and Keyes, "Structure of Psychological Well-Being Revisited," 1995)

Self-Acceptance

High-scorer: possesses a positive attitude toward the self; acknowledges and accepts multiple aspects of self, including bad qualities; feels positive about past life.

Low scorer: feels dissatisfied with self, is disappointed with what has occurred in past life, is troubled about certain personal qualities, wishes to be different than what he or she is.

Positive relations with others

High scorer: has warm satisfying, trusting relationships with others; is concerned about the welfare of others; capable of strong empathy, affection and intimacy; understands give and take of human relationships.

Low scorer: has few close, trusting relationships with others; finds it difficult to be warm, open, and concerned about others; is isolated and frustrated in interpersonal relationships; not willing to make compromises to sustain important ties with others.

Autonomy

High scorer: is self-determining and independent, able to resist social pressures to think and act in certain ways, regulates behavior from within, evaluates self by personal standards.

Low scorer: is concerned about the expectations and evaluations of others, relies on judgments of others to make important decisions, conforms to social pressures to think and act in certain ways.

Environmental mastery

High scorer: has a sense of mastery and competence in managing the environment, controls complex array of external activities, makes effective use of surrounding opportunities, able to choose or create contexts suitable to personal needs and values.

Low scorer: has difficulty managing everyday affairs, feels unable to change or improve surrounding context, is unaware of surrounding opportunities, lacks sense of control over external world.

Purpose in life

High scorer: has goals in life and a sense of directedness, feels there is a meaning to present and past life, holds beliefs that give life purpose, has aims and objectives for living.

Lower scorer: lacks a sense of meaning in life; has few goals or aims, lack sense of directness; does not see purpose in past life; has no outlooks or beliefs that give life meaning.

Personal growth

High scorer: has a feeling of continued development, sees self as growing and expanding, is open to new experiences, has sense of realizing his or her potential, sees improvement in self and behavior over time, is changing in ways that reflect more self-knowledge and effectiveness.

Low scorer: has a sense of personal stagnation, lacks sense of improvement or expansion over time, feels bored and uninterested with life, feels unable to develop new attitudes or behavior.

A person who scores high on the said six dimensions has psychological well-being. Lower scorers do not have psychological well-being.

Corey L.M. Keyes went a step further in expanding the concept of well-being. This author maintains (2002) that when assessing how well they function, people take into account not only emotional but also the psychological and social aspects of their life. In other words, there are three kinds of well-being: *emotional* well-being, *psychological* well-being and *social* well-being. Each of these forms of well-being has its own characteristics or symptoms.

There is no doubt that in its expanded form, that is, as the unity of emotional, psychological and social well-being, SWB seems closer to mental health than is the case when only affective SWB (happiness) is taken into consideration.

Subjective Well-being and Mental Health

There is a strong tendency within the context of positive psychology, to equate SWB and mental health. In a good number of cases the most prominent positive psychologists did not express any doubt that SWB and mental health is the same thing. For example, Keyes, one the leading experts in the field of SWB, quite unequivocally equates SWB and mental health. Thus, he writes: "Mental health may be operationalized as syndrome of symptoms of an individual's subjective well-being" (2002). He writes along the same lines in the same paper: "Mental health is best operationalized as syndrome that combines symptoms of emotional well-being with symptoms of psychological and social well-being" (2002). Here is one more citation which shows that Keyes equates SWB and mental health: "Research now supports the hypothesis that health is not merely the absence of illness, it is also the presence of higher levels of subjective well-being" (2006).

This equation of SWB and mental health is essential for further consideration of positive psychology view of mental health.[9]

It is worth stressing out that irrespective of whether we sign up more with the hedonic or the eudaimonic stream of SWB, happiness is the most important part of SWB. "Although it is probably not the case that even individuals who focus primarily on happiness view it as the definitive aspect of the good life, it is clear that happiness, positive emotion, and life satisfaction are all typical outcome measures in many studies of well-being" (King, 2001)

If happiness is a substantial feature of SWB, then it is a key component of mental health as well. Briefly said, one cannot be mentally sound if she or he is not happy.

And what does it mean to be happy? It means countless things. The common point of numerous definitions of happiness—in an explicit or implicit form—is that happiness is an affective state. Regardless of whether you feel happy because you are well off or because you are not hungry or because you are in love or because you have experienced epiphany or because you have devoted yourself completely to God or because you made a breakthrough in science—your happiness is always primarily an affective state. Whenever one feels over the moon emphatically pleasant emotions permeate them. There is no such a thing as non-affective, non-emotional happiness.

Operational Definition of Mental Health
on the Basis of Subjective Well-being

In the paper "Mental illness or mental health? Investigating axioms of the complete state model of health" (2005) Keyes contends that "nearly half a century has yielded as many as 13 symptoms (i.e. measures) of mental health that, when factor analyzed, represent either the latent structure of hedonic well-being or *eudaimonic* well-being."

The author defines complete mental health as the absence of mental illness and the presence of flourishing.

He was the first to articulate an operational definition of mental health which is modeled after DSM-III-R approach to diagnosing major depressive disorder. As is obvious from "Symptoms description" (Table 2.2), emotional, psychological and social well-being were included into his "Categorical Diagnosis of Mental Health." Since this is the only operational definition of mental health so far, it is worth presenting it *in toto*.

What do different scores at Keyes' categorical diagnosis of mental health indicate? There are three degree of mental health: *flourishing* (mentally healthy), *moderately mentally healthy*, and *languishing*.

To be diagnosed as *flourishing* individuals must exhibit high levels on one of the two scales of hedonic well being and high levels on 6 of the 11 scales of positive functioning.

Table 2.2
Categorical Diagnosis of Mental Health (i.e., Flourishing)
(Keyes, "Mental Illness and/or Mental Health? Investigating Axioms of the Complete State of Health," 2005)

Diagnostic Criteria	Symptom Description
Hedonia: requires high level on at least one symptom scale (Symptoms 1 or 2) *Positive functioning*: requires high level on six or more symptom scales (Symptoms 3-13)	1. Regularly cheerful, in good spirit, happy, calm and peaceful, satisfied and full of life (*positive affect past 30 days*) 2. Feels happy or satisfied with life overall or domains of life (*avowed happiness or avowed life satisfaction*)[a] 3. Hold positive attitudes toward oneself and past life and concedes and accepts varied aspects of self (*self-acceptance*) 4. Has positive attitude toward others while acknowledging and accepting people's differences and complexity (*social acceptance*) 5. Shows insight into own potential, sense of development, and open to new and challenging experiences (*personal growth*)

Table 2.2 (continued)

Diagnostic Criteria	Symptom Description
	6. Believes that people, social groups, and society have potential and can evolve or grow positively (*social actualization*)
	7. Holds goals and beliefs that affirms sense of direction in life and feels that life has a purpose and meaning (*purpose in life*)
	8. Feels that one's life is useful to society and the output of his or her own activities are valued by or valuable to others (*social contribution*)
	9. Exhibits capability to manage complex environment, and can choose or manage and mold environments to suit needs (*environmental mastery*)
	10. Interested in society or social life; feels society and culture are intelligible, somewhat logical, predictable, and meaningful (*social coherence*)
	11. Exhibits self-direction that is often guided by his or her own socially accepted and conventional internal standards and resists unsavory social pressures (*autonomy*)
	12. Has warms, satisfying, trusting personal relationships and is capable of empathy and intimacy (*positive relations with others*)
	13. Has a sense of belonging to a community and derives comfort and support from community (*social integration*)

[a] Life domains may include employment and marriage or close interpersonal relationship (e.g., parenting)

To be diagnosed as *languishing* in life, individuals must exhibit low levels on one of the two scales of hedonic well-being and low levels on 6 of the 11 scales of positive functioning.

Moderately mentally healthy do not fit criteria the criteria for either flourishing or languishing in life.

It is of note that the results of a study (2005) Keyes carried out using "Categorical Diagnosis of Mental Health" show that most adults who were free of mental disorders 12 months prior to the study were moderately mentally healthy (about six out of ten). Few adults (about two out of ten) were flourishing or completely mental healthy. The same number of adults were mentally unhealthy (languishing).

A Critique of the Equating of
Subjective Well-being and Mental Health

The fundamental question relating to associating SWB, i.e., happiness and mental health, is whether such an association is well founded; how much, if at all, it is warranted? In other words, is happiness the key component of mental health?

I have serious reservations about this kind of association. Such an association is highly debatable, to say the very least.

Critique can be leveled at many aspects of the equating SWB and mental health. I will focus on the following issues:

- The tyranny of happiness;
- Is a happy life a real life;
- Unlike mental health happiness is a subjective phenomenon;
- Happiness and the correct perception of the reality;
- Happiness is a potential source of creative work;
- The relation between SWB, adjustment, and normality;
- Subjective ill-being rather than subjective well-being as a possible indicator of mental health,
- Learned optimism (happiness).

Let us now see why, in my opinion, happiness is not the defining characteristic of mental health.

The Tyranny of Happiness

In her recently published book *Smile or Die. How Positive Thinking Fooled America and the World* Barbara Ehrenreich claims that in the twentieth century systematic positive thinking and feeling happy about oneself had gone mainstream in the U.S. "gaining purchase within such powerful belief systems as nationalism and also doing its best to make itself indispensable to capitalism" (2009: 4). She also says that positivity is not so much something people should seek, it is not so much a preferred condition or mood, either, as it is a part of the dominant ideology in the United States.

Despite a growing anti-American sentiment across the board it seems that the tyranny of happiness has spread to the rest of the world. Positive thinking and feeling happy has gone global. It became *must have* or *must feel*. People are preoccupied not only with how to be happy but also with how to be happier. To paraphrase Mark Twain, to be happy has become as mandatory as it is to pay tax and to die. If you do not see the world in rosy colours, if you are negative about something or somebody, if you are afraid that the worst case scenario could come true, and consequently are more than concerned, something is wrong with you. You should cheer up and see the bright side of the street. The point is: nothing but the bright side of the street.

It is not that only popular culture has been permeated by the tyranny of positive thinking. As rightly noted by Barbara S. Held, Barry N. Wish Professor of Psychology and Social Studies at Bowdoin College in Main, "our professional culture is saturated with the view that we must think positive thoughts, we must cultivate positive emotions and attitudes, and we must play to our strengths to be happy, healthy, and wise (2004)."

No matter how a bad lot has befallen you, which disease you have been diagnosed with, or how serious losses you have recently suffered, you should think positive. There is no better remedy for your plight, for the outcome of your disease, for managing hard times caused by the losses, than to think positive. And if you, for whatever reason, are not able to transcend distress you should feel guilty. And feeling guilty could not help but make your suffering even worse. That is what Held calls "adding insult to injury."

Now, let us go back to the above mentioned association of SWB (happiness) and mental health. Does happiness as something that is mandatory suggest that mental health should also be mandatory?

I do not think that mental health should be, officially or unofficially, declared compulsory. Needless to say, it is good to be mentally healthy; in any case, it is better to be mentally healthy than to be mentally disordered. Further on, it is not only in your own interest but also in the interest of the society that you are mentally healthy. In that sense it is highly recommended that you undertake activities aimed at preserving or upgrading you mental health. However, mental health should not be perceived as something which is constraining. You should not be, to put it that way, forced into mental health the way people are nowadays compelled to be happy. Mental health is a matter of informed consent. You should be provided information about the benefits of mental health, but it is up to you whether or not you will follow given advices.

Briefly said, people should be given information about what to do to be mentally healthy, but they should not perceive as mandatory measures aimed at improving mental health. Indeed, one way to make mental health more attractive is to posit that once you are mentally healthy you will be happy or happier. But, such an assertion does not match reality. The truth is that you can be mentally healthy without being happy.

One may remark that the tyranny of happiness is of recent date and that far-fledging and over-encompassing conclusions should not be drawn on the basis of a recent phenomenon. The tyranny of happiness is of a recent origin, but so is positive psychology's equating of happiness and mental health.

Is a Happy Life a Real Life?

It can sound like a truism, but life is not meant to be happy. Nevertheless, it is worth reminding positive psychologists of this truth nevertheless.

Life implies sadness and joyfulness, enchantment and disenchantment, despair and elation. The combination of these mental states gives flavor to life. It is the salt of life.

Can you imagine a lady or a gentleman who would be happy all her or his life through? Such a happy life might be achieved at the price of cowardly more than courageously turning a blind eye to life as it is, which, in fact, means at the price of being in denial.

There is another route leading to long-life happiness. You can suffer from chronic mania or hypomania, or your intelligence can be, mildly said, not the best. Either way you will enjoy a distorted outlook on life, which will probably make you feel happy or happier about yourself.

Finally, if you are not keen of burying your head in the sand, nor are you suffering from chronic (hypo)mania, nor is your general cognitive capacity in an unenviable state, there are still two opportunities left to achieve happiness. You can do charity work and approach a psychologist who will treat you by cognitive therapy. These two last options (charity work and cognitive therapy)—as he reader will see in the text below—are the key component parts of Seligman's recipe for positive thinking, for (learned) optimism and happiness.

The thrust of my argument is that a happy life is a life which is out of step with the real life. A happy life is a counterfeit life.

Ivo Andric, Nobel Prize winner for Literature, once said that happiness is something that does not last long. I would add that happiness comes and goes, and it comes when least expected.

One can remark that just because life is not good, our duty is to eliminate or belittle the bad sides of life and enlarge the good ones, to get bad days shorter and good days longer. After all, that is what people from time immemorial have been struggling to achieve; to make more room for happiness; to make positive affect prevail over negative affect, to become satisfied with their own life.

However, such a dream—because it is a dream more than anything else—is by and large elusive as most dreams are. For thousands of years people have been endeavouring to make them happy or less miserable. And what is the result? No one would dare to claim that, today, people are happier than they were for example in ancient Athens or sixteenth–century Paris for they have always been as happy as unhappy. It does indicate that life is not meant to be either good or bad, and that no matter how a noble exercise is to be more or less permanently after happiness, to achieve eternal happiness on earth, such an exercise is doomed to fail.

And if, hypothetically speaking, long-life happiness was achieved and happy people were somehow generated, would we or should we look at such apparently blissful people as mentally healthy? The answer is in the negative. Such humans would be less than human. Their life would be a parody of life. And most likely they themselves would soon become sick and tired of such a happy life and would start envying those who are not short of bad experiences.

Mental health should not be conceived in such a way that it betrays the complexity and diversity of human nature. And humans—to repeat it—are not meant to lead a happy life. Although we now and then curse our destiny, when we put our life in perspective we cannot help but infer that the life we have had has been quite a savoury combination of happy and unhappy moments.

Subjective Well-being Perspective on Mental Health is Subjectivist

In assessing the state of an individual's mental health, positive psychologists completely rely on self-reporting.

Respondents are asked to either verbally or in written form say how they feel and how they evaluate their functioning. No other instrument of assessing respondents' SWB (mental health) is applied. It holds for the hedonic and eudaimonic stream of SWB alike.

This means that, in SWB perspective, mental health is viewed as an entirely subjective phenomenon. People are mentally healthy if they say that they feel great and if they evaluate their functioning as very positive. This virtually means that no one except the subject whose mental health is in question is entitled to say whether they are mentally healthy or not.

Such an approach is understandable and warranted with regard to how the subject feels. "Although self-report has certainly been criticized, the use of self-report is essential in the study of happiness" (Kashdan, Biswas-Diner, King, 2008.) No one can tell how I feel except for myself. "There is no better way to gauge someone's positive experiences, life satisfaction, self-determination, and meaning in life than to directly ask about them" (Kashdan, Biswas-Diener, King, 2008).

However, it is questionable whether an individual's subjective estimation of their functioning alone should be regarded as relevant in evaluating their mental health. For example, a person's estimation of their ability to manage a complex environment or to have insight into their own potential often does not match reality. People cannot help but be at least a bit biased in rating their cited and other abilities. And it is just this discrepancy between their estimation of their abilities and the real state of their abilities that indicates that either the respective individual is biased, or that their perception of themselves is not correct (which comes down to the same), or that something is "wrong with their mind."

We cannot grasp the mentioned discrepancy if in our evaluation of our mental health we solely rely on our evaluation of ourselves, on how we feel, on how we estimate our psychological and social well-being. Briefly said, someone other than a person whose mental health is being evaluated should participate in the evaluation and eventually make the assessment.

Indeed, the respective individual's view of themselves should not be ignored in the evaluation process; however, it should not be the only criterion of their mental health either.

That is the first point. The second point is that, apart from a person's verbal behavior, apart from what they say about themselves, their (in the largest sense of the word) behavior should be taken into account in the evaluation of their mental health.

We cannot do without taking into consideration a person's behavior while assessing whether or not they are mentally disordered, and if yes, which kind of disorder they suffer from. As stated by Kendell, "most contemporary classifications of psychiatric disorders are largely based on clinical symptoms, a term which is usually assumed to include abnormalities of subjective experience elicited by questioning and *abnormalities of behaviour observed by the examiner or described to him by others*, in addition to the symptoms of which the patient actually complains" (1988: 208-209, my emphasis).

The same holds for the mental health assessment.

Leaving the evaluation of a person's mental condition solely in that person's hands, as the equation of SWB and mental health, and more broadly, positive psychology view of mental health does, is unwarranted and unacceptable.

Ed Diener, Suh Eunkook, and Shigehiro Oishi, the advocates of the *hedonic* view of mental health, seem to be aware of the danger of the subjectivization of the assessment of mental health, if SWB is used as the only measure of mental health. They write: "In the field of SWB a person's beliefs about his or her own well-being are of paramount importance. Naturally, this approach has both advantages and disadvantages. Although it gives ultimate authority to our respondents, it also means that SWB cannot be a consummate definition of mental health.... Thus a psychologist will usually consider measures in addition to SWB in evaluating a person's mental health" (1997).

So long as, in addition to SWB, other measures are not used in the evaluation of a person's mental health SWB perspective on mental health will remain emphatically *subjectivist*. It denies mental health and mentally healthy individual, for that matter, as an objective datum. It turns out that mental health exists only in individuals' feelings about themselves and the world, and in their evaluations of their functioning.

One of the most important fallouts of such an approach to mental health is that the assessment of the reliability and/or validity of the diagnosis of mental health and individual mental health states are out of question. Such an assessment becomes a mission impossible.

Happiness and the Correct Perception of Reality

Now the question arises does the correct perception of reality, which is "often treated as the *sine qua non* for reality adaptation" (Jahoda, 1958: 50), and "which appears so self-evident ... that many authors present the criterion in an almost axiomatic fashion" (Jahoda, 1958: 49-50) go with hedonic enjoyment.

In explaining what criteria have to be met by a person who perceives and evaluates their life and the quality of their function in life in order to be qualified as flourishing, i.e., mentally healthy, Keyes says, as stated, that such an individual must exhibit high levels on one of the two scales of hedonic well-being and high levels on six of the 11 scales of positive functioning. Let us focus on the first, hedonic criterion. A happy person has to be either "regularly cheerful, in good spirits, happy, calm and peaceful, satisfied, and full of life (*positive affect past 30 days*)," or to "feel happy or satisfied with the life overall or domains of life" (avowed happiness or avowed life satisfaction).

Briefly said, hedonic enjoyment, or happiness, includes mood which is above base line. When a person feels happy they are delighted, they feel on top of the world.

And what the correct perception of reality is? "As a rule, the perception of reality is called mentally healthy when what the individual sees corresponds to what is actually there," writes Jahoda (1958: 49).

Without analyzing in depth what "reality" is, a topic primarily dealt with by philosophers, it is worth examining the *relation between happiness and the correct perception of reality*.

It goes without saying that the one who is happy is not depressed. So the cited question of the relation between the correct perception of the reality and happiness can be rephrased as follows: do people who are happy or those who are depressed have the correct perception of reality?

Mentally ill people are said to be ill because, among other things, they have a distorted view of reality. Thereby those who are mentally sound are supposed to have an accurate perception of reality.

If happiness and mental health are the same, as positive psychologists claim, then happy people should have a correct perception of reality. Do they have it?

Shelly E. Taylor and Jonathon D. Brown may help us in answering this question. These two scholars published the paper "Illusion and well-being: A social psychological perspective on mental health," in 1988. The paper upset the psychological community, in particularly those who deal with the mental health issue.

The starting point of the authors is the widespread belief that a correct perception of oneself and the world are essential element of mental health. Against this backdrop, they reviewed evidence indicating that most people exhibit positive illusions in three important domains: (a) They view themselves in unrealistically positive terms; (b) they believe that they have greater control over environmental events than is actually the case; and they hold views of the future that are more rosy than base-rate data can justify (Taylor and Brown, 1994).[10]

Before going into details regarding the findings of these two scholars it is of note that illusions are enclosed in human's existence. One might say that illusions help people to survive. They make everyday life less rough, they embellish our view of the world, they produce meaning so needed to our existence. Yet they do so by falsifying "what is actually there."

Asked to tell what kind of person they are, the majority of people enumerate their positive and negative sides. Yet, as a rule, the former outweigh the latter. In addition, people more easily recall circumstances in which their positive features were exhibited than if and when their imperfections were visible. Asked whether they are better or worse than the putative average man, they have no doubt whatsoever that they are better than the average. This shows, among other things, how unrealistic they are, for if the majority of people are above the average, then what does make the average. Finally, the fact that other people praise us lesser than we do does testify that something is wrong with how we look at ourselves.

It is interesting that depressed people do not have such illusions. They do not think they have more good than bad sides; nor do they think they are better than the average; finally, their self-perception squares with how other people see them.

Furthermore, the majority of people believe they can control events over which they have no control at all.

Again, depressed people do not share such deceptive views. Their estimation of when and how they can influence events is right.

Finally, a number of studies referred to by Taylor and Brown show that people are more oriented towards the future than towards the present and the past. In addition, their view of the future is fairly optimistic. Even when there are no grounds—and I am afraid to say that that is most often the case—people believe that the future would be bright. In fact, they see the future the way they would like it to be. However, since a mere wish cannot determine the future, people's beliefs that they would feel more comfortable or less unhappy about themselves in the months and years to come is nothing but an illusion.

Depressed people do not suffer from such illusion, either.[11]

On the basis of the foregoing, it turns out that it is depressed people rather than those who are not depressed who have a correct perception of the reality. In any case, happy people would be the last ones to have a correct perception of the reality. Thus, if happy people had a distorted view of reality, how could they be regarded as mentally healthy?

And still another question: how could those who have an incorrect perception of reality be able to manage a complex environment and/or show insight into their own potential, which are two scales of positive functioning presented in Keyes's operational definition of mental health? The incorrect perception of the reality hampers proper management of a complex environment and makes insight into one's own potential difficult to achieve.

Martin E.P. Seligman, whose views of mental health and SWB will be discussed later in the text, could not dodge the question: given the association between depression and the correct perception of reality, how much is *depressive realism* (more accurately, the realism of depressed people) good for mental health; how much it is shared by mentally healthy people. He found an evasive answer in the notion of *flexible optimism* (unlike *blind optimism*) (1992: 172-174). Being aware that, born or learned, optimists do not excel in perceiving the reality, and at the same time keen on promoting optimism, Seligman chose the syntagma *flexible optimism*. May be the term *corrected optimism* will be more appropriate.

In my view, terms such as *flexible optimism* and *benign illusions* are not the right answer to the question—how to negotiate an incorrect perception of reality, SWB (optimism) and mental health. I will deal with this question later in the text.

If the so-called ordinary people who are supposed to have mostly balanced basic mood do not perceive themselves and the world correctly, how could those people whose basic mood is higher than the average have a correct perception of themselves and the world? It is quite known that those who are happy are not reliable people, due to their tendency to over-rate their capabilities, to see themselves as more attractive, more praise-worthy than they are, and to ignore everything that could question the accuracy of their self-perception and their perception of the world.

So the question arises as to whether we should regard as mentally healthy those who are unreliable and who due to the prevalence of positive over negative affect nurture an inaccurate view of themselves and the future? I do not think we should.

Unhappiness as a Potential Source of Creative Work

It was Stefan Zweig who once said—scolding us a bit for our ignorance—that we are not aware how much we owe to those who have felt crestfallen for most of their life. Zweig was referring to great creators in general, and great artists in particular.

This view is shared by Robert L. Woolfolk, a psychologist, who writes: "Actually, it turns out that many of the individuals we admire most were negative thinkers, if not depressive." Then he adds: "Many of the most important products of Western civilization have required negative thinking. In other times and places, great cultures incorporated in their worldviews elements of what I am calling negative psychology" (2002).

Indeed, if you read the biography of great poets and novelists you easily grasp in how many cases they were unhappy, how deep doubts tormented their mind, how much they were unable to find peace of mind, how unsuccessful they were in managing their private matters. Even while creating—and the moments of creation are considered as the only moments of their enjoyment, not to mention happiness—great artists are plagued by discontent, by questions of whether they managed to express what they intended to say, whether they found out the most appropriate form to convey their vision, their nightmares, their specific way of looking at people and the world.

Happy life is not the field on which creative work grows. It does not provide valuable insights. Leo Tolstoy wrote at the very beginning of his novel *Anna Karenina* that all happy families are happy in the same way and that each unhappy family is unhappy in its unique way. My guess is that if you read this Tolstoy's sentence in the following way, you will get it right. Happy families and happy people are not worth of special attention. Once you meet a happy man—if there is such a creature—you know what all happy people look like. In so far happy people are much less engaging than unhappy people (Kecmanovic, 2010).

The uniqueness of individual experience meaning the difference among people in regard to how they feel, how they think, how they relate to themselves and other people—this is what life renders so interesting and exciting. I have in mind not only the matchlessness of my own experience, awareness that I am unlike any other human being but also knowledge that other people are also unique in their own way. And the longer one lives the more she or he unveils that unhappiness is an unavoidable and at times a dear life companion, a potential source of inspiration, and a royal route to a larger-than-life knowledge about the life.

In the light of what I just said I am wondering whether it would be fair and founded to say that unhappy people are mentally ill people or that they are not mentally sound? Or, to put it another way, is it proper to contend that happiness and mental health come down to the same, that the first is the key part of the latter, and that the latter cannot do without the former as its dominant element?

Finally, should we say that, irrespective of how much we owe to great artists, we should not regard them mentally sound due to the mere fact that, in a good number of cases, and for a good number of years, they felt more unhappy than happy?

After all, this question refers not only to artists but also to all those people whose unhappiness incited them to do praiseworthy things which they probably would not have done had they been in high mood most of their life.

Subjective Well-being, Adjustment, and Normality

A person may have the hedonic well-being for reasons other than because they are mentally healthy. For example, to have or not to have the hedonic well-being may have to do with expectations—how low or high they are. For example, according to the Eurobarometer Survey, more than two-thirds of Danes report being very satisfied with their life, a figure that has held steady for more than 30 years. What is the secret of the Danish bliss? Expectations. Danes have low expectations, and so "year after year they are pleasantly surprised to find out that not everything is rotten in the state of Denmark," says James W. Vaupel, a demographer who has investigated Danish bliss (Wener, 2009).

Expectations have to do with goals. The more quickly and more fully we are able to achieve our goals, the more we will be cheerful and in good spirits, the more we will feel happy or satisfied with life overall or domains of life (Carver and Scheier, 1990). Thus goals and their realization are the crux. Telic theories claim that SWB is gained when goals are reached (Diener, 1984)

Are the goals subjective or objective? Both. Society determines and shapes most of those goals which seem to be purely subjective. Society does it either directly or indirectly, i.e., through an individual's interiorization of social goals. Society defines goals that are socially worthy and is expected to provide socially adequate means for the realization of socially honorable goals. The more congruent socially worthy goals and the means for their realization are in a given society, the more individuals will be able to realize those goals, and correspondingly the more individuals will feel happy with life overall, meaning with themselves and reality.[12]

Individuals feel delighted because they are able to effectuate goals that are as much theirs as they are social by using socially sanctioned measures. It would appear that the correspondence of social values and social means, and their availability, is a fertile soil on which SWB, primarily the hedonic part of it, grows.

It is of note that the concept of the congruity of socially defined goals and socially authorized means implicitly puts the hedonic component of SWB, and mental health for that matter, on the same footing with mental normality.

Let me explain this important implication of the hedonic well-being which comes from the life in a society where social (personal) goals (values) can be achieved by socially approved means.

What does it mean when it is said that the more fully an individual realizes socially defined goals by resorting to socially acknowledged means the more they feel contented? The assumption of such an assertion is that it does not matter what social values are in question, nor does it matter what socially approved means are. Individuals feel good because they are able to achieve socially valued goals (which they experience as their own goals) by socially approved instruments. In other words, they feel good because they are well adjusted. The adjustment to the given society is another name for striving to realize social goals by making use of approved social means. Thus, it is not surprising that the adjustment appears as important part of many definitions of mental health. For example, W.W. Boehm (1955) writes: "Mental health is a condition and level of social functioning which is socially acceptable and personally satisfying" (1955). Karl Menninger shares this view: "Let us define mental health as the adjustment of human beings to the world and to each other with a maximum of effectiveness and happiness" (1947). The definition of mental health in various dictionaries also implies the *adjustment* as the key element of mental health.[13]

To question the nature of social goals and approved measures is merely beyond the point. The adjustment matters. So does happiness.

So much about mental health as adjustment to the given society, so much about mental health as normality, because the adjustment to the given society is what normality is all about.

However, is normality the same as mental health? Hardly.

Every society launches its image of what a good life looks like. In the era of globalization, the image of a good life has also been globalized, i.e., spread across the world. Nevertheless, the image of good life to some degree varies from one country to another, from one regime to another, from one culture to another. Either tradition or those who are in power—such as the most affluent, political leaders, business, or religious leaders—determine or co-determine the image of the good life. Indeed, those in power keep on saying that the image of the good life they promote—the ideas of those who rule are always the ruling ideas, someone said—is in tune with real human needs, with the human nature. Yet, throughout the history, the interests of a particular group of people have always been behind the image of a good life that has been advanced and cultivated. As for the rest of the population, meaning the greatest majority of people, they do not stop doing their best to lead a life that is closest to the public picture of the good life. They feel happy when they succeed, and unhappy when they do not, in living in accordance with the public image of a good life.

Should we consider mentally healthy those who feel happy because they have accommodated their life to the public image of a good life, an image created by the political and financial interests of those in power?

Ryff and Keyes write: "History provides countless examples of those who lived ugly, unjust, and pointless lives, and who were nonetheless happy" (1995). That is deadly true. And have those who "lived ugly, unjust, and pointless lives" been mentally healthy? Since they strived to realize social goals, which they have recognized as their own, even correspondent to their both universal human and unique individual potentials, and since they felt happy, they should be, according to those who put SWB and mental health on the same footing, mentally healthy. That is what happens with mental health when it is reduced to happiness.[14]

Can Subjective Ill-being Rather than Subjective Well-being Be the Sign of Mental Health?

The character of social and personal goals, the satisfaction of which leads to SWB should be taken into account, say the protagonists of critical social theory (Max Horkheimer, Erich Fromm, Herbert Marcuse and others). Through ideologization, society, i.e., those who are in power, makes people believe that false needs are real human needs (See the definition of *true* and *false* needs in the text below). They do it because they benefit if people invest energy and time in satisfying false needs, i.e., if people accept at face value the dominant social goals and socially ap-proved means; in a word, if people are normal. However, normal people are not mentally healthy people, insist critical social theoreticians. People are healthy if they manage to grasp the game, if they distinguish true needs from false needs, and say that people should be devoted only to the satisfaction of truly human needs. Such people feel unhappy about themselves and the social reality.

They feel unhappy about themselves because as the members of a given society they willy-nilly, at least to a certain degree, partake in the satisfaction of fake needs, and because the satisfaction of such needs makes them feel empty and discontented. They are unhappy with the social reality because it is opposed to any change that includes the affirmation of new social values and means aimed at creating better opportunities for the realization of real human needs.

Now needs have come in the focus of our attention. I will return to the notion of needs. At this moment I wish to stress that although different needs and their realization can be treated as equivalent in terms of their ability to produce SWB, which is the position of telic approaches, the question is whether equating SWB and mental health is appropriate, bearing in mind the character of needs whose realization leads to SWB?

People react by anger, discontent, and aggressiveness if they cannot realize their needs (*frustration-aggressiveness hypothesis*). Their inability to realize their needs can be intrinsic and extrinsic. Let us focus for the moment on the extrinsic causes.

Through ideologization, and at times by resorting to the use of brute force, society opposes the realization of those needs which it regards as antisocial. Those who govern, be they political parties, interest groups, democratic majority, or a dictator, see as antisocial, illegal, and illegitimate those goals whose realization presupposes a significant change in social values and social practice, and thereby carries the risk of a change of the regime, of a change in the power hierarchy.

If people react by getting angry, by a sense of discomfort, and unhappiness to such a reality, could not that serve as a sign that they are critical of the social reality as it is, regardless of whether they are ready to make a step further and try to make it more congruent to real human needs? History teaches us that discontent precedes and ensues from a critical attitude towards the social reality. It precedes a critical attitude towards the social reality since some people—those whose needs have not been totally ideologized—feel uncomfortable and frustrated because they cannot fulfill real human needs. A portion of those people are aware that the character of social reality has to do with their sense of frustration and general uneasiness. Others do not. Discontent ensues from a critical attitude towards the social reality because people are perplexed when they become aware of how difficult is to change social reality, to make it congruent with real human needs.

If mental health is conceptualized in terms of the realization of real human needs, or at least as awareness of them, and endeavors to satisfy them, then it is not subjective well-being but rather *subjective ill-being* that is a mark of mental health.[15]

If—in the context of critical social theory—SWB stops being a key element of mental health—the question arises whether people could feel happy because they are unhappy. In other words, could they by content-ment, and even happiness, react to discontent caused by awareness that the social environment in which they live is unfriendly towards true hu-mane needs? Could they feel good because they managed to see through the veil knit of indoctrinations, manipulations, and ideologization.

They feel proud of themselves because they understand that mental normality as compliance with the existing social reality does not help them get closer to mental health; rather, it prevents them from being mentally healthy.

Scrutiny of the individual/society relationship is fundamentally missing from positive psychologists' concept of well-being and for that matter of mental health. I refer specifically to how an individual relates to dominant social values and practices.

Both Marie Jahoda, and Carol D. Ryff and Corey L.M. Keyes men-tioned this aspect (individual/society relationship) of mental health but only in passing, i.e., they did not envisage its importance for mental health, and therefore did not elaborate on it. Thus, when Jahoda dis-cusses meeting situational requirements and adjustment as the elements (criteria) of mental health, she indicates that these issues question healthiness of the environment to which individuals adjust by meeting its requirements. However, Jahoda dismisses further discussion of this question by the following words. She is explicit: "To speak of situations as healthy means stretching the meaning of the concept beyond permis-sible limits" (1958: 58).

I do not agree with Jahoda. I am of the opinion that the consideration of the individual/society relationship, and in particular the examination of the society within which an individual self-actualizes, feels happy and positively functions, cannot and must not be deleted whenever pondering mental health, its origin and manifestations.

Ryff and Keyes also did not pay due attention to an individual' critical view of the given society as one of the symptoms of their mental health.

When they were describing autonomy as one of the six dimensions of a healthy individual they mentioned "ability to resist social pressure to think and act in certain ways" (1995). And in "Categorical Diagnosis of Mental Health" (Table 2.1), Keyes describes an autonomous individual as an individual who exhibits self-direction that is often guided by his or her own socially accepted and conventional internal standards and *resists unsavory social pressures.*

However, the notion of "ability to resists social pressure to think and act in certain ways," or "to resist unsavory social pressures," does not indicate why the individual should resist social pressure. Should they resist social pressure just for the sake of their autonomy, or because the given social reality is not congruent with real human needs and impedes their realization?

To illustrate how much the character of the social reality should be taken into consideration in the discussion about mental health, and why an only apparently critical view of the existing social reality is more misleading than eliminating social reality from mental health equation I will draw the reader's attention to the notion of *acquired or learned optimism.* Optimism and SWB, it is worth adding, are frequently considered as the same.

Learned Optimism

Could those who are not born optimists acquire optimism, meaning mental health? Could people learn how to be optimists and by the same token how to be mentally healthy?

Martin E.P. Seligman, one the most prominent American psychologists, and the former president of the American Psychological Association, contends that we can learn to be optimists. *Learned Optimism: How to Change Your Mind and Your Life* (first published in 1991) is the title of one of his most popular books.

SWB of those who are not born optimists may be generated in various ways. Thus, according to Seligman (2002: 61), if you wish to increase your happiness level by changing external circumstances you should first, live in a wealthy democracy, not in an impoverished dictatorship, second, get married, third, avoid negative events and negative emotions, fourth, acquire a rich social network, and fifth, get religion.

The cited conditions that reportedly generate SWB deserve critical consideration.

Does the mere fact that the U.S. citizens live in an affluent and democratic country, regardless of numerous circumstances that, to say the very least, seriously spoil their life enjoyment, suffice to make the

U.S. citizens meet one of the criteria of a happy existence? It is of note that SWB reports have not changed at all in wealthy nations such as the United States, Japan, and France as they have gained more income over the last 20 years (Diener, 1995).

Also, for the sake of preserving the outweighing of positive over negative emotions, should people think twice before attending funeral ceremonies in particular when a loved one is going to be buried? I do not think so. "Thus under some condition (e.g., the death of a loved one) a person would be considered to be more fully functioning, and, ultimately, to have greater well-being if he or she experienced rather than avoided the negative feeling of sadness" (Ryan and Deci, 2001).

As for the relationship between religion and SWB there are reports that indicate that religious attendances have a positive impact on SWB (for example, Ellison, 1991). However, there also are reports which say the opposite. For example, Philip Brown and Brian Tierney (2009) found a strong negative relationship between religious participation and subjective well-being "in a rich multivariate logistic framework that control for demographics, health and disabilities, living arrangements, wealth and income, lifestyle and social networks, and location."

According to Seligman, there are some other actions that we should undertake in order for positive affect to prevail in us. Thus, if we wish to be (learned) optimists we should do the following. First, we have to stop be self-centered. The culture of "maximal I" should be corrected by paying (more) attention to the community, primarily to those living in the same community as we do.

What does this kind of attention shift look like in practical terms?

Seligman (1992: 289) writes that you should put aside 5 percent of last year's taxable income to give away. A portion of time you spent on pleasurable activities (watching a rented movie, hunting on fall weekends, shopping for new shoes, and so on) you should devote to the well-being of others or of the community at large (helping in a soup kitchen, visiting AIDS patients, cleaning the public park, and so on). Moreover, you should spend three hours per week "talking to the homeless and giving money to the ones in true need." Spend three hours weekly in writing "fan letters to people who could use your praise and mend-your-ways letters to people and organizations you detest. Follow up with letters to politicians...." Finally, "teach you children how to give things away."

Thus paying attention to the community at large and the needs of the community members would be, according to Seligman, the first sort of activities to be undertaken so as to enhance people's SWB.[16]

Cognitive therapy is the second sort of activities that is designed for making people happy or happier. Those who use cognitive therapy techniques increase their SWB. What does it virtually mean? (1992: 89-90)

First, "learn to recognize the automatic thoughts flitting through your consciousness at the times when you feel worst." In the course of cognitive therapy you become aware that your automatic thoughts are but the explanations you give to yourself as to why you feel bad. Such explanations then spread all over your personality and present you as a bad person. And that is not the whole story. Due to the wrong explicatory style you believe that you will never get better.

Second, you have to "learn to dispute the automatic thoughts by marshalling contrary evidence." And even those who are in low mood can find at least a few proofs that they are not totally lost. Focus on such evidence.

Third, you have to learn "to make different explanation, called retributions, and use them to dispute your automatic thoughts." In other words, try to diversify your explanatory styles meaning try to find some other explanation for what is going in you and around you. Automatic thoughts in which you present yourself in the worst possible light replace by thoughts about how you have felt, from one occasion to the other, bad and good.

Fourth, "learn how to distract yourself from depressing thoughts."

Fifth, "learn to recognize and question the depression-sowing assumptions governing so much of what you do."

Briefly said, if you wish to have SWB you should implement the key principles of cognitive therapy. If, in addition, you devote energy, money and time to charity work, you are likely to be in good mood, even in very good mood. And by the same token you will be mentally healthy.

This entire project of increasing the likelihood of having SWB seems to me, mildly said, naive. This project had been shaped—I assume—under the influence of many circumstances. First, the awareness that, even from a psychological point of view, the claim that there is no society but only individuals—the claim made by Margaret Thatcher and neoconservative ideologues—is not founded.[17] Second, the awareness that the belief that each and every individual is autonomous, and that what they are going to do with themselves and for themselves depends but on them.[18] (Cognitive therapists say: you have to work on yourself, you have to change your way of thinking, to correct you explanatory style.) Third, the belief that ("in spite of everything") American society is the best society. It provides everyone countless opportunities, it is democratic and affluent. Thus, there is no need for any radical change aimed, for example, at a fairer distribution of wealth. More charity work and more cognitive therapy will suffice to make people happier, to enjoy SWB, i.e., to be happy and mentally healthy.

Seligman's own words testify that this is what he had in mind while giving recipes as to how to reduce depression and increase SWB among people at large.

"The fundamental change in the field of psychology is intimately related to a fundamental change in our own psychology. For the first time in history—because of technology and mass production and distribution, and for another reasons—large numbers of people are able to have a significant measure of choice and therefore of personal control over their lives. Not the least of those choices concerns our own habits of thinking. By and large people have welcomed that control. We belong to a society that grants to its individual members powers that have never had before, a society that takes individuals' pleasures and pains very seriously, that exalts the self and deem personal fulfillment a legitimate goal, an almost sacred right" (1992: 9-10).

Aren't these words reminiscent of the best days of Soviet propaganda?!

It is highly questionable, to say the very least, whether people who strictly follow Seligman's advices about how to become an optimist, that is, to have SWB, are likely to become mentally healthy, as well.

Cognitive therapy for masses or mass cognitive therapy propagated by Seligman as the best way to get rid of depression, become happy, i.e., increase SWB, cannot be of much help to people who would like to be mentally healthy or healthier. To be mentally healthy or healthier is more than to fight depression, decrease self-centeredness, devote time and money to the community, and doing charity work. It is, among other things, to be critical of the given society; not the way Seligman is, indeed.

It is fair to say that Martin E. Seligman is not the only scholar who has got the ambition to make people happy or happier—and healthy or healthier, for that matter—through programs designed to improve their well-being. For example, Robert C. Cloninger, Professor of Psychiatry at Washington University, in St. Louis, recently (2004, 2006) joined the club.

Cloninger maintains (2006) that psychiatry should make a substantial contribution to improving average levels of happiness both of mentally sound and mentally disordered people. According to him, "despite vast expenditures on psychotropic drugs and extensive efforts to manualize psychotropic methods, there has been as yet no substantial improvement in average levels of happiness and well-being in general populations, as well documented in Western societies like in the United States."

This is a strange way of reasoning. How could the average level of happiness and well-being in the *general population* be improved by psychotropic drugs and psychotherapy? Did Cloninger expect that people's resorting to Prozac in their search for happiness will increase people's SWB? Or that various variants of psychotherapy will have the same effect? Just to remind the reader that Cloninger is talking about the average level of happiness and well-being in the *general population*.

Furthermore, Cloninger writes that although "the treatment of mental disorders has been improved with the introduction of many medications and psychotherapy techniques … available treatment are … associated with frequent dropout, relapse, and recurrence of illness." Such a state of affairs has resulted "in persistent residual symptoms of disease and distress, as well as low levels of life satisfaction and well-being."

The assumption is that there would be less non-response and non-adherence to medication, and fewer intolerable side-effects, if mentally ill were happier. And how might such a goal be achieved?

"Fortunately," Clinger replies, "recent work on well-being has shown that it is possible to improve character, increase well-being, and thereby reduce disability in the general population, and in most, if not all, mental disorders." Cloninger continues, "the methods of improving well-being can be understood working on the development of future branches of mental self-government that can be measured as character traits using Temperament and Character Inventory (TCI). These three TCI are called self-directedness (i.e., responsible, purposeful, and resourceful), cooperativeness (i.e., tolerant, helpful, compassionate) and self-transcendence (i.e. intuitive, judicious, spiritual)." Those who score high in all these character traits have frequent positive emotions (i.e., happy, joyful, satisfied, optimistic).

Cloninger has developed a psychotherapy program that involves a sequence of 15 intervention modules to guide a person along the path to well-being. "These are described as scripts of a dialogue with a patient going thought therapy to become more healthy and happy."

Several questions arise in regard to Cloninger's design to improve people's well-being and happiness. I will mention just few of them.

How could such a psychotherapeutic treatment be applied to general population that includes millions of individuals? Moreover, where would one find the huge quantity of therapists needed for the implementation of such a program? No matter how well designed, does therapeutic treatment suffice to provide people a better quality of life, and to make them happier, or less desperate, or should a change in some aspects of social-political environment they live in be included in such a noble endeavor? Or Cloninger believes that individuals' SWB has nothing to do with the character of social context in which people live and work, and love, indeed.

As for mentally ill people, those who have dealt with them for years cannot help but pose the question as to whether seriously mentally disordered people are amenable to psychotherapeutic treatment with some modules comprising, for example, observing and elevating your thoughts, charting your maturity and integration, contemplation of mysteries.

Concluding my critique of positive psychology view of mental health, it is worth reiterating some points. The view of mental health in SWB perspective is subjectivist. The eudaimonic well-being is so broadly and loosely defined that it is open to various interpretations. Happiness, i.e., the hedonic well-being does not go with the correct perception of reality, which is considered as one of the key criteria for mental health. The adjustment, another element that appears in many definition of mental health, conceived of both as making use of socially approved means for attaining socially defined goals and as a sense of enjoyment it provides, is the same as normality. However, normality and mental health cannot be put on the same footing for mental health includes a critical view of the social reality. In accordance with this feature of mental health, subjective ill-being rather than subjective well-being could be considered as the mark of mental health. Finally, it has been shown why learned happiness in Seligman's interpretation is a far cry from mental health. Also, Cloninger's ideas about improving average level of happiness in general populations have been questioned.

Carol D. Ryff and Burton H. Singer write that "positive mental health is not, in the final analysis, a medical question but rather is a fundamentally philosophical issue..." (1998). Those who favor the humanistic-philosophical approach have been saying the same thing for long time.

Humanistic-Philosophical Approach to Mental Health

Authentic human nature and true human needs are in the focus of those who define mental health in humanistic-philosophical terms. For them, a mentally healthy individual is the epitome of what humans should be like. Only someone who is devoted to the realization of true human needs can be said to be mentally healthy.

Viewed in a humanistic-philosophical perspective, mental health is an ideal. There is no, and there cannot be, an individual who is mentally healthy to the full. The mentally healthy individual only exists as an ideal which people strive or, more accurately, should strive to reach.

There are many barriers on the way to mental health. First, the milieu people live in can be, and most often is, structured in such a way that it prevents people from becoming aware of their true needs, and if they become cognizant of them, it thwarts their realization. Or lets them realize their true needs in a distorted way. Second, an individual's psychological make-up, the state of their mental condition can hinders them from becoming aware of true human needs, and/or to realize them.

In some cases, these two sets of reasons for not being able to become aware of real human needs and to realize them are interlinked and mutually conditioned.

Now I will focus on the concepts about specific human needs and potentials as articulated by Erich Fromm, Herbert Marcuse, and Abraham Maslow. I have chosen those authors as the representatives of the humanistic psychological orientation and critical social theory, respectively.

Each of them looks at human needs in their own way, and each of them, when deliberating about human nature, directly or indirectly, deals with mental health as well.

Fromm dubs *normative humanism* his conceptual position. He maintains that mental health is achieved if man develops into full maturity according to the characteristics and laws of human nature. Fromm admits that we cannot yet give a satisfactory definition of man in a psychological sense, and that our task is to "recognize the laws inherent in human nature and the inherent goals for its development and unfolding" (1954). Fromm does not talk about what an individual feels to be his or her needs—"because even the most pathological aims can be felt subjectively as that which the person wants most"—but rather about what true human needs are objectively, "as they can be ascertained by the study of man."

It is the kind of relationship between the individual and society, in a particular epoch, that mostly determines the realization of which human needs will be banned or thwarted. And to date all societies have to some degree forestalled the realization of true human needs. "Since no society so far, including our own," Fromm maintains, "has created the conditions for the full realization of man, the main task is essentially one of critical evaluation of society, which must be combined with the constructive attempt of considering which socio-economic forms would be more in accordance with man's nature and needs" (1954).

Marcuse on his part differentiates true and false humane needs. The latter are the product of social interests rather than interests having to do with human nature.

When talking about self-actualization as one of the key human specificities, Maslow much less than Fromm and Marcuse sees it in the light of the individual-society relationship.

Erich Fromm, psychologist and philosopher, who was the member of the Frankfurt's school, holds that there are five specific human needs, which are the expression of the *condition humaine*. He described these needs in his book *Sane Society*, first published in 1955. Here are the specific human needs, according to Fromm.

A. *Relatedness vs. narcissism.* "The necessity to unite with other living beings, to be related to them, is an imperative need on the fulfillment of which man's sanity depends." (1968: 30)

B. *Transcendence—creativeness vs. destructiveness.* Man is thrown into this world without his knowledge, consent or will, writes Fromm, and he is removed from it again without his knowledge, consent or will. "But being endowed with reason and imagination, he cannot be content with the passive role of the creature.... He is driven by the urge to transcend the role of the creature, the accidentalness and passivity of his existence, by becoming a 'creator'" (1968: 36). The creation, Fromm adds, presupposes love for that which one creates. And what does happen if hey cannot create, if they cannot love? "There is another answer to this need for transcendence: If I cannot create life, I can destroy it" (1968: 37).

C. *Rootedness—brotherliness vs. incest.* Today, people feel rooted when they belong to a particular ethnic or national group. However, ethnonational rootedness potentially turns people against each other. "Only when man succeeds in developing his reason and love further than he has done so far," Fromm writes, "only when he can build a world based on human solidarity and justice, only when he can feel rooted in the experience of universal brotherliness, will he have found a new, human form or rootedness, will he have transformed his world into a truly human home" (1968: 60).

D. *Sense of identity—individuality vs. herd conformity.* The notion of mental health is closely linked to a truly individual sense of identity. "Since I cannot remain sane without a sense of "I", I am driven to do almost anything to acquire this sense" (1968: 63). Sometimes people acquire a sense of identity by being one of the herd. They do it by sacrificing their own thoughts, by surrendering their individuality. Such a sense of identity is an illusory one.

E. *The need for a frame of orientation and devotion—reason vs. irrationality.* Fromm maintains that the need for a frame of orientation and devotion exists on two levels. "The first and the more fundamental need is to have *some* frame of reference, regardless of whether it is true or false. Unless man has such a subjectively satisfactory frame of orientation, he cannot live sanely" (1968: 65, emphasis in original) Beliefs such as for example animism, totemism, or Buddhism provide this kind of frame of reference. They give meaning to human existence, and procure an explanation of what the world is about. "On the second level the need is to be in touch with reality by reason, to grasp the world objectively" (1968: 65).

There are many ways in which the realization of specific human needs might be thwarted. Let us start from *relatedness vs. narcissism*.

People quite often intrumentalize other human beings. They see them as a means to realize their own goals rather than a goal that is valuable in itself. So long as they are successful in literally using other individuals in order to realize their own goals, people feel happy about themselves and the world. They have SWB in spite of the fact that in their case the relatedness need takes the form of a perverted need for relatedness as an instrument of exploiting other people.

Let us now have a look at transcendence-creativeness vs. destructiveness need. Today, a great number of jobs do not require a minimum of invention, let alone creativeness. Jobs are reduced to monitoring machines' work (people are an appendix to machines), or to a more or less mechanical repetition of a few actions or movements. Many clerks spent a good number of working hours in filling out forms, checking out whether all needed forms have been submitted, and the like.

Millions of people do such, mildly said, non-creative, dulling jobs on a day-to-day basis.

How things are going with the rootedness-brotherliness vs. incest need?

Conflicting interests of various countries, various corporations, of the members of different ethnic and national groups, prevent people from developing solidarity with humanity, which is a substantial aspect of this need. Few people in today's world share the sense of belonging to all other people, of being the same despite all the differences. The point is that most people fulfill the rootedness-brotherliness vs. incest need by feeling very close to co-nationals and co-ethnics, to those with whom they share the same faith, rather than by feeling part of the human race.[19]

And again, all those people who fulfill their rootedness-brotherliness need in a perverted, sort of incestuous way, are not short of feeling good about themselves.

What I said in regard to the rootedness-brotherliness need holds for the identity-individuality vs. herd conformity need, as well. Today, ethnic, national, religious, tribal identities provide people identity. This sort of identity determines, or at times even replaces, their personal identity. And still they feel happy with being short of a personal identity, with melting their personal identity into the identity of their collective.

The framework of orientation and devotion vs. irrationality need corresponds to a unifying outlook on life that Marie Jahoda (1958: 39-40) describes as one of the features of mentally healthy people.

Commitment to long-term goals, which is one of the characteristics of mental health could also be related to the frame of orientation and devotion vs. irrationality need.

What, today, are the long-term goals of millions of people. They yearn for accumulating ever bigger wealth in the shortest possible term. They are driven by acquisitiveness and competition. The dominant political and economic model today not only allows but also encourages citizens, Peter Singer, a philosopher and ethicist, writes (2003: 19), to make the pursuit of their own interest, understood largely in terms of material wealth, the chief goals of their life. A good number of them are obsessed with expounding their religion to as many regions and countries as possible. Besides, in a good number of cases they are determined to, directly or indirectly, exterminate those who do not share their faith. They dream about doing all they can for their ethno-national group and/or religious collective.

And all the same they feel good about themselves.

So the question arises could people who fulfill negative sides of specific human needs and all along feel happy about themselves and the world, i.e., have SWB, be regarded mentally healthy. Could those who are destructive, narcissistic, uprooted, conformists, and irrational, be considered mentally healthy? The answer is in the negative, if you are in favor of a humanistic-anthropological view of mental health.

So far, I have referred on several occasions to *true* and *false* needs. This is the right place to say what is meant by these notions. There is no better way to do so than to cite Marcuse who uses these terms.

In his book *One-Dimensional Man* (first published in 1964) Herbert Marcuse makes a clear distinction between *true* and *false* needs. Our contemporaries are busy with the satisfaction of false rather than truly human needs. Marcuse makes a clear distinction between true and false needs. False "are those which are superimposed upon the individual by particular social interests in his repression: the needs which perpetuate toil, aggressiveness, misery, and injustice" (2007: 6). No matter how much such needs may have become the individual's own, Marcuse continues, "reproduced and fortified by the conditions of his existence; no matter how much he identifies himself with them and finds himself in their satisfaction, they continue to be what they were from the beginning—products of a society whose dominant interest demands repression (2007: 15)."

On the other hand true needs are those needs that are determined by the individual and reinforce individuality and creativity. "But as historical standards, they do not only vary according to area and stage of development, they also can be defined only in (greater or lesser) *contradiction* to the prevailing ones" (2007: 8).

Could those who enjoy "euphoria in unhappiness" (Marcuse's term) be considered mentally healthy? Hardly. Could they be regarded as happy? Possibly. After all, they say they are happy.

How does Abraham Maslow, the originator of humanistic psychology, portray human nature, and the characteristics of mentally healthy people?

Maslow asserts (1968: 3-8) that such a thing as human nature exists. He equates human nature and inner self.

Self-actualization, a key notion in Maslow's vocabulary, implies the realization of potentials encompassed by inner self. According to Maslow, "fully human persons are the actualization of what many human beings could be" (1968: 163). The problem is, however, that "the inner nature is not strong and is easily overcome by habit, cultural pressure, and wrong attitudes towards it" (1968: 4).

Maslow adds that healthy people have the following clinically observed characteristics: superior perception of reality, increased acceptance of self and others, increased spontaneity, increase in problem-centering, increased detachment and desire for privacy, increased autonomy and resistance to enculturation, greater freshness of appreciation, higher frequency of peak experiences, increased identification with the human species, changed interpersonal relations, more democratic character structure, greatly increased creativity, certain changes in value system (1968: 26).

I would draw the reader's attention to the characteristic of mentally healthy people that Maslow dubbed "increased autonomy and resistance to enculturation." This characteristic of mentally healthy people implies not only their resistance to the imposition of cultural standards that do not assist people in realizing their human potentials, their inner self, but also their striving to overcome internal forces that impede the realization of human potentials. The description of an authentic individual provided by Maslow testifies that this is what he meant by "increased autonomy and resistance to enculturation." "An authentic person implies a new relation to his society, and indeed, to society in general. He not only transcends himself in various ways; he also transcends his culture. He resists enculturation. He becomes more detached from his culture and from his society" (1968: 11-12).

How many people all over the world are able to transcend themselves and culture they are born in and live in, and resist enculturation? A small, a very small number, indeed. Adaptation to the milieu, i.e., acceptance of the dominant social standard is the only possible form of relatedness to society for the majority of people.

And is adapting to the given social (political) environment the manifestation of mental health, or mental health itself? Maslow's answer reads: "Adjustment is, very definitely, not necessarily synonymous with psychological health" (1968: 211).

This short survey of the opinions of humanistic psychologists and critical social theorists about mental health shows that a great many people today either do not fulfill real human needs, or only fulfill false needs, or fulfill negative sides of specific human needs, or are not able to perform self-actualization. Hence they are not mentally healthy because they do not live and work in tune with the needs and dictates of the *condition humaine*.

Yet a large body of research indicates that the majority of people have SWB. They are happy about themselves and the world. For example, according to Gallup (Caroll, 2007), most Americans say they are generally happy, with a slim majority saying they are "very happy." Another research (Myers, 2000) showed that Americans are not the only people who feel extremely happy. Research findings have consistently revealed that the majority of people all over the world score well above the neutral point on measures of life satisfaction (Diener and Diener, 1996). Slum dwellers in Calcutta are also happy about themselves and the world (Biswas-Diener and Diener, 2001).

So what do we have here? On the one hand, people do not live and work in tune with their specific positive human needs. They do not fulfill their real human needs, they are short of self-actualization, and, on the other, still feel happy. Fromm dubbed this phenomenon *pathology of normality*, and features of those who exhibit conformist behavior *socially patterned defects*.

The point is that those who are in power manage through ideologization and indoctrination to force people to want to do what they have to do, and to make them feel happy about a lifestyle which they should have. In other words, the way they behave, activities they undertake and possessions they have or yearn to have is that kind of behavior, of *being* and of *have*, which is in the interest of those who hold power in the given society. This is the main reason why people are so committed to the satisfaction of false needs and oblivious of their real needs which originate in human nature.

Many questions arise. Can the real human needs become irrelevant: people ignore them, or suppress them, or pay lip service to them, and such an attitude towards their real needs, towards needs that are the expression of the *condition humaine*, does not make people unhappy? Is ideologization of all aspects of human existence so powerful that people virtually believe that they live in the best of all possible worlds, no matter what the society they live in is like? Do people have very low expectations, easy-to-achieve goals and therefore they feel happy? Do people easily get used to the *status quo*, no matter what it is like, and do not want to bother assuming a critical view of it?

Since we are dealing in this text primarily with mental health, the crucial question is: can people who betray the *condition humaine* be mentally healthy?

As states in the text above, the answer of humanistic psychologists and critical social theorists is in the negative.

The three discussed approaches to mental health (the clinical-prag-matic, the positive psychology view of mental health, and the human-istic-philosophical approach to mental health) differ from one another. To make the differences among them more conspicuous I will briefly compare the major features of each of them.

Clinical-Pragmatic, Positive Psychology, and Humanistic-Philosophical Approach to Mental Health: A Comparison

The advocates of these three concepts agree only on one thing: a person cannot be mentally healthy if they are mentally disordered. They more or less disagree on all other points.

Adjustment to the given society. According to the first concept, men-tally healthy people are well adjusted. The same holds for the second concept. The proponents of the third concept claim that a mentally healthy person is not, and cannot be well adjusted.

Dominant emotions. Those who use the first concept do not pay at-tention to the emotional state of those who are mentally sound. Positive psychologists claim that happiness is the key feature of mentally healthy people. Advocates of the humanistic-philosophical approach implicitly designate subjective ill-being (discontent) rather than subjective well-being (contentment) as the basic mood of mentally healthy people.

Real and false needs. Those who believe that mental health is the absence of mental disorder do not care about real and false needs, the least of all about distinguishing them. Positive psychologists behold that the origin of happiness is irrelevant; whether it comes from fulfilling real or false needs, or from the satisfaction of any other need. Happi-ness matters, no matter where it comes from. Advocates of the critical social theory maintain that only those who distinguish real and false needs and who make efforts to satisfy the former rather than the latter are mentally healthy.

Dimensional/categorical conceptualization of mental health. Advo-cates of the clinical-pragmatic approach to mental health view mental health as a distinct category. A person is either mentally disordered or mentally sound. Positive psychologists define mental health dimen-sionally—from pure languishing to moderately mentally healthy to completely mentally healthy. Even though they do not talk about mental health in terms of category or dimension, they seem more inclined to conceptualize mental health dimensionally. So are those who favor a humanistic-philosophical view of mental health.

How many people are mentally healthy? The implicit assumption of those who sign up to the view that mental health is the absence of mental disorder is that majority of people are mentally healthy. This view is shared by positive psychologists. Those who regard mental health in a humanistic-philosophical perspective think that the majority of people are not mentally healthy.

Mental health: an objective or subjective category. Those who favor clinical-pragmatic view of mental health do not consider mental health as objective or subjective. As they in most cases do believe that mental disorder is objective, the guess is that they see mental health as objective too. The positive psychology view of mental health is subjective, even subjectivist. People themselves report how they feel, and how they evaluate their life. I would argue that the humanistic-philosophical view of mental health is objective. The gauge of mental health is first, people's awareness about how much time and energy they spend in satisfying false needs, second, how big efforts people make to change the social reality so as to make it more congruent with real human needs. Once we agree on what real and false needs are, mental health, in humanistic-philosophical perspective, is not a subjective category. Real, authentic human needs are an essential part of *human nature* and its derivative too.

A Possible Definition of Mental Health

After critically reviewing three today dominant concepts of mental health I am expected to provide a definition of mental health that at the very least does not comprise the deficiencies of the concepts I have inspected.

Here is a possible definition of a mentally healthy person that is closest to my view of mental health.

- They are critical of themselves.
- They are truly interested in other people (their needs, concerns, aspirations, and so on), and make efforts to understand them.
- They have a sense of directness (in life).
- Their (inner) mental conflicts, and/or affect, and/or manipulations on the part of those in power, do not distort their perception of reality.
- While endeavoring to realize their intrinsic potentialities (self-actualization), they recognize those of them which, realistically or potentially, harm other people, and manage not to give them free reins.
- They identify and speak out against those aspects of the existing social-political-economic organization that induce and facilitate foremost those human needs which can be beneficial only to those in power.

The first three criteria are mainly correspondent to two characteristics of well-being (self-acceptance, purpose in life) and to some degree to one characteristic of well-being (purpose in life) set out in "Definitions of Theory-Guided Dimensions of Well-being" (Ryff and Keyes, 1995)

Now, I am going to give a bit larger account of the aforesaid defining characteristics of mental health.

Mentally healthy people do not turn a blind eye to those aspects of their personality that either they and/or other people consider as evil. They do not tend to rationalize those sides of their personality. In other words, they are critical of themselves.

Also, mentally healthy people are not self-centered to the point of being oblivious to other people. Quite the opposite. They are genuinely interested in other people, in their concerns, aspirations, and suffering. Besides, they respect the fact that people differ in terms of their needs, preferences, and animosities; by the same token they do not expect other people to think and behave the way they want them to think and behave.

Mentally healthy people have projection of themselves onto the future. They do not live from one day to another, careless of what the future will bring. They see meaning in life.

People's perception of reality can be distorted for many reasons and in various ways. Our inner conflicts, our affective state as well as the interest of those in power are most often to blame for our deformed view of what is going on within us and in the society. Mentally healthy people are successful in resisting the influence of the mentioned reality-distorting factors; at least to such a degree that their view of reality is less deformed than the view of those who are less healthy or unhealthy.

Irrespective of how we define mental health, no one of its component parts should include doing harm to other people. *Harm* is here conceived of in a broad sense—from physical harm to restraining other people's freedom to using other people for one's own benefit.

While working on their mental health, i.e., doing their best to be mentally healthy (or mentally healthier) people have to keep in mind that such efforts should not be accompanied by, and/or result in, doing harm to other persons. Otherwise they run the risk of becoming less healthy than they were. It is vital to underscore the importance of this aspect of mental health because mental health is not healthy if it includes maliciously harming other people. I will give two examples of how maliciously harming other people may be an integral part of subjective well-being as well of so much acclaimed self-realization.

For example, if we say that mental health is equal to subjective well-being, and that subjective well-being is equal to happiness, then we must acknowledge that there are people who can be happy only when ill-treating a particular person or a group of people. Furthermore, if we assert that self-realization, i.e., the realization of one's own potentialities is an important component part of mental health—as well as one of the basic human needs—we have to admit that destructiveness, cruelty, malice, and the like are also inherent human potentialities.

I do not think that Abraham Maslow is right when he writes (1986: 3) that destructiveness, sadism, cruelty, and malice are not intrinsic; that they rather seem to be violent reaction against frustration of our intrinsic needs, emotions, and capacities. Probably, the aforesaid activities aimed at harming other people are both intrinsic and a reaction to having our intrinsic needs thwarted.

The point I want to make is that neither happiness that is produced by ill-treating a particular person (or a group of person) nor the realization of intrinsic potentialities such as destructiveness, cruelty, malice and the like can be considered a component part of mental health or mental health itself because they include doing harm to other people.

In addition, mentally healthy people are aware of their intrinsic potentialities and strive to realize them. Yet, in doing so they are watchful to those potentialities the realization of which will, realistically or potentially, harm other people, and they do whatever needed to prevent the actualization of such potentialities.

Eventually, mentally healthy people do not nurture illusions about the society they live in. They take a critical stance towards it, and keep on pointing at those aspects of the existing social-economic-political situation that impede the fulfillment of human needs, with the exception of those needs which are either false or are in a broad sense harmful to other people.

My definition of mental health is polythetic the same as is my definition of mental disorder that I presented in chapter 1. To be mentally healthy one has to fulfill all six criteria for a mentally healthy person. Of course, the degree to which one fulfils the aforesaid criteria differs from one person to another. This fact lays the ground for classification of mentally healthy states.

Classification of Mentally Healthy States

As Melvin Sabshin noted (1989), psychiatrists have shown small interest in the nuances of mental health. In fact, psychiatrists look at mental health as a whole, unwilling or unable to see that there is more than one mental health (state). Consequently they do not attempt to produce a classification of mental health states.

Daniel Offer and Melvin Sabshin have taken the first steps aimed at classifying mental health states. They have done it in the context of their arguing for the formation of a new science, which they have dubbed *normatology*,[20] i.e., the science of the normal (1966, 1991).

It is of note that a would-be classification of mental health states is not the same as the classification of personality types. Briefly said, personality types are not supposed to match individual mental health states.

Given the existence of different approaches to mental health it is hard to even imagine the classification of mental health states that would be of the type one size fits all. There should be as many classifications of mental health states as there are approaches to the definition of mental health.

For example, the clinical-pragmatic classification of mental health states might be effectuated on the basis of characteristics of a mentally healthy individual. To those who use the clinical-pragmatic approach to mental health mental health is equal to the absence of mental disorder. However, those who are not mentally disordered differ a lot from one person to another. They are not the same in regard to many features; for example, in regard to the state of their individual mental functions.

Thus, mentally healthy people could be classified according to the state of their individual mental functions. All mental functions are not developed to the same degree in all people. Some people have more or less undeveloped or impaired one or more mental functions. Others excel in a specified activity that requires highly developed one or more particular mental functions. For example, some people have awe-inspiring memory, some are strongly determined in whatever activities they undertake, some are exceptionally skilful in social communication. These kinds of differences could be used as one or more principles of the classification of mentally healthy people.

Positive psychologists' operational definition of mental health cannot be of much help in classifying mental health states because in the context of positive psychology mental health does not exist as an objective category. If, however, subjectivist definition of mental health is accepted as useful, the classification of mental health states could be articulated on the basis of people's proneness to react by contentment or happiness to particular events or situations. Or on the basis of how quickly they react by happiness to these or those events or situations. Or on the basis of how long they stay happy afterwards.

As to the humanistic-philosophical concept of mental health the classification of mental health states could be made according to the following criteria: "critical of the social milieu they live in but unable to make a clear distinction between real and false human needs," "critical of the given social milieu, and able to distinguish real and false human needs," "willing to take steps so as to make the given social milieu less human unfriendly," "taking steps aimed at transforming the given social reality in way that will make the realization of real human needs less unfeasible."

Moreover, the classification of mental health states could be constructed on the basis of any of six component parts of my definition of mental health; for example, on the basis of how much a particular person is critical of themselves; how much they are truly interested in other people; how much is distorted their view of reality, and so on.

Also, resilience to various unsettling events and circumstances could be used as a criterion on which a classification may be based.

It is of vital importance to note that the same as mental disorder, i.e., variants of mental disorder, mental health, i.e., mental health states are not a stable, fixed phenomenon. Indeed, some of them are more resistant to change, others more tend to fluctuate. Besides, some more interfere with a person's private and/or social life, others do it less or not at all. Some cause a person's suffering, others do it to a lesser degree, or make people happy about themselves.

The creation of the classification of mental health states would be of much help in legitimizing the provision of mental health services to those in need. Mentally healthy people do require psychological-psychiatric assistance when they have problems in living they cannot cope with, or have difficulty to cope with; when they have difficulties in handling day-to-day hassles, difficulties that impair quality of their life and life-enjoyment; when their overall managing capacity is in decline, and so on.[21]

Legitimization of the delivery of mental health services to mentally healthy people—and the classification of mental health states would be of much help in that regard—would have a positive impact on health insurance companies, on psychiatrists, clinical psychologists, and mentally healthy people who require psychological-psychiatric assistance.

Hopefully the legitimization of the provision of mental care to mentally healthy people would incite insurance agencies to cover the bill for services provided to mentally healthy people. Therefore, clinical psychologists and psychiatrists should no longer need to pathologize mentally healthy states in order to get reimbursed for services provided to mentally healthy people. By the same token, they would be more ready to provide assistance to those mentally healthy people who are in need.

Mentally healthy people would then not be as hesitant as they are today to approach a clinical psychologist or psychiatrist. They would be less fearful that the clinical psychologist or psychiatrist will label them mentally disordered. Also they would be less anxious that the psychiatrist or clinical psychologist would proclaim them mentally healthy and therefore not in need of psychological-psychiatric assistance. Hopefully, a number of so-called premorbid disorders would be recognized and duly treated.

The problem is, however, that, as stated, it is not possible to construct such a classification of mental health states that would be operative within each concept of mental health. As a result, the co-existence of different classifications of mental health states would be the only available option. And that is the recipe for growing misunderstandings among providers of mental care, for never-ending discussions about which concept of mental health is more reliable, and closer to the "very nature" of mental health.

That is how the existence of more than one legitimate concept of mental health jeopardizes endeavors to put the large mental health field in order, to clear conceptual clouds hovering over it, and provide assistance to those mentally healthy people who require psychological-psychiatric care.

Conclusion

Psychiatrists' interest in mental health does not match the importance of the notion of mental health for psychiatric theory and practice.

Widespread belief that psychiatrists should only deal with mental disorders and never cross the boundaries of psychiatry as a medical discipline are two main reasons why psychiatrists do not pay (enough) attention to mental health.

Whoever tries to define mental health faces up to countless conceptual difficulties not easy to address. Unlike mental disorder, mental health is common: we are mentally healthy, mental health is all around us. Being an integral part or the commonest denominator of our daily existence, mental health evades definition. Mental health thwarts attempts to conceptually squeeze it into a definition. The same as life does. On the other hand, mental health could be considered as an ideal. We are never as much mentally healthy as we should be. In this case the notion of mental health is closely linked to the nature of the most cherished value, be it human nature, real human needs, the individual's autonomy, her or his ability to love and work (Freud), or something else.

I have identified three approaches to mental health definition: clinical-pragmatic, positive psychologists', and humanistic-philosophical.

According to the clinical-pragmatic concept there is mental health where there is no mental disorder. This concept is not plausible because it defines mental health in negative way—as the absence of mental disorder.

Positive psychologists link mental health to SWB. However, someone who is mentally healthy need not have SWB, the same as no one is mentally healthy due to having SWB.

Those who favor the humanistic-philosophical approach read mental health in terms of authentic human needs and self-actualization. For them, a mentally healthy individual is a person who does not yield to dominant social values and practices because they are aware that such values and practice serve interests of those in power.

There is no way to reconcile the cited concepts of mental health. They have so few common points that their convergence is out if question.

Back in 1978 Martin Hoffman contended that "it would seem that our difficulty in defining 'mental health' is due precisely to the fact that it is not properly a scientific term." Then he added that "in fact, it can only be meaningful when *ultimate values* have already been postulated by some extra-scientific (e.g. religious, cultural) means" (my emphasis).

Indeed, we will never agree on the nature of *ultimate values*. We cannot even agree on what is the *condition humaine*, and what *real human needs* are. I submitted for consideration the reading of the *condition humaine* and *real human needs* in terms of a few proponents of humanistic psychology and critical social theory. My choice itself is not value-free. It reflects my theoretical and practical preferences.

So what will the future bring? My guess is that the protagonists of each concept will stick to the basic principles of their favorite concept. Clinicians will stay happy with the definition of mental health which is neither more nor less than the absence of mental disorder. Positive psychologists will not stop deliberating about the various aspects of the association of SWB and mental health. Those who argue that a critical view of the given social milieu should be a key element of the definition of a mentally healthy will not change their mind.

As with the definition of mental disorder, the definition of mental health is still elusive. The fact that mental health is defined in different contexts and for different purposes makes the definition of mental health even more difficult to define than mental disorder. Unlike mental disorder that can be regarded as a *terminus technicus* of psychiatry, mental health can be defined, and is most often defined, within philosophical, psychological, and psychiatric frame of reference. Definitions of mental health made in the cited contexts do not have much in common except for the absence of mental disorder as the absolute condition for a mental state to be considered mentally healthy.

The lack of a widely agreed-up definition of mental health is and will be in years to come a stumbling block on the way to a classification of mental health states that might transcend individual approaches to this phenomenon.

Psychiatrists need an agreed-upon definition of mental health. The same as they need a widely accepted definition of mental disorder. There are no hints that such definitions will be produced any time soon. Since mental disorder and mental health are fundamental notions in psychiatry, psychiatrists should, if nothing else, joint deliberations about theoretical and practical problems that have to be negotiated to answer the question what mental disorder and mental health are.

Notes

1. David Freides explains his position as follows: "A truly objective solution to the problem of defining normality when one is concerned with something more than average existing traits and behaviors, when one seeks to embody a particular conception of what man may be, is impossible to attain" (1960).

2. Commenting on the fact that psychiatrists deal more with mental disorders than with mental health, Martin E.P. Seligman (2002) notes that the National Institute for Mental Health (NIMH), set up in 1947, in Bethesda, Maryland, should be renamed as the National Institute for Mental Disorders.

3. For example, mental disorder and mental health are defined in the following way in "Mental Health Fact Sheet" of the "Mental Health Council of Australia." "A mental disorder is a diagnosable illness that significantly interferes with an individual's cognitive, emotional or social abilities. Mental disorders are of different types and degrees of severity and some of the major mental disorders perceived to be public health issues are depression, anxiety, substance use disorders, psychoses and dementia.... A mental health problem also interferes with a person's cognitive, emotional or social abilities, but to a lesser extent than a mental disorder. Mental health problems are more common mental complaints and include the mental ill health temporarily experienced as a reaction to life stressors. Mental health problems are less severe and of shorter duration than mental disorders, but may develop into mental disorders. The distinction between mental health problems and mental disorders is not well defined and is made on the basis of the severity and duration of the symptoms" (The MHCA's Web is www.mhca.org.au).

4. Mental health is not the absence of mental disorder the same as mental health is not the absence of positive mental health. Dorothy C. Conrad (1952) uses the notion *negative health* and *nonhealth* to designate those mental health states which are not beyond the frontiers of mere social existence ("some form of vegetating").

5. Aubrey Lewis writes: "The serviceable criterion commonly employed to define mental health is absence of mental illness. This shifts the difficulty, and slightly lessens it" (1967: 183). The question is, where does this criterion "commonly used to define mental health" shift the difficulty to, and how does such a criterion lessen the difficulty in defining mental health.

6. Kennon M. Sheldon and Laura A. King (2001) defined positive psychology as follows: "It is nothing more than the scientific study of ordinary human strengths and virtues. Positive psychology revisits 'the average person', with an interest in finding out what works, what is right, and what is improving. It asks, 'What is the nature of the effectively functioning human being, who successfully applies evolved adaptations and learned skills. And how can psychologists explain the fact that, despite all the difficulties, the majority of people manage to live lives of dignity and purpose?'"

7. There are always positive and negative emotions in every man. The question is which ones outweigh others, and for how long.

   Barbara L. Fredrickson has an interesting observation regarding the dynamic of the relationship between positive and negative emotions. Fredrickson dubs *positivity ratios* the ratio of people's good and bad feelings. However paradoxical it may sound, negative emotions have a greater impact on SWB than positive emotions. There is so-called negativity bias: bad is stronger than good. Positive affect is taken for granted. It is more habitual, more everyday than bad affect. Therefore it is not recommendable to have 1:1 ratio between positive and negative affect. When the ration is 1:1 people feel pretty miserable because, as stated, negative emotions stronger influence our mood than positive emotions. The clue is either to increase positive emotions or to reduce negative ones, or to do both.

   Fredrickson has found that in about two thirds of people the range of positive and negative affect is from 3:1 to 11:1 in favor of positive affect. When the ratio is 2:1 or 1:1 people are depressive. Yet when the ratio is more than 13:1 people are more than elated, which cannot be the ideal of mental health.

   Thus the goal is to realize the dominance of positive over negative affect, and to shift the ratio from "danger zones" 3:1 or 4:1 towards 8:1 or 9:1 in favor of positive emotions.

8. The adjective *eudaimonic* is derived from the Greek noun *eudaimonia*. Aristotle in *Nicomachean Ethics* describes eudaimonia as the highest of all goods achievable by human action. It has been translated as happiness. Ryff (1989) is of the opinion that *eudaimonia* has more to do with feelings related to the realization of one's potential; in other words, happiness is not be the correct translation of *eudaimonia*.

9. Ed Diener, Enkook M. Suh and Shigehito Oishi are less ready to equalize SWB and mental health. They somewhat leave the question open. "Although we cannot say whether high SWB is essential for mental health, we can say that most people consider it to be a desirable condition" (1997).

10. In the papers "Do positive illusions foster mental health? An examination of the Taylor and Brown formulation" (1994a) and "Positive illusions and well-being revisited: Separating fiction from facts" (1994b) C. Randall Colvin and Jack Block criticized the paper "Illusion and well-being. A social-psychological perspective on mental health" (1988) by Shelley E. Taylor and Jonathon D. Brown. Taylor and Brown addressed the criticisms made by Taylor and Brown in the same issue of *Psychological Bulletin*. Finally, Colvin and Block in the same issue of the journal,

concluded that "the differing interpretations of the relation between positive illusions and well-being held by Taylor and Brown and by us cannot be reconciled."

11. The relation between realism and depression can be observed in another way, too. Thus the question may be raised whether a correct perception of oneself and reality is a risk factor for depression. See Aloy, L., Clemens, C. 1992. "Illusion of control: Invulnerability to negative affect and depressive symptoms after laboratory and natural stressors," *Journal of Abnormal Psychology* 101: 234-245.

12. Max Weber (see Shils and Finch, 1949), and Robert K. Merton (1968) have written extensively about the relation between social goals and socially approved means for reaching them.

13. To use socially approved means to achieve social goals is what social adjustment is all about. Thus it is not surprising that, in dictionaries, *mental health* is defined as adjustment: satisfactory adjustment, adequate adjustment.

    Here are definitions of mental health that can be found in three dictionaries (http://dictionary.reference.com/browse/mental+health)

    Mental health is (1) A state of emotional and psychological well-being in which an individual is able to use his or her cognitive and emotional capabilities, *function in society*, and *meet the ordinary demands of everyday life*, (2) a branch of medicine that deals with the achievement and maintenance of psychological well-being, and (3) a person's overall emotional and mental condition (my emphasis).

    Dictionary of English Language. Fourth Edition, Houghton Mifflin, 2009.

    Mental health is (1) a psychological well-being and *satisfactory adjustment to society* and to ordinary demands of life, (2) the field of medicine concerned with the maintenance or achievement of such well-being and adjustment (my emphasis).

    Based on *Random House Dictionary*, Random House, 2009.

    Mental health is the condition of being sound mentally and emotionally that is characterized by the absence of mental disorder (as neurosis or psychosis) and by *adequate adjustment* especially as feeling comfortable about oneself, positive feelings and others, and ability to meet the demands of life (my emphasis).

    Merriam-Webster's Medical Dictionary, Merriam-Webster 2002

14. In this context, it is worth mentioning Devereux's view of mental health, that is, of a mentally healthy individual. "It is hardly necessary to add that a passive and uncritical acceptance of the highly dereistic and unhealthy culture in which one happens to live is not a criterion of psychological health and mature adjustment but a sign of pathological passivity and dependence. The healthy individual simply recognizes the objective reality of the 'sick' society in which he must live without introjecting it uncritically. Instead, he will seek to survive in it long enough to modify this cultural reality in the direction of greater reasonableness and an increased efficiency on the human level" (1980: 83-84).

15. George Devereux notes that an individual's shunning the introjection of norms of a sick society results in their discomfort and feeling of isolation. "In order to escape from this 'double life' (he or she is rational enough to adjust overtly to a sick society *without also introjecting its norms*), an individual has two choices: either to engage in an ill-timed and therefore self-destructive rebellion or to accept basically uncongenial norms and become a fanatic as a defensive reaction" (1980: 5, emphasis in the original).

    In my view, it is not appropriate to denote a society as sick. Unless used metaphorically, the notion of sickness should be reserved for individuals' pathological manifestations rather than for characterization of groups, in particular large groups such as a society.

16. It is not clear whether Martin E.P. Seligman, by advocating the provision of assistance to the community, is keen on correcting individualism, which is "a quintes-

sentially American thing" (Oyserman, Coon, Kemmelmeier, 2002), or recommends a mix of individualism and collectivism as a recipe for SWB. If the latter is the case, then such a mix is a mission impossible. Individualism and collectivism are founded on fundamentally different premises.

17. It is of note that greediness and selfishness (self-centeredness) of high ranking managers and financial experts is being blamed for financial meltdown that hit the world in October 2008. The most recent introduction of ethics in many business schools curricula in the United States, the country that is regarded the birth place of the financial crash, does indicate that much more should be done so as to keep human tendency to pay attention only to oneself under control. The charity work proposed by Seligman will not be of any help in that regard.

18. Barbara Ehrenreich, in her latest book entitled *Bright-Sided: How the Relentless Promotion of Positive Thinking has Undermined America* (2009), argues that "positivity is not so much our (American, D.K.) condition or our mood as it is part of our ideology—the way we explain the world and think we ought to function within it. That ideology is 'positive thinking'." She mentions a few reasons for that kind of ideology. First, "positive thinking supposedly not only makes us feel optimistic but actually makes happy outcomes more likely. If you expect things to get better, they will." Second, "the practice of positive thinking is an effort to pump up this belief in the face of much contradictory evidence.... Positive thinking may be a quintessentially American activity, associated in our minds with both individual and national success, but it is driven by our terrible insecurity.... We have the highest percentage of our population incarcerated, and the greatest level of inequality in wealth and income. We are plagued by gun violence and racked by personal debts." Third, "if early capitalism was inhospitable to positive thinking, 'late' capitalism, or consumer capitalism, is far more congenial, depending as it does on the individual's hunger for more and the firm's imperative of growth. The consumer culture encourages individuals to want more—cars, larger homes, television sets, cell phones, gadgets of all kinds—and positive thinking is ready at hand to tell them they deserve more and can have it if they really want it and are willing to make efforts to get it." Fourth, "positive thinking has made itself useful as an apology for the crueler aspects of the market economy. It optimism is the key to material success, and if you can achieve an optimistic outlook through the discipline of positive thinking, then there is no excuse for failure." (http://www.nytimes.com/2009/10/10/books/excerpt-bright-dised.html)

19. Gillian Brock and Quentin D. Atkinson (2008) argue that those needs that nationalism—and any form of groupism, I would add—is said to satisfy can be met by cosmopolitanism as well. However, they do not provide any explanation for the dominance of nationalist ideas and sentiments over the cosmopolitan ones. In other words, they are short of answering the question as to why in *real life* commitment to nationalist ideas and behavior by and far outweighs commitment to cosmopolitanism.

20. The term *salutogenesis* is synonymous with *normatology*. *Salutogenesis* is a term coined by Aaron Antonovsky, a Professor of Medical Sociology at the Hebrew University of Jerusalem/Hadassah. It designates investigations about the nature and origin of health. The word *salutogenesis* comes from the Latin *salus* which means health, and the Greek *genesis* meaning origin.

21. Mental health professionals have three roles. First, their key role is to treat people with mental disorder. Second, they should be available to help those who are not mentally disordered but have difficulties in coping with stress and distress. Third, they should help people to enhance human potential (Klerman and Schecher, 1981).

3

Physical Diseases and Mental Disorders: Should They Be Differentiated?

> *Long indeed is the road to be traveled before we*
> *can hope to reach a definition of mental-cum-physi-*
> *cal health, which is objective, scientific and wholly*
> *free of social-value-judgments; and before we shall*
> *be able, consistently and without qualification, to*
> *treat mental and physical disorders on exactly the*
> *same footing.*
>
> Barbara Wootton, 1959

Lay people will not say that pneumonia is a mental disorder and schizophrenia a physical disorder. They never make such mistakes. The difference between physical diseases and mental disorders constitutes *tacit knowledge* in Michael Polanyi's terminology.

Yet in recent times, opinions have been voiced that physical diseases and mental disorder are the same.[1] Only the adjective "mental" may suggest that there is some difference between them, but this adjective cannot justify the consideration that physical diseases and mental disorders are different phenomena, the argumnet goes.

As the reader will see later in the text, such views have been promoted by a number of renown psychiatrists (for example, Martin Roth, Robert E. Kendell) as well as by the authors of DSMs, which is much more notable because this diagnostic and classificatory system has been acknowledged as the "most scientific" all across the world.

When discussing how similar or different physical diseases and mental disorders are, there are three questions that should be answered.

Have physical diseases and mental disorders always been the same but we have not been aware of that, and therefore have not perceived them as such? In other words, the perception of these phenomena did not match their very nature.

Have physical diseases and mental disorders been different for a long time, and only recently become similar to one another; so similar that today we should not distinguish between them?

Does today's knowledge about physical diseases and mental disorders tell us that there is no difference between them?

There is no doubt that physical diseases and mental disorders have not changed over time, although there are new physical diseases, the same as there have been some changes in the clinical picture of some mental disorders. For example, today catatonic forms of Schizophrenic Disorder are quite rare. The same holds for those forms of hysteria (today called Conversive Disorder) which were dominant one hundred years ago. The course and symptoms of some mental disorders have changed. They are not the same as they were in the pre-neuroleptic era.

However, neither physical diseases nor mental disorders have, in fact, changed. Thus the only thing that might have changed is either our perception of what we recognize as particular disorders, or our knowledge about them.

The perception of a phenomenon and knowledge about it can be closely correlated. Thus new knowledge about that phenomenon shapes our perception of it. However, more often than is supposed, the way we observe things, beings, and situations is a function of the observers' interests, or the specific circumstances under which we perceive them rather than our knowledge about them.

Therefore, the proper question is as follows: which circumstances prompted a number of distinguished psychiatrists to assert that we should put physical diseases and mental disorders in the same basket although, as stated, the majority of people consider for example gangrenous changes of legs and emphatically heightened affect to be quite different occurrences.

Reasons for Equating Physical Diseases and Mental Disorders

On the basis of the arguments for equating physical diseases and mental disorders proposed by DSMs as well as by Robert E. Kendell (2001) guess is that progress made in neuroscience, mounting knowledge about the functioning of the central nervous system, made them believe that it was high time to say that physical diseases and mental disorders are the same.

I will now present the view of Martin Roth, the late Professor of Psychiatry at Cambridge University, UK, and the view of Robert E. Kendell, the late Professor of Psychiatry at Edinburgh University, UK.

In the book *The Reality of Mental Illness* (1986), which he coauthored with Jerome Kroll, Roth writes: "To be precise, even the term 'mental illness' is a misnomer; it is based upon an outdated distinction between body and mind that remains a philosophical, but not a biological dilemma. All illnesses eventually interfere with functioning in psychological, social, economic and physical spheres, place the affected person at a biological disadvantage, bring suffering to self and others, are present at times without the ill person recognizing it, have acute and chronic forms, and are associated with increased mortality" (1986: 26).

Robert E. Kendell, one of the most vociferous advocates of the idea that any differentiation between physical diseases and mental disorders is a false dichotomy, went so far in negating that physical diseases and mental disorders are distinct that he required the elimination of the term "mental disorder" altogether. Thus in the first chapter of the book *Companion to Psychiatric Studies*, that he coedited with A.K. Zealley, he consistently uses the terms "psychiatric illness" and "psychiatric disorder" instead of "mental disorder." According to Kendell, the terms "psychiatric illness" and "psychiatric disorder" "imply simply that the conditions in question are usually treated by doctors with a psychiatric training" (1993: 5). In fact, Kendell is concerned about the negative impact that the use of the terms "mental disorder" and "mental illness" has had on medical and lay attitudes. "The implications of the terms mental illness and mental disorder are ... seriously misleading, and have had a baneful influence on medical and lay attitudes for nearly 20 years" (1993: 5).

Kendell in a later published text writes: "Not only is the distinction between mental and physical illness ill-founded and incompatible with contemporary understanding of disease, it is also damaging to the long-term interests of patients themselves" (2001).[2]

Such a view, as rightly noted by Mark A. Turner (2003), relies on the assertions made by Carl Gustav Hempel. By his deductive-nomological model of scientific explication (1948, 1965) this scholar exercised crucial influence on the development of DSMs.

Hence, it is no wonder that the authors of DSMs share the views of Roth and Kendell about the need to equate physical diseases and mental disorders. They contest that it is difficult do make a distinction between "physical disease" and "mental disorder": "Although this volume is titled the *Diagnostic and Statistical Manual of Mental Disorders,* the term *mental disorder* unfortunately implies a distinction between 'mental' disorders and 'physical' disorders that is a reductionistic anachronism of mind/body dualism. A compelling literature documents that there is much 'physical' in mental disorders and much 'mental' in 'physical''disorders. The problems raised by the term 'mental' disorders has been much clearer than its solution, and, unfortunately, the term persists in the title of DSM-IV because we have not found an appropriate substitute" (1994: XXI).[3]

Here are some other possible reasons for making no distinction between physical diseases and mental disorders.

First, psychiatry is a medical discipline. All medical disciplines deal with physical diseases. The fact that psychiatrists deal with mental disorders, the argument goes, should not be a reason for considering them as different from other disorders dealt with by specialists other than psychiatrists.

This view is flawed. Regardless of how medical psychiatry is, psychiatry is *not only* a medical discipline or, more accurately, it is *more than* a medical discipline. Psychiatry could be said to be midway between natural sciences and the humanities.

Second, the *likeness argument* is seen as a means of resolving the issue of is there such a thing as mental disorder. The argument goes, if putative mental disorders have the same features as those disorders which are universally accepted as diseases (such as pneumonia), mental disorders exist. Thus the likeness argument is more about attesting the existence of mental disorder than about how similar or dissimilar physical diseases and mental disorders are. Their (dis)similarity is used to confirm or refute mental disorder.

Neil Pickering (2003) labels the *paradigm* and the *generic* approaches the two main versions of the likeness argument. According to the former, the notion of mental health must match the notion of physical disease as a physiological condition, and "physiological medicine should be viewed as the paradigm health discipline" (Boorse, 1976). According to the latter, in defining physical diseases and mental disorders there is no reference to physiological processes. The same criteria apply to both. "It is in virtue of this impartiality between the physical and mental" that this approach is generic. The paradigm approach might be regarded as partial in so far as it assumes the ontological status of physical disease as unequivocal. Mental disorder is a disorder if it is like physical disease. So making mental disorder like physical disease, or equating the former and the latter is a way to equally rank them.

Richard G.T. Gips opposes the view underlining the likeness argument that "talk of mental illnesses would seem to one to be the more valid the more one accepts the view that mental illnesses are ultimately physical illnesses." In Gips's opinion, "if one is attached to the concept of mental illness, the worst thing to do … is to suppose that it requires some kind of justification, a justification to be found by comparing it to what is counted as illness in a quite different order of reality" (2003).

Third, it is believed that the stigma of mental illness will be eliminated if mental disorder is treated like any other disease. This belief is groundless. The medicalization of mental disorders does not result in the attenuation or neutralization of negative responses to people with mental illness. It just leads to the expansion of the stigma to psychiatry itself (Guimon, Fischer, and Sartorious, 19996: VIII).

Recently Anthony F. Jorm and Elizabeth Oh (2009), on the basis of a meta-analysis of the studies carried out so as to assess whether medical or psychosocial causal explanation have a greater influence on the stigma of mental illness, concluded that the findings are consistent: varying (biological versus psychosocial) causal explanation has no effect on social distance from a mentally ill person. And social distance is not only a dimension of the stigma but also one of the measures of how strong is the stigma.[4]

Fourth, to get more government money for mental health care could be one of the reasons for equating physical diseases and mental disorders.

"Health dollars" are unequally distributed. As a rule, mental health care is given a disproportionately small amount due to deeply entrenched beliefs that investment in mental health care gives smaller return than investment in other medical disciplines.

Thus those who are keen on changing such a state of affairs in regard to the distribution of "health dollars" claim that mental disorder is like any other disorder. By doing so they wish to prompt those who hold the purse strings to give more money to mental health care. If there is no difference between physical diseases and mental disorders why should health dollars be distributed unequally, that is the rationale behind the claim that physical diseases and mental disorders are the same.

For example, at a conference on mental health, held in the White House on June 7, 1999, organized by Hillary Rodham Clinton, then the first lady, and Steven Hyman, then director of the National Institute for Mental Health, Clinton said: "This is an historic conference, but it is more than that: it's a real signal to our nation that we must do whatever it takes not only to remove the stigma from mental illness, but to begin treating mental illness as the illness it is on a parity with other illnesses. And we have to understand more about the progress that has been made scientifically that has really led us to this point" (2000: 38).

However well intentioned Clinton's words were, the progress that has been made in brain research does not provide sufficient reason to equate physical diseases and mental disorders.

Anticipating what I will elaborate in detail later in the text, I wish to stress that people with physical diseases and people with mental disorders live in non-identical worlds. The mentally disordered live in two different worlds at the same time. The first is the world of the organism. The second is the world of values and meanings. So long as there are mental disorders, regardless of whether their origin turns out to be physical or something else, they will manifoldly transcend their organic foundation.

I do not want to be misunderstood, values and meanings alike are not unknown in the world of physical disease. Nevertheless, values and meanings are much more relevant in the genesis of mental disorders and their interpretation than in the formation and explanation of physical diseases. "There is no problem ... for disease concepts in acute physical medicine: a hearth attack, in itself and for the person concerned is a bad condition for everyone. Here our values are shared. But in psychiatry ... we are concerned, typically, with desires, beliefs, emotions, motivations, and so forth, areas of experience and behavior in which human values are, characteristically and legitimately, *diverse*" (Fulford, 2001, emphasis in original).

In this chapter, I will set out how knowledge is acquired in somatic medicine and psychological medicine. Then I will explain in which regards physical diseases and mental disorders are different. They differ in terms of their etiology, clinical picture and diagnostics, as well as in regard to their social meaning.

Knowledge in Somatic and Psychological Medicine: How to Acquire It?

The scientific status of psychiatric knowledge has been discussed for decades. "There has always been a longstanding debate on truth, method and the scientific status of psychiatric knowledge, and questions about the possibility of true knowledge in psychiatry are inherent to psychiatric thinking" (Denys, 2007). What is debatable is the very possibility of psychiatric knowledge about values and meaning, on the one hand, and objective data, on the other, since they are intertwined in the diagnostics and treatment of mental disorders. "This is a frustrating situation, but it seems an unavoidable one, since we must somehow integrate data ranging from the biochemical to the sociological and we must form an appreciation of man as both subject and object, as both agent and organism" (McHugh and Slavney, 1983: 11).

The question which is not yet properly answered is how to reconcile subjective interpretation and scientific explanation. Hence it is no wonder that there is no such thing as a coherent psychiatric epistemology, a set of mutually meaningfully related concepts underlying psychiatric knowledge.[5]

The crux of the matter is that psychiatrists have to have medical knowledge, but this does not suffice to be a psychiatrist.

The specific nature of humans' mental life requires a specific method of acquiring knowledge about the origin and nature of mental disorders. Methods used to acquire knowledge about physical diseases differ from the methods that are applied in the process of gaining knowledge about mental disorders.

Since they deal with *mental* disorders, psychiatrists have to make use of those methods that are suitable to the *mental side* of mental disorders, but also methods befitting the *physical side* of mental disorders. On the other hand, medical specialists other than psychiatrists do not need to accord equal weight to the *mental* and the *physical* of physical diseases because the mental is not in the focus of their interest. That is why *methodic pluralism* is unavoidable and necessary in psychiatry.

What is meant by the notion of methodic pluralism is the application of two different methods—the *hypothetical-deductive method*, which is the key method in natural sciences, and the *hermeneutic-interpretative method*, which is specific to humanities.[6]

Authors have dubbed these methods differently. For example, German philosopher Wilhelm Windelband speaks about the *nomothetic* and *ideographic* approach, and Karl Jaspers, German psychiatrist-turned-philosopher, about *causal explanation* and *meaningful understanding*.

It would not be fair to say that medical specialists other than psychiatrists are not interested in the mental life of their patients. Their primary focus, however, is on the physical, organic, physical, and biological. Of course, it is good for medical experts, who are not psychiatrists, not to ignore the *mens* of their patients. But the therapeutic efficacy of, for example, an ophthalmologist or orthopedic surgeon will not be significantly affected if they pay little or no attention to the mental life of their patients. Such an approach will most likely cause patients' mental suffering, but they will fully benefit from the diagnostic skill and efficacy of therapeutic intervention provided by those medical people who do not care about their patients' *mens*.

Since methodic pluralism reflects the specificity of psychiatry, that is, how distinct psychiatry is from other medical disciplines, I will present the peculiarities of each method that psychiatrists use, or should use, relying on the description of them provided by Paul R. McHugh and Philip R. Slavney in their book *The Perspectives of Psychiatry* (1983: 5-25).

Hypothetic-Deductive Method

The goal of those who use this method is to gradually advance from the formulation of a hypothesis, through testing the hypothesis (confirming or refuting it) till the formulation of principles, theories, or even laws.

Within this approach the whole is dissected into its parts which are suitable for quantification.

The object of research is to assess whether there is a correlation between a dependent variable (for example, Schizophrenic Disorder) and independent variables (for example, the social class of subjects, the number of blood relatives suffering from the same disorder, season of birth). The statistical method is used to see whether there is a correlation between variables. The degree of correlation is formulated as the degree of risk of falling ill from a particular disorder.

If, under equal circumstances, the same method is used, the same results should be obtained.

Testing the correlation between still untested independent variables and a dependent variable increases knowledge about the subject-matter.

Psychiatrists owe a great deal of knowledge to this approach. For example, they know that people who talk about taking their life are more likely to attempt suicide. Or that the closer one is related in family terms to a patient suffering from Schizophrenic Disorder, the more chances they have of developing the same kind of disorder.

Hermeneutic-Interpretative Approach

The basic principle of this approach is that the contents of consciousness cannot be regarded "simply as events emerging from brain mechanisms but also as the products of a person with hopes, desires, and intentions—the products of a person with a life story" (1983: 19).

The aim of using this method is to assess how the feelings and thoughts of a person come from their other feelings and thoughts. The starting point is that there are always subjective, experiential reasons why people feel as they feel, why they think as they think, why they are obsessed with this or that.

"At its simplest application, this method comprehends how feelings are derived from events: grief from loss, homesickness from departure, happiness from fulfillment. By its extension we sense why the responses of a given individual are coherent for him, how they grow out of the nexus between his personality and the way he views his circumstances.... The furthest extension of this method suggests how someone's personality might itself have been formed by prior experiences..." (1983: 20).

Psychiatrists put themselves into their patient's shoes. They try to find in their own "experiential arsenal" some similarity, something common with the patient's experiences, feelings, thoughts. Psychiatrists are considered as more skilful the more they are able to empathize with the patient, to partake in their experiences, to share them. And the better they understand the patient's mental problems the more they are able to provide them assistance.

There is no generalization within this approach. If the psychiatrist manages to establish a meaningful relation between a particular event and the patient's (emotional or any other) response to it, this relation presents as self-evident. There is no need to test it, to analyze it.

It is essential to keep in mind the reaches and limitations of each of these methods—*explication* and *understanding*. The use of either of them does not enable us to know all we should know about mental disorders. In the approach to people with mental illness each of these methods is limited and insufficient, but necessary at the same time.

In conclusion, the methods that should be used when approaching people with physical diseases and mental disorders are an important aspect of the difference between those two kinds of pathological phenomena. Only explanation, typical for natural sciences, is valid in the approach to physical diseases. Both explanation and understanding, hypothetic-deductive and hermeneutic-interpretative methods are necessary when approaching people with mental illness. The method of understanding is emblematic for the humanities. Explanation and understanding are fundamentally different.

Thus psychiatry and other medical disciplines differ not only in regard to their subject-matter but also in terms of the methods they use. And the difference between psychiatry and other medical disciplines reflects the difference between mental disorders and physical diseases and vice versa.

By comparing the etiology, clinical picture and diagnosis of physical diseases and mental disorders I will additionally substantiate my claim that they significantly differ.

Etiology

There are four key differences between physical diseases and mental disorders in terms of etiology: the role played by biological (physical) and social-psychological factors in the etiology of physical diseases and mental disorders; knowledge about the cause of physical diseases and mental disorders; the transformation of the mental into the physical, and vice versa, and the etiology of physical diseases and mental disorders in the context of different psychiatric models.

The Role Played by Biological (Physical) and Social-Psychological Factors in the Genesis of Physical Disease and Mental Disorders

There is such a huge body of data demonstrating the role played by biological (physical), psychological and social variables in the engenderment and shaping of both physical diseases and mental disorders, that it would be senseless to argue that physical diseases are caused only by physical, and mental disorders only by social-psychological factors.

Few physical diseases, along with their biological causation, have not been to some degree conditioned, or at least triggered by social-psychological influences. On the other hand, the science of human genetics has recently made such remarkable progress that one cannot turn a blind eye on hereditary factors in the formation of mental disorders. Furthermore, functional MRI provides even more insight into how the brain operates.

Thus, the general assertion reads: the same agents (biological-physical, psychological, social) give rise to both physical diseases and mental disorders. And that is where the similarities between the etiology of physical diseases and mental disorders begin and end.

If we take one step further from this general statement, the differences between physical diseases and mental disorders start to emerge. Even though, as stated, biological (physical), psychological, and social agents participate in the formation of both physical diseases and mental disorders, physical-biological factors are comparatively more responsible for the genesis of physical diseases just as social-psychological factors are comparatively more relevant in the etiology of mental disorders than in the etiology of physical diseases.

Of course, as stated, it is groundless to claim that all physical diseases are caused by physical-biological and all mental disorders by social-psychological factors. I am talking only about dominant etiological determination.

Closest to the mark seems to be the following view of the relationship between the biological (physical) and psychological (social) in health and pathological states. Functional occurrences in the brain and other parts of the body are the basis of both mental and organic-physiological activities. Regulation systems in the organism are extremely complex and integrated, which virtually means that the activities of any organ influence the activities of all other organs.

The same is valid for mental activities. Someone's memory functions influence their orientation in time and space, and with regard to other persons. Emotions also impact memory. For example, depressive patients complain of poor memory (pseudo-dementia of depressed people). Furthermore, emotions, in particular short-term and strong emotions, influence thinking, perception. Motivation increases or decreases the degree of concentration. And so on.

These observations should be complemented by the following claims. Biological (physical) and mental activities are closely correlated and mutually conditioned. Occurrences in parts of the body other than the brain influence the brain, the same as brain functions affect the functions of all other individual organs.

With due respect to the interconnectedness of all organs' functions, it is fair to say, that is, to repeat that, *in the genesis of physical diseases the role played by physical-biological factors outweighs the role played by psychological-social factors; on the other hand, physical-biological, psychological and social factors mostly equally participate in the etiology of mental disorders.*

This is an important difference between physical diseases and mental disorders with regard to the etiology.

Knowledge about the Causes
of Physical Diseases and Mental Disorders

There is a huge disproportion in our knowledge about the causes of physical diseases and mental disorders. We know much more about the causation of physical diseases than about the causation of mental disorders.[7]

The brain is the locus of the origin of psyche. That is a general statement very few psychiatrists, regardless of their general conceptual orientation, would be keen to dismiss nowadays. So far, however, this general assertion has not proved to be of much help in tracing the origin of the majority of mental disorders. Joseph Glenmullen, clinical instructor in psychiatry at Harvard Medical School, wrote: "In medicine, strict criteria exist for calling a condition a disease. In addition to a predictable cluster of symptoms, the cause of the symptoms or some understanding of their physiology must be established.... Psychiatry is unique among medical specialties in that ... we do not yet have proof either of the cause or the physiology for any psychiatric diagnosis.... In recent decades, we have had no shortage of alleged biochemical imbalances for psychiatric conditions. Diligent though these attempts have been, not one has been proved. It has just been opposite" (2000: 192-3). This view has been shared by many scholars (for example, Valenstein, 1998).

Unlike in psychiatry, the causes of a great many physical diseases have been revealed.

The Transformation of the Physical into the Mental, and Vice Versa

The relation between the physical and mental is an important issue in any discussion about the differences between the etiology of physical diseases and mental disorders.

A question that cannot be dodged while considering the pathogenesis of physical diseases and mental disorders is as follows: how does it happen that the neuro-electrical, biochemical, and other material processes produce feelings, thoughts, memory, cognition? How does subjective experience arise from neural computation? How do two substantially different phenomena: the material (neurotransmitters, neural associations) and the mental (thoughts, affection, memories) relate to one another? In particular, how does the former get transformed (translated) into the latter?

Psychiatrists may say that it is a philosophical question, and that is not up to them to deal with it. Yet, no matter how much they ignore the fundamental question of the nature of the relationship between the material and the mental, and, for that matter, between the brain and the mind, it is a question which, as long as it remains unanswered, casts a long shadow on an increasing biological knowledge base for understanding the physical origins of mental disorders. The question relates to the fundamental discontinuity in the hierarchical sequence of psychiatric explanation that makes the relationship between such issues as metabolism, on the one hand, and trust or distrust, on the other, obscure (McHugh and Slavney, 1982).

To be aware of that question means to be cognizant of hard-to-surmount hurdles psychiatrists have to face in their day-to-day practice. "As contemporary philosophers have stressed, the irreducible subjectivity of consciousness defies description in non-mental terms.... Hence the language of psychology and the language of biology involve two different levels of discourse when working with a patient" (Gabbard and Kay, 2001).

Today, neurophysiologists and neuropsychologists explain how the physical-biological is transformed into the mental. However, one thing is explication, and another thing is understanding.

Indeed, the transformation of the mental into the physical-biological is not as difficult to comprehend as it is the transformation of the physical-biological into the mental because some mental occurrences have visible organic-physiological correlates. For example, when you are in the grips of fear you get pale, your heart is pounding, your pulse rate accelerates, your mouth is dry. The observation that it is not as difficult to understand the translation of the mental into the physical-biological primarily refers to those mental states or functions that are accompanied with some sort of emotion, and, as it is known, emotions are said to be mid-way between the mental and physiological (biological).

The idea of the transformation of the material into the mental is at the heart of the acknowledgment that the brain is the birthplace of the psyche, and of the notion that biological changes underpin mental disorders; and still such transformation is beyond our comprehension. Psychiatrists and clinical psychologists behave in clinical practice as if there is nothing obscure in regard to the relation of the physical (biological) and the mental. However, they are short of answers when asked how alleged brain (dis)functions cause Pathological Jealousy, which is one form of Delusional Disorder. "In fairness, ignorance over how the brain, the primary source of all aspects of mental life, evokes either healthy or unhealthy psychological events hinders a more essential etiopathic classificatory system for psychiatry" (McHugh, 2005).

Things are quite different when the etiology of physical diseases is in question. No one is at pains to understand how physical pathology produces the signs of, for example, bacterial pneumonia, or uremia, or diabetes mellitus. Physical-biological occurrences have physical-biological effects.

Difficulties in understanding the transformation of the physical (biological) into the mental, as well as discordant explications of that process, feed into the doubts of some people that a distortion of particular neuro-physiological processes underlies mental disorders.[8]

This is the third key difference between the etiology of physical diseases and mental disorders.

Psychiatric Models and the Etiology of Physical Diseases and Mental Disorders

There is one more point of difference between the etiology of physical diseases and mental disorders. There are as many etiologies of mental disorders as there are psychiatric models. That is not the case with the etiology of physical diseases because physical medicine does not have as many legitimate concepts as there are in psychiatry.

One can argue that differences in conceptualizing the etiology of mental disorders come from differences among psychiatric models, and that there is actually only one etiology of mental disorders. Psychiatrists, however, are not ready to give credit to such a view. Advocates of each single general model in psychiatry are adamant: their model is the best one and therefore binding for all those who strive to find the causes of mental disorder. By the same token, no one knows what the supposed right etiology of mental disorder would be; what would *three-partisan* view of the etiology of mental disorders be like, to put it that way.

The fact that each psychiatric general concept has its own language—and "the different courses in psychiatry are ... more separating than the languages of different countries are" (Langenbach, 1993)—is an additional obstacle on the way to a unified psychiatric theory. "Although most medical specialties are unified by their discourse, psychiatry is not" (Langenbach, 1993)

I will discuss at length various general models in psychiatry in the chapter titled "Conceptual Cacophony in Psychiatry." Therefore I will only sketch the main features of each of the three major psychiatric models here.

The *medical (disease) model* regards mental malfunction as a consequence of physical and biological changes primarily in the brain, but in some other organs as well. The proponents of the *psychological model* argue that mental occurrences (unconscious, wrong explicatory schemata, wrong habits) underpin mental disorders. According to the *social model* mental illness is related to social factors.

Given the multitude of conceptual approaches in psychiatry it is no wonder that psychiatrists, depending on their conceptual orientation, find relevant, i.e., the most important etiological agents of a particular mental disorder either in physical pathology, or in unconscious forces, or bad habits, or wrong explicatory schemata, or in social influences.

This is not the case with health professionals in fields other than psychiatry. In most instances they share the same conceptual approach. When a person has, for example, pneumonia or uremia, virtually all the specialists in internal medicine from whom they seek help will explain the origin of the signs and symptoms of these diseases in more or less the same way.

In that sense, Tanya M. Luhrmann rightly notes: "It matters a great deal how a psychiatrist is taught to look at mental illness, because the 'how' cannot be clearly separated from the 'what' of the disease. To understand the psychiatric way of seeing, we have to proceed knowing that what counts as 'fact' is a tinted window onto the world you cannot look outside to see" (2000: 10).

It seems that K.W.M. Fulford and Anthony Colombo give a true picture of the attitudes of psychiatrists towards psychiatric models. "Asked directly, most mental health professionals, notwithstanding the current dominance of the 'medical model,' will claim that their understanding of mental disorder reflects a balanced 'biopsychosocial model'. In their respective professional discourses, though, in professional journals, in research priorities, in training curricula, and so forth, they give very different weights to different ways of understanding mental disorder" (2004).

In conclusion, the review of the difference between the etiology of physical diseases and mental disorders shows that they do significantly differ. Physical (biological) agents play a more important role in the etiology of physical diseases than psychological and social-cultural factors. Furthermore, the transformation of the physical (biological) into the mental, which is the basis of the assumption that physical (biological) changes underpin mental disorders is still vague, most often difficult to understand. Yet, the transformation of the physical-biological into the physical-biological, a process that is on the basis of many physical diseases, is quite comprehensible. Finally, the etiology of mental disorders is differently viewed within the context of different psychiatric models. On the other hand, in most cases there is no discordance among medical specialists other than psychiatrists in regard to the etiology of a great number of physical diseases.

Clinical Picture

In relation to their clinical picture, the major difference between physical diseases and mental disorders is that physical diseases manifest through primarily physical signs, whereas mental symptoms are the dominant manifestation of mental disorders.

Mental Disorders Present with Mostly Mental Symptoms,
and Physical Diseases with Mostly Physical-Biological Signs

This is the view of a great number of scholars who deal with establishing the difference between physical diseases and mental disorder. Thus Michael S. Moore (1980) writes that a person's symptoms rather than their causes determine whether that person has mental disorder or physical disease. Charles M. Culver and Bernard Gert share this view. "Mental maladies are distinguished from physical maladies primarily by the types of symptoms of evils that characterize them. Though etiology plays some role, as does the type of treatment that is effective in relieving the symptoms or curing the maladie, it is the dominant symptoms that play the largest role in determining whether we regard a person as having a physical or mental maladie" (1982: 88).

It other words, a disorder is mental if the symptoms which constitute that disorder are *primarily* mental symptoms. Attention should be given to *primarily* meaning dominantly. It is noteworthy that Robert L. Spitzer and Joanne Endicott also mention this *primarily* in their definition of mental disorder, presented in a paper published two years before the publication of DSM-III, in which there is a definition of generic mental disorder. "A mental disorder is a medical disorder whose manifestations are *primarily* signs or symptoms of a psychological (behavioral) nature..." (1978, my emphasis).

Why is *primarily* important? Because few physical diseases have no mental symptoms as well, the same as neurological signs can be found in a number of mental disorders.

Now the question might be raised: what about those clinical pictures which have nearly the same number of mental symptoms and physical signs? Are these physical diseases or mental disorders?

As stated, mental symptoms and physical signs appear in a good number of physical diseases and mental disorders. The question is always the same: what dominates the clinical picture—physical signs or mental symptoms. If the number of the former and the latter is nearly equal, underlying disturbances are usually dubbed *neuropsychiatric*. That is the case of Huntington's disease, Parkinson's disease, some forms of dementia, some types of epilepsy, etc. These kinds of disturbances are most often described in both psychiatric and neurological textbooks.[9]

If we look at the history of psychiatry and neurology, it is easy to grasp that as soon as the organic basis of an up-to-then psychiatric disorder was identified, it started to be considered as neurological or neuropsychiatric. This "change in the nature" of some mental disorders results from the wrong premise that the kind of etiology rather than the clinical picture decides, if a particular maladie will be classified as mental disorder or as physical disease. Also, the flawed concept that an unknown organic basis is the major characteristic of mental disorder prepares these maladies to be transferred from psychiatric into neurological or neuropsychiatric once their organic foundation is identified.

Hypothetically, the ultimate consequence of the opinion that when the organic basis of a maladie is identified it ceases to exist as a mental disorder, is that if one day the organic underpinning of the majority or of all mental symptoms is revealed, there will be no need for psychiatry because there will be no more mental disorders. All mental disorders will be renamed as neurological or maybe neuropsychiatric.

Still another point. Both the practice of proclaiming as neurological those mental disorders whose organic foundation was detected, and the concept about mental disorders whose major specificity is that their cause is unknown, speak in favor of the much-disputed views of Thomas S. Szasz.

Thomas S. Szasz, Emeritus Professor of Psychiatry in Syracuse, New York State, has argued for years that there is no such a thing as mental disorder. It does not exist because there is no organic basis of such a kind of disorder. According to Szasz (1961), a cluster of symptoms or signs cannot be considered as physical disease or mental disorder if their organic foundation is unknown. If they do have such a foundation, then they are neurological diseases rather than mental disorders. Those maladies which are usually called mental disorders, Szasz argues, are nothing but problems in living, which are for moral and political reasons renamed as mental disorders.

In 1961, when Szasz launched his idea about the myth of mental illness, he—I am confident—could not surmise that his claim that a disorder whose organic foundation is known is not a mental disorder would be authenticated by the current practice of renaming as neurological those disorders whose organic foundation is discovered.

In contrast to Szasz and today's practice of renaming as neurological those disorders whose organic ground is revealed, I am of the opinion that mental disorders are both those disorders whose organic foundation is unknown and those disorders whose organic basis is revealed. They are mental disorders so long as mental symptoms rather than physical signs dominate the clinical picture.

Those who disagree with my opinion might cite some cases which apparently contradict the view that a disorder is a mental disorder due to the dominance of mental symptoms in the clinical picture. I will now consider those exceptions that seemingly challenge my view.

Apparent Exceptions

The following disorders might be adduced as exceptions to the rule: first, Psychophysiological Disorders, which were previously called Psychophysical Disorders, and second, Somatization Disorder and Conversion Disorder. These last two kinds of disorder are now subsumed under Somatiform Disorders.

Why could psychophysiological disorders and somatiform disorders contradict the statement that the kind of clinical picture determines the kind of disorder? Because physiological signs, functional and structural changes, rather than psychological-behavioral symptoms prevail in the clinical picture of these mental disorders. However, only apparently.

Here are the arguments aimed at confirming the accuracy of my position. Psychophysiological (or Psychophysical) disorders (for example, essential hypertension, ulcerative colitis, stomach ulcer, asthma, neurodermatitis, hyperthyreosis) have for some time been presented in textbooks of internal medicine and other respective medical disciplines rather than in psychiatric textbooks. There are no operational definitions of these disorders in DSM-IV. This last fact, among others, testifies that these are not perceived as mental disorders.

And what about Somatiform Disorders? According to the definition of Somatization Disorder presented in DSM-IV, "The essential feature of Somatization Disorder is a pattern of recurring, multiple, clinically significant physical complaints.... The multiple physical complaints cannot be fully explained by any known general medical condition or the direct effects of some substance. If they occur in the presence of a general medical condition, the physical complaints or resulting social and occupational impairment are in excess of what would be expected from the history, physical examination, or laboratory tests. There must be a history of pain related to at least four different sites (e.g., head, abdomen, back, joints, extremities, chest, rectum) or functions (e.g., menstruation, sexual intercourse, urination). There also must be a history of at least two gastrointestinal symptoms other than pain.... There must be a history of at least one sexual or reproductive symptom other than pain.... Finally, there must also be a history of at least one symptom other than pain that suggests a neurological condition" (1994: 446).

Among associated features and disorders it is mentioned that people who have this kind of disorder "usually describe their complaints in colorful, exaggerated terms," and that "prominent anxiety and depressed mood are very common" (1994: 446).

If we take a closer look at the cited clinical picture of Somatization Disorder, it is easy to grasp that, in fact, mental symptoms rather than physical signs dominate in the clinical picture of this kind of disorder. Pain which prevails in the clinical picture is both an objective and subjective phenomenon. Furthermore, patients describe their problems in "colorful, exaggerated terms," which also indicates their more subjective than objective origin. Among mandatory symptoms there are plenty of those which are mid-way between physiological and mental (for example, nausea, abdominal bloating, sexual indifference). Finally, physical difficulties are more often accompanied by "prominent anxiety symptoms and depressed mood" than is the case with physical diseases.

Conversion Disorder is also, only at first sight, a disorder in which objective signs rather than mental symptoms dominate the clinical picture. I say "only at first sight" because psychogenic paralysis of one or more limbs, psychogenic blindness, deafness, or aphonia, as the most frequent symptoms of this kind of disorder, are not objective but rather subjective phenomena. They are only apparently objective signs.

In conclusion, Somatization Disorder and Conversion Disorder cannot be taken as an argument against the assertion that physical (physiological) signs prevail in the clinical picture of physical diseases whereas mental symptoms prevail in the clinical picture of mental disorders.

The Role of Personality in Shaping the Clinical Picture

The role played by the personality in shaping the manifestations of physical diseases and mental disorders is an additional point of difference between the two.

The truth is that the personality affects various aspects of physical diseases and mental disorders; for example, someone's perception of either is heavily influenced by their personal vulnerability; early conditioning; socioeconomic status; environmental stress and emotional arousal. In turn, the perception of one's disease or disorder, and consequent personal attitude towards them, affects their course, outcome and primarily the extent of disability.

Yet, the personality plays a more important role in the engenderment and shaping of mental disorders than physical diseases. The influence of the personality on the transformation of structural-functional changes of some organ(s) (for example, inflammation, degeneration, hyper- or hypofunction) into physical signs (for example, edema, cough, high body temperature, the change of urine's color, tremor, intense sweating, difficulty in swallowing) is not significant, if at all.

That does not hold for mental disorders. The personality of the patient is involved in the process of creating the clinical picture even before the appearance of the first symptoms of the disorder. How is that? A good number of mental disturbances originate in the particular psychological make-up of the individual. Furthermore, it is personality which struggles to counter the menacing mental imbalance at the very beginning of mental illness. Since mental defensive mechanisms are an integral part of the personality, it is the personality which tries to accommodate the developing mental disorder, to establish a sort of co-existence of the individual and the disturbing mental symptoms. By doing so the personality abundantly tailors the clinical picture of mental disorder. Hence the symptoms of a mental disorder are an amalgam of putative physical-biological pathology, psychological dysfuntion, and coping mechanisms of that particular individual (Kecmanovic, 2006).

The patient's reaction to their mental disturbance is also an integral part of their disorder. So much so that in many cases it is hard to tell what are genuine symptoms of the disorder and what is the individual's reaction to them, so closely are they interwoven.

The more important role that the personality plays in shaping the clinical picture of mental symptoms rather than of physical diseases makes the clinical picture of mental disorders more individualized, more personalized, meaning more different from one person to another than is the case with physical diseases. For example, the signs of pneumonia, or uremia, or a fracture of femur are more similar from one patient to another than are the symptoms of people suffering from Schizophrenic Disorder, or from Dysthymia, or Generalized Anxiety Disorder. In brief, the personality colors the symptoms of mental disorder more than the signs of physical diseases. It does color the patient's reaction to a particular physical disease, but it does not tint the objective signs of physical diseases.

That is why many doctors in medical disciplines other than psychiatry tend to pay lip service to the patient's reaction to their disease. The signs of the disease matter; they determine the doctor's treatment. In psychiatry, however, doctors have to accord due weight to the patient's personality, to their defense and coping mechanisms, to their reaction to mental disturbance because all of them are an integral part of the manifestations of a particular disorder. Therefore it is virtually impossible not to take them into consideration in the treatment of that particular patient.

Co-determination of the clinical picture by genuine symptoms of a particular disorder, on the one hand, and the personality's coping and defense mechanisms (if a distinction between them is appropriate) on the other, additionally impedes diagnosing of mental disorders. Making a diagnosis is particularly difficult when the genuine symptoms of the disorder have not fully developed, and the manifestations of the personality's struggle to prevent them from emerging dominate the clinical picture. Making a diagnosis is (even more) difficult because the manifestations of the personality's fighting the symptoms of emerging disorder are often in the grey zone between the normal and pathological. Therefore, quite often the following question should be answered: is something wrong with the personality, or is what we see the symptoms of a mental disorder?

The greater role of the personality in shaping the clinical picture of mental disorders is one of the reasons why diagnosing them is more demanding than diagnosing physical diseases. Aubrey Lewis, the late Professor of Psychiatry at London University, one of the most prominent figures of the Institute of Psychiatry, Maudsley Hospital, noted this difference in diagnosing the former and the latter: "Physiological functions can be (thus) designated and judged far more satisfactorily than the psychological. We can, therefore, usually tell whether an individual is physically healthy, but we cannot tell with the same confidence and consensus of many observers, whether he is mentally ill" (1953).

There is still one interesting aspect of the relation between the personality and mental disorder. The impairment of one or more mental functions (for example, perception, memory, emotions, volitional functions) is one of the key elements of mental disorders. And all mental functions, more accurately, their unique combination constitutes the personality, makes one person different from another. What constitutes our personal specificity, our discreteness and distinctiveness, is not our bones, liver, kidneys, lungs, etc. but rather our personality. As Christopher Boorse wittingly noted: Even unconscious ideas and desires are still more ours than guts movements are ours (1975).[10]

Thus when someone develops a mental disorder it is believed that their personality has fallen ill. Mental illness seems to affect the core of people, their personality.

That is not the case with physical diseases. They are not as connected with someone's personality as are mental disorders. If you fall ill from pneumonia, or diabetes, or if you get lung cancer, no one will suspect that it has to do with your personality, or that your personality has fallen ill along with your body.

Indeed, there are attempts at establishing the relationship between someone's personality type and the physical disease they contract. Thus type A personality and type B personality have been identified. The former is characterized by competitiveness, assertiveness, by striving to be successful in life and business, to complete all duties on time, by obsessive personality traits. This type of personality is said to be more prone than the rest of the population to heart problems. Type B personality is easy going, laid back. They are not competitive, and do not care much whether or not they complete their duties on time. Those who have this type of personality are said to have lower chances of having heart problems than those having A type personality.

Also it is believed that there are more specific personality types among those who suffer from a particular form of Psychophysiological Disorders (Psychophysical Disorder). For example, obsessive-compulsive personality traits are said to be associated with high blood pressure.

This kind of linking the personality and physical diseases is, however, limited to only a small number of diseases and personality types. In the case of mental disorders virtually every disorder is regarded as having to do with the personality insofar as every disorder goes with the impairment of some mental functions which constitute the personality.

In conclusion, it is obvious that the personality plays a much bigger role in the engenderment and shaping of mental disorders than physical diseases. The personality's coping and defense mechanisms have a greater influence on the genesis and character of the clinical picture of mental disorders than that of physical diseases. Finally, mental disorders seem to affect the personality more than physical diseases do.

Diagnosis

Can differences be established between diagnosing physical diseases and mental disorders?

First of all, there are serious arguments against diagnosing mental disorders, arguments that are not valid in physical medicine. I will mention but three arguments. First, the diagnosis of a mental disorder is not of much help if we want to learn more about the intimate aspects of a particular person's mental suffering; about how they experience the impairment of this or that mental function, which is usually accompanied by a reduction in overall mental capacity; about their experience of negative attitudes of other people towards them, and such an experience is somewhat incorporated in the clinical picture; about the defense mechanisms they prefer to use, and so on. Briefly, the diagnosis of a mental disorder does not open the door to an individual's subjective, experiential microcosm. It does not even say which symptoms the respective individual has because those who have the same diagnosis may have a good number of different symptoms. Thus, the diagnosis of a mental disorder conceals more than it discloses.

Second, psychiatric diagnosis has negative social connotations. Once a person gets a psychiatric diagnosis they are not regarded the same way as they were before they were diagnosed. The stigma of mental illness either makes or deepens the chasm between the mentally ill and the milieu. In this sense—one might say—the stigma of mental disorder, and psychiatric diagnosis for that matter, has a negative impact on the course and outcome of a mental disorder.

Third, "diagnoses ... inherently ignore the conditions of persons who fail to meet criteria for 'caseness'" (Horwitz, 2002b). Over time, criteria for diagnosing particular mental disorders change. No matter how uncertain and changeable criteria for mental disorders are, whenever they are defined, all those people who have symptoms but do not meet criteria for any particular disorder are left out; they are not on the radar of psychiatrists' attention. Thereby a good number of those who do need psychiatric assistance do not get it. They have to wait until a new classification is constructed, in which their symptoms will may be meet criteria of a new, or of an old, newly designed disorder.

Most of these arguments against diagnosis in psychological medicine do not hold in physical medicine; maybe except for the third one.

And are there some advantages, some positive sides of psychiatric diagnosis? There are, and they are the same as those in physical medicine. Here are some of them.

If there were no diagnosis, health workers would have a great deal of difficulty in communicating with each other, exchanging information about a particular patient. Without diagnosis we would not know the prevalence and incidence of a particular disease or disorder in a specific region. Without diagnosis it would not be possible to conduct research on individual aspects of diseases and know the effects of a particular type of treatment.

Diagnostic Procedure in Somatic and Psychological Medicine

Physical diseases are diagnosed on the grounds of the history of disease, medical checkups aimed at finding the objective signs of a disease, as well as on the grounds of laboratory tests. Yet mental disorders are diagnosed on the basis of the history of the illness, what the client says about their mental problems, about how they experience themselves, people around them, and on the basis of observations of the behavior of the person in question. Information about the client provided by those who know them might be of help in the diagnostic procedure.

There is a distinct difference between diagnosing physical diseases and mental disorders. In diagnosing physical diseases the focus is on objective pathological changes (body changes and test findings). The extent and the kind of assessed changes play a major role in the diagnostic process, in reaching a conclusion as to whether the respective client is ill, and if yes, which kind of disease they suffer from.

In psychological medicine, diagnostic procedure is different. Various and numerous subjective elements play a much more important role in diagnosing mental disorders than in diagnosing physical diseases.

Table 3.1 presents the basic elements and circumstances that play a role in diagnosing mental disorders. On the basis of the elements and circumstances that are presented in Table 3.1, it is easy to grasp the difference between diagnosing physical diseases and mental disorders.

In somatic medicine, depending on the doctor's skills, their knowledge and experience, they will detect objective signs of a change that suggest that the client might suffer from a particular disease and will ask for particular tests to be carried out. Furthermore, in somatic medicine, an increasing number of diseases are diagnosed based on test results (laboratory tests, imaging techniques, and so on). The subjective of the patient and the subjective of the doctor play a decreasing role in diagnosing physical diseases due to ever more sophisticated investigation techniques and the fact that diagnoses in physical medicine are quite often etiological. In other words, since the cause of a great number of diseases has been discovered, in a good number of cases the diagnosis is made when the cause of the disease is found, be it specific structural and functional alterations, or one or more particular pathological agents.

Table 3.1
Some Elements of the Diagnostic Procedure in Psychiatry

What the psychiatrist perceives as diagnostically important in the patient's verbal and non-verbal behavior
How the psychiatrist interprets what they perceive as diagnostically important in the patient's verbal and non-verbal behavior
Which criteria of the mentally normal and psychopathological are used by the psychiatrist when considering a patient's manifestations as psychopathological
Which psychiatric model the psychiatrist relies on in the diagnostic procedure
Whether the psychiatrist in the diagnostic procedure uses the definitions of mental disorders presented in some official classifications of mental disorders, rely on their own definitions, their "sixth" sense, and the like
If the psychiatrist uses an official classification of mental disorders, which classification it is

Diagnosing mental disorder is more complex. Circumstances under which a client approaches a psychiatrist; how they relate to the psychiatrist; their interest in being or not being diagnosed as suffering from a mental disorder; their image about what a mental patient looks like, what they say, how they behave; their dominant defense mechanisms—all these factors and circumstances constitute a filter for what a patient actually experiences, what they think, what they aspire to, what they wish or do not wish, and so on.

The existence of various psychiatric models further complicates diagnosing mental disorders and makes the result of the diagnostic process even more uncertain. What a psychiatrist recognizes as important in diagnostic terms depends on their favorite psychiatric model. For example, things that will be diagnostically relevant to a psychiatrist who embraces the medical model will be of no interest to a psychiatrist who considers the psychological model as the only model worth espousing.

On the other hand, in somatic medicine, conceptual approaches are not as different from one another and their existence does not substantially impede the diagnostic procedure.

Some other circumstances also determine psychiatrists' diagnostic perception. What a psychiatrist will recognize as diagnostically notable depends on, first, their definition of mental disorder, and second, on their concept of the cluster of which symptoms (how intense they are, how long they have been manifested) makes the diagnosis of a particular mental disorder more correct than the diagnosis of some other disorder. In practical terms, it means that psychiatrists' diagnostic perception depends on the diagnostic and classificatory system they favor.

But if the psychiatrist does not follow to the letter the guidelines or the prescriptions of operational definitions—and a good number of them do not—they rely on "psychiatric intuition," on the "sixth sense," which is very difficult to define, indeed.

It is difficult to believe that a doctor today would diagnose any physical disease relying solely on intuition or the sixth sense.

And that is not the end of the story. Psychiatrists—like laypeople, after all—disagree on whether and how much a person is depressed, for example, whether and how much they are anxious; whether and how much their affect is blunted, whether and how much they are distressed, and so on.

It is particularly difficult to agree on whether the impairment of a particular mental function is mild or more than mild. And the extent of the impairment of one or more mental functions, the same as the extent of internal psychological dysfunction, and the extent of distress, play a significant role in evaluating whether a person is mentally disordered or not.

Doctors in medical disciplines other than psychiatry do not bother with such questions. They rely on test findings. And in most cases tests comprise cutoff point (i.e., the level of a particular substance in urine or blood; how high is blood pressure; how dense and large are particular areas of the brain imaged by CT or MRI) that tell what is and what is not within normal limits.

Psychiatry is far from such diagnostic precision. For example, if somebody says that they hear voices although there is not any source of voice within earshot, there is no diagnostic procedure that would be able to confirm or dismiss the client's allegations. The same holds for visual hallucinations. Yet both auditory and visual hallucinations are diagnostically relevant.

Apart from hallucinations, delusions are considered to be another indicator that the people who produce them might be psychotic. Can the client's allegations that someone is chasing them, tapping their phone conversations, hatching a plot against them, putting poison into the tea they order in a café, be verified? No, they cannot. People can tell a lie, they can fake that they feel extremely affected by the "fact" that they are the target of other people's ill intentions, and they can keep on doing it in spite of evidence to the contrary. The psychiatrist cannot be certain whether the patient is malingering or telling the truth, that is, whether they really have delusions or do not have them. If the patient sets about behaving in accordance with the dictate of the "delusions" (or delusions), if they begin living them: they notify the police about people who threaten them, and take other necessary steps so as to protect themselves, the psychiatrist is more likely to take the patient's delusions as genuine. But even then they cannot be certain that faked delusions are not involved.

There is still another issue that indicates just how different diagnostic procedures are in physical and psychological medicine.

Physically ill and mentally ill people differ in terms of the awareness of their disturbance, in particular when their disturbance has fully developed. Patients who have a fully developed clinical picture of heart failure, or kidney failure, or those who are in the terminal phase of lung cancer, are very rarely unaware that something is wrong, very wrong with their health. They simply cannot but be aware that their health is going downhill.

That is not the case for acutely psychotic people. (If people with mental illness can be ranked according to the degree of seriousness of their disturbance, acutely psychotic patients would be on the top.) They lack insight into what is going on with them, they are not aware that they are ill. That is one of the main reasons why they do not seek help, and if forcibly taken to a psychiatrist, are reluctant to be treated. They are far too seriously mentally ill to be able to know that they are mentally ill.

As stated, a seriously physically ill patient cannot suffer from that kind of "blind spot"—and if they do, it occurs extremely rarely.

From what has been said about the differences in the diagnostic procedures in physical and psychological medicine, it turns out that the subjective of the psychiatrist and the subjective of mentally ill people play a much more significant role in diagnosing mental disorders than in diagnosing physical diseases. And that subjective factor paves the way to substantial disagreements among psychiatrists, dilemmas and controversies in psychiatry. The reliability of the diagnosis of mental disorder is one of these contested topics.

Reliability of Mental Disorder Diagnoses

Reliability indicates the degree of agreement among psychiatrists in regard to the diagnosis of the disturbance of a particular patient. The degree of reliability can be measured in different ways. Usually, a few psychiatrists will interview one or more patients and then diagnose the mental problems of each one of them. The degree of concordance among psychiatrists in regard to the diagnosis of each patient is the gauge of its reliability.

The psychiatric community was taken by surprise when Robert E. Kendell, John E. Cooper and others published the results of the examination of psychiatric diagnostic practice on either side of the Atlantic in 1971.[11] After interviewing the same patients, psychiatrists in New York City diagnosed the patients' mental problems as indicative of Schizophrenic Disorder twice as frequently as their colleagues in London who said that the patients diagnosed as suffering from Schizophrenic Disorder by the American psychiatrists actually suffered from Depressive Disorder, Personality Disorder, and Neurotic Disorder.

These findings rang the alarm. The question was raised: can we trust psychiatrists? What is psychiatric diagnosis all about? Does it really suffice to cross the Atlantic to have the same mental troubles diagnosed differently?

The courts and health insurance companies also exercised pressure on psychiatrists to do something to increase the reliability of the diagnosis of mental disorder. The courts did not know what to do when confronted with the opposing opinions of psychiatrists regarding the mental status of one and the same person who committed an offence, or someone who claimed compensation for sustained injuries and associated mental suffering. Health insurance companies had the same problems: how to know what kind of disorder a patient has who wants to get insurance or be paid off? What is the point of providing preferential treatment for a particular mental disorder if psychiatrists do not agree on the kind of disorder the patents suffer from?

Requests for the greater reliability of psychiatric diagnoses came from psychiatric researchers as well. They posed the question: how could research be conducted into the origin of this or that mental disorder, or an assessment made of the efficacy of a particular psychiatric treatment, if due to low reliability of psychiatric diagnosis no one was sure whether the subjects in the experimental group suffered from the same kind of disorder.

Moreover, the critics of psychiatry, antipsychiatrists in particular, played on the low reliability of psychiatric diagnosis in order to show that arbitrariness is in the heart of psychiatry, that such a thing as mental illness does not exist at all, and that psychiatric discourse has no other purpose than to provide legitimacy to those psychiatrists who label as mental disorder all socially, politically above all, undesirable ways of behaving and believing. Psychiatrists who were keen on countering such claims by the critics of psychiatry were more than interested in having the reliability of psychiatric diagnosis enhanced.

Those dealing with the public health aspects of mental disorders were also concerned. How could the incidence or prevalence of mental disorders, or of a particular mental disorder, be assessed; how could the association between a particular mental disorder and some biological or social factors be established, if there was no agreement on the diagnosis of the mental problems of people in the selected sample.

Some regarded the increased reliability of psychiatric diagnosis as an opportunity to mend the fragmentation of psychiatry. The existence of many psychiatric models was believed to be one of the reasons why it was difficult to increase the reliability of psychiatric diagnosis. Where there are many different conceptions about the nature and origin of mental disorder, it is not easy to create such a diagnostic-classification system that would be instrumental in increasing the reliability of psychiatric diagnosis.

All these factors and circumstances spurred psychiatrists to set down to thinking seriously about what should be done to enhance the reliability of psychiatric diagnosis.

The following measures were undertaken. First, in order to minimize or exclude altogether subjective interpretations of a patient's symptoms psychiatrists are asked to only rely on observable symptoms. Second, as different ways of interviewing the patient on the part of different psychiatrists might be one of the reasons for the low reliability, the interviewing process was standardized. Psychiatrists were trained to conduct interviews in the same structured way. Third, psychiatrists were asked to use the same definitions of particular psychopathological phenomena. Fourth, in the third edition of the Diagnostic and Statistical Manual of

Mental Disorders (1980) mental disorders were defined by means of operational definitions.

Did all these measures result in the higher reliability of psychiatric diagnosis? Yes and no.

According to the opinion of Stuart A. Kirk and Herb Kutchins based on an analysis of a great many studies of the reliability of particular psychiatric diagnoses, carried out after 1980, the problem of the low reliability of psychiatric diagnosis has not been resolved. It is just not on the agenda any longer, which gives the impression that the problem has been fixed. "Are mental health clinicians now much less likely to disagree about diagnoses than in the past?," ask these authors, and reply: "If the available evidence is examined more carefully, the answer to these critical questions is either No or We do not know" (1992:141).

Gordon Parker, Professor of Psychiatry at New South Wales University in Sydney, writes (2008) that the claims of the authors of DSMs that these classifications have a high reliability have never been confirmed.

Yet Robert E. Kendell and Assen Jablensky maintain that "the reliability of psychiatrists' diagnoses was dramatically improved, at least in research settings in which structured interviews were used, by the introduction of explicit definitions and decision rules in DSM-III and in the ICD-10 Diagnostic Criteria for Research" (2003).

The closest to the mark seems to be the assertion that if the reliability of psychiatric diagnoses has been enhanced in the post DSMs era, it has been achieved only in research settings. But psychiatric practice does not take place in such settings. In fact, psychiatric research constitutes only a small portion of psychiatric activities.

There are still many unresolved problems as far as the reliability of psychiatric diagnosis is concerned. Even when they are willing to comply with the definitions of individual psychopathological phenomena, this does not mean that all psychiatrists will identify the same mental manifestations as normal or pathological. Even if they accept the same definition of, e.g., depressive mood, there will always be differences among psychiatrists as to whether a particular patient is depressed at all, and whether their depression has pathological proportions.

Efforts were made to resolve this difficulty. Groups of psychiatrists were trained to get as close as possible in their evaluations of whether a patient presented one or more psychopathological phenomena, and if yes, how intense they were. This training was initially designed for those who are involved in research projects. Later on some students of psychiatry underwent this kind of training in order to make the way they evaluate a patient's mental condition more uniform.

However, it is hard to believe that most psychiatrists or all psychiatrists can be trained to evaluate in the same way whether a patient is, e.g., anxious; whether their basic mood is a bit high, and how much; whether and how much their affect is blunted, and so on. It is possible to achieve such a goal but only after the intensive training of those who are going to take part in some specific research. But these are only specific circumstances, and any conclusions that could be drawn from them cannot be generalized.

In addition, a small number of psychiatrists conduct the interview in a standardized way in their day-to-day practice. As Alex Spiegel noted " (...) structured interviews do not always have much in common with the conversations that take place in therapists' offices, and since the publication of the DSM-III, in 1980, no major study has been able to demonstrate a substantive improvement in reliability in those less formal settings" (2005).[12]

On the basis of my own experience, I must admit that Spiegel is very close to the mark. Psychiatrists "in less formal settings" quite often do not conduct the interview in a standardized way and do not follow the DSMs guidelines.

It is of particular importance to point out that when two psychiatrists do not agree upon the kind of mental problems of a particular patient, no criterion exists that could say which psychiatrist was right and which one was wrong. That is why psychiatrists use to say that the time rather than themselves will establish the *right* diagnosis.

Phil Brown (1987, 1989), from Harvard Medical School, concedes that in day-to-day clinical practice psychiatrists are sparing in their use of the standardized diagnostic methods including the operational definitions of mental disorders.

Prompted by psychiatrists' "diagnostic behavior" he observed, Brown made the distinction between *psychiatric technique* and *psychiatric work* (1990).

Psychiatric technique includes the formalization of the classification, the standardized diagnostic techniques, rating scales, and wherever possible, the quantification of psychopathological phenomena. *Psychiatric technique* is rarely used in everyday psychiatric practice, which Brown dubs *psychiatric work*.

Many reasons might be enumerated for why psychiatrists do more *psychiatric work* than they use *psychiatric technique*: psychiatrists' belief that psychopathological phenomena cannot be formalized let alone quantified; the conviction that personal experience is of the greatest help in the diagnostic process; the need to complete the diagnostic procedure as soon as possible; tacit antagonism between academic psychiatry which created *psychiatric technique*, and the majority of psychiatrists who do *psychiatric work*.

Furthermore, doubts were raised as to whether the structure of operational definitions was instrumental to achieving higher reliability of psychiatric diagnoses. The operational definitions of the majority of mental disorders include many symptoms. The diagnosis of a particular disorder can be made if the patient has a fixed number of all the listed symptoms; for example at least five out of nine cited symptoms. In some cases it is also mentioned how long the symptoms should be present to make a diagnosis.

Michael M. Chang and T. George Bidder slightly caricatured the DSM's operational definitions of mental disorders, in particular the requirement that the patient has a fixed number of all listed symptoms: "At the current state of psychiatric knowledge, grouping patients according to selected properties rather than in terms of their total phenomenology is analogous to classifying a car by observing any four of the following eight properties: wheels, motors, headlight, radio, seats, body, windshield wipers, and exhaust system. While the object with four of these properties might well be a car, it might also be an airplane, a helicopter, a derrick, and a tunnel driller" (1985).

Sticking with one diagnostic-classification system so as to make reliability of psychiatric diagnosis higher implies that the correctness of that particular system is not questioned; it should be taken at face value. To question the "truthfulness" of a particular diagnostic and classification system means to ask about its validity. And that should not be done. In that sense the motto of all endeavors to increase the reliability of mental disorder runs as follows: It does not matter what it is that we agree upon. It matters that we agree.

Desubjectivization: The Price of Efforts to Increase the Reliability of Psychiatric Diagnosis

Tim Thornton writes (2007: 178) that desubjectivization of the diagnostician and patient is one of the prices of the efforts to increase the reliability of psychiatric diagnosis. A classificatory judgment is valid if it can be characterized using the resources of only a dehumanized natural scientific standpoint, fully independent of human interests. I would say that the same is valid for a diagnostician's judgment.

The ambition of the authors of DSMs was to reach this kind of classificatory and diagnostic judgment. Did they manage to do so, and at what price?

Indeed, mental disorder occurs in the subjective and objective sphere. This fact, as stated, is the source of not only diagnostic but also other controversies and dilemmas in psychiatry. To put the objective sphere in brackets means to renounce efforts to increase the reliability of psychiatric diagnosis. To exclude the subjective sphere means to falsify the nature of mental disorders.[13]

The DSMs have not resolved this controversy.

I will point out a number of fall-outs of the DSM's formalization of diagnostic procedure, that is, its reliance on operational diagnostic criteria in general, and on only observable, objective data in particular: in spite on DSM's reliance on only observable phenomena, non-observable, meaning subjective phenomena, such as for example delusions could not be excluded from diagnostic criteria; given the complex relationship between a patient's subjective and objective, the diagnostician's interpretation of this relationship, i.e., the diagnostician's subjective could not be prevented from playing its part in the diagnostic process; the importance of so-called intuitive diagnosis has been completely discarded, and there has been an increase in "psychiatric comorbidity."[14]

First, in order to omit different interpretations of the psychopathological phenomena provided by the protagonists of different psychiatric models, the authors of DSMs have confined diagnostic procedure to what is visible in the clinical picture, to what is objective, not susceptible to the diagnostician's interpretation. That is what they claim to have done, at the very least. However, contrary to their claim, they list, among others, a sense of despair, of helplessness, delusions, hallucinations, low self-esteem as the symptoms of the operational definitions. Are these symptoms accessible to the eye of a diagnostician; are they observable? How can they be visible, objective? How could a psychiatrist know that someone's self-confidence has dropped if they did their best to conceal it, not to show it in how they relate to themselves and other people, if their behavior has not changed in tune with their self-perception, and if they are reluctant to talk about how low they rate themselves?

Paul R. McHugh writes that Spitzer so as to increase the reliability of mental disorders "picked those features that were *observable*, such as hallucinations and delusions, and insisted they be so defined that any psychiatrist could confidently recognize them" (2005). However, how can a psychiatrist observe someone's hallucinations or delusions if the patient does not verbalize them, and/or if their behavior has not changed in accordance with the content of the hallucinations and delusions? Just to remind the reader that as far as physical-biological diseases are concerned virtually a great number of their signs, including those that are not traceable from outside, can be traced down by modern diagnostic techniques.

Second, if they only focus on the patient's behavior while attempting to make diagnosis, can psychiatrists refrain from interpreting the meaning of this or that kind of behavior, from endeavoring to detect which mental contents are behind a specific form of the patient's behavior?

Psychiatrists do not know—and how could they know?—which kind of relationship there is between subjective experience and objective behavior in the case of a particular patient. Since there is no rule governing the correspondence of specific experience and its behavioral expression—if there is always a behavioral expression of a particular experience at all—psychiatrists cannot help but make assumptions about the meaning that a specific behavior hides or reveals. By doing so they interpret, decipher, translate (Wiggins and Schwartz, 1994: 92). And each one does it in a different way or slightly different way at best. They thereby betray the sacred principle of objectivity which is the foundation of the DSMs. In other words, while interpreting psychiatrists use a hermeneutic-interpretative method, which the authors of the DSMs struggled to exclude from their classifications, and thereby make them more reliable than the previous ones (Spitzer, M., 1988).

Third, the authors of the DSMs do not even mention the importance of intuitive diagnosis in psychiatry. They could not do so because it ran counter to their ambition to increase the reliability of psychiatric diagnosis by eliminating, among others, all issues that are not objective; and intuition is a subjective phenomenon par excellence. Yet, by doing so the authors of the DSMs lost sight of how significant a role intuition may play in making a diagnosis. Here are a few examples.

The entire clinical picture is not the same as the sum of its individual elements. For example, a cluster of mental symptoms such as affective bluntness, the loss of interest in people and matters, the feeling that other people can read our thoughts, the phenomenon of thought withdrawal, may prompt a psychiatrist to suspect that the person who presents with these symptoms might suffer from Schizophrenic Disorder. But psychiatrists in some instances do not make this diagnosis until they grasp the *psychopathological gestalt* which either corroborates this diagnosis or makes psychiatrists doubt that it is schizophrenia. And they need experience and intuition to grasp the psychopathological gestalt.

In addition, in many a case when the cited symptoms are absent, or are not fully developed, psychiatrists still say that it might be a case of Schizophrenic Disorder. How and why? Because there is such a thing as a specific way in which schizophrenic patients relate to themselves and others which incites psychiatrists, when they recognize or, more accurately, feel it, to say that that particular person could suffer from schizophrenia. Henricus Cornelius Rümke, the late Professor of Psychiatry in Utrecht, Netherlands, coined (1941) the term *praecox feeling* to denote a markedly subjective feeling or intuition that the schizophrenic patient induces in the diagnostician.[15] Without referring to it, many psychiatrists rely on it in diagnosing schizophrenia.

Fourth, as Maj points out (2005), the old clinical descriptions laid emphasis on the various clinical aspects, "whereas in current operational definitions the various clinical features are usually given the same weight." Consequently "traditional clinical descriptions encouraged differential diagnoses, whereas current operational definitions encourage multiple diagnoses, probably in part because they are less able to convey the "'essence' of each diagnostic entity."[16]

Fifth, DSMs are focused on the symptoms rather than on the patient's narrative. As a result psychiatrists are progressively loosing interest in experiential dimensions of mentally ill people, i.e., in psychopathology. "We have lost not only our curiosity about how a psychotic patient thinks, but also our abilities to observe. This is a major unanticipated consequence of this most empirical of all diagnostic systems" (Tucker, 1988).

In concluding, there are numerous reasons why the reliability of psychiatric diagnosis should be increased. The ambition of the authors of the DSMs was to do so. There is no conclusive evidence that the DSMs managed to achieve such a goal except in research settings.[17]

Any attempt to increase the reliability of the diagnosis of mental disorders comes across hurdles that are hard to overcome. The hurdles have been erected by the specific nature of the mental disorder, the fact that mental illness exists in two worlds: the world of the subjective (meanings, values), and the world of the objective (biological grounding of mental disorders, the behavior of people with mental illness) as well as the fact that etiological diagnoses of mental disorders are unknown.

The controversies and dilemmas faced by anyone who is determined to carry out the noble goal of increasing the reliability of psychiatric diagnosis wait to be resolved.[18]

As the majority of diagnoses in physical medicine are etiological medical specialists other than psychiatrists do not have to bother with the mentioned issues; in any case, much less than psychiatrists do.

Now I would like to turn the reader's attention to the validity of psychiatric diagnosis, and mental disorder, for that matter.

Validity of Psychiatric Diagnosis

The reliability of diagnoses and of the entire diagnostic and classification system is not a goal in itself. It does not serve itself. The true purpose of increasing the reliability of mental disorder diagnoses is to establish the validity of mental disorders' diagnoses and the validity of classification of mental disorders.

What is the validity of the diagnosis of a particular disorder? When the diagnosis is valid, it cannot be put in question. When it is valid it is in accordance with reality or with nature, which, roughly speaking, boils down to the same thing. And do those phenomena which we identify as mental disorders correspond to "real" processes occurring in nature (reality)? It seems too optimistic or the expression of naiveté to hope that there is a correspondence between the segments of reality and the diagnostic categories we use to define individual mental disorders (Parnas and Zahavi, 2002: 137).

It follows from what I said about the validity of mental disorders that it is extremely significant not only for diagnostics and classifications of mental disorders but also for psychiatry itself.

There are several sorts of validity of diagnostic categories. Usually the mention is made of four forms of validity: *construct validity* which indicates a coherent, explicit group of key characteristics of a particular disorder; *content validity*, a notion that comprises the verifiable observations by means of which the existence of a specific disorder can be proved; *concurrent validity* which says that the diagnosis of a particular disorder can be verified using independent procedures like biological and psychological tests, and *predictive validity* on the basis of which the course and outcome of a disorder can be predicted. In psychiatry, concurrent and predictive validity are most widely used.

Have the measures that have been undertaken to increase the reliability of the diagnosis of mental disorders resulted in its increased validity. The answer is in the negative.

This is the view of scholars who particularly deal with the reliability and validity of the diagnosis of mental disorders. For example, David J. Kupfer, Michael B. First, and Darryl Regier, in the "Preface" to the book *Research Agendas for DSM-V* (2002), write that as far as the reliability of classifications is concerned, psychiatry in the last few decades has made a step of one hundred miles, but as for validity virtually nothing has been achieved. Bill Fulford, Tim Thornton and George Graham assert in *Oxford Textbook of Philosophy and Psychiatry* that the hope was that "reliability would lead on to validity. But this has not happened" (2006: 323). And Allan V. Horvitz and Jerome C. Wakefield note that "just creating a reliable system that has clear rules that everybody can follow does not ensure even an approximation of validity" (2007: 100).

It was the text "Establishment of Diagnostic Validity in Psychiatric Illness: Its Application to Schizophrenia" (1970) by Eli Robins and Samuel B. Guze, from Washington University, St. Louis, that initiated the discussion about the validity of diagnostic categories in psychiatry. They were the first to define criteria for the validity of psychiatric diagnostic categories.

Robins and Guze begin their paper by stating that "since Bleuler psychiatrists have recognized that the diagnosis of schizophrenia includes a number of different disorders." In order to establish the difference between the disorders covered by the notion of schizophrenia, and following their long-term efforts aimed at constructing a valid classification of mental disorders, the cited authors defined five phases of validation of a particular diagnostic concept: clinical description, laboratory studies, delimitation from other disorders, follow-up studies, and family studies.

This paper laid the groundwork for further research of the validity of psychiatric diagnoses.

After its publication there were some other attempts to define the criteria of validity of diagnoses in psychiatry. Thus, for example Kenneth S. Kendler (1980) has to a certain extent expanded Robins and Guze's criteria of validity. Kendler distributed the criteria of validity into three groups: *Antecedent validators* (familial aggregation, premorbid personality, and precipitating factors), *concurrent validators* (psychological tests), *predictive validators* (diagnostic consistency over time, rates of relapse and recovery, and response to treatment).

In "The Validation of Psychiatric Diagnosis: New Model and Approaches" (1995), Nancy C. Andreasen writes that "the validation of psychiatric diagnosis is evolving and maturing as the neuroscience base that supports our discipline also evolves and matures" (1995). Therefore she proposes "a second structural program for the validation of psychiatric diagnosis." (The first one is the mentioned one of Robins and Guze.) This second program emphasizes "an additional group of validators that can be used to link symptoms and diagnoses to their neural substrates." There are many of these external validators: molecular genetics and molecular biology, neurochemistry, neuroanatomy, neurophysiology, functional imaging techniques.

Andreasen, one of the most vocal proponents of the medical model in psychiatry, did not pay due attention to two questions. First, she writes: "Once a reliable method is applied to define symptoms or delineate a potential diagnostic category or dimensions of psychopathology, the variables can then be validated by examining their relationships to external measures, which can provide a link to mechanisms or etiology or both." So far, a reliable method to differentiate psychiatric syndromes (or potential psychiatric categories) has not been found. As Kendell and Jablensky (2003) pointed out, "several attempts have been made to demonstrate natural boundaries between related syndromes or between a common syndrome such as major depressive and normality.... Most such attempts have ended in failure." Thus, if we follow the sequence of procedures suggested by Andreasen: a reliable method to differentiate psychiatric syndromes; the validation of these syndromes by external validators, and as a result a link to mechanisms or etiology or both, it turns out that the first step, or the first link is missing. As we are short of a reliable method of clearly delineating psychiatric syndromes or mental disorders, other proposed sequences become questionable, or more accurately, unfeasible. Second, Andreasen mentions Huntington's disease, and the mental retardation associated with phenylketonuria or fragile X syndrome as an example of a successfully established link between abnormalities in genes and mental illnesses. The truth is, as Kendell and Jablensky (2003) underlined, that abnormality in genes in people suffering from those disorders could have been identified "because at the conceptual level at which they are defined, they are clearly different from other superficially similar conditions." However, that is not the case with most mental illnesses. At the conceptual level at which they are defined, they are not clearly differentiated from other more or less similar conditions.

Andreasen has established a sequence of procedures that should be completed up to the final point which represents the identification of a pathogenic mechanism of the formation of a mental disorder, or the identification of its etiology, or both.

And yet no one who deals with the validity problem has said any-thing about whether all validity criteria should be met in order to have a mental disorder or psychiatric syndrome validated. In addition, it has not been mentioned whether all validation criteria have the same weight, whether some of them are more and some others less important for having a concept validated. For example, if we take Robins and Guze's criteria, should the same validation significance (validation weight) be attributed to family studies as to delimitation from other disorders, or clinical description?

Readers of the previous pages have easily come to the conclusion that the debate about the validity of psychiatrists' diagnoses implies more questions than definite answers, more unresolved problems than solutions, more inconclusive than conclusive evidence.

Yet one thing is for sure. The identified organic-functional basis of a particular mental syndrome or disorder is the proof of the validity of the concept of that syndrome or disorder; its verification, confirmation. In other words, only an etiological diagnosis is a valid diagnosis.

It seems simple, and self-evident. However, it is not.

The first thing that comes to mind are difficulties in detecting the un-equivocal organic foundation of a particular disorder. These difficulties are extremely serious, indeed. This time another sort of difficulty is the case in point. Kendell and Jablensky fully elaborated that other sort of difficulty in validating the concept of a mental syndrome or disorder. They did it in the paper entitled "Distinguishing between the validity and utility of psychiatric diagnoses" (2003). The fact that the paper has been cited several hundred times since its publication indicates that the psychiatric community has recognized its importance. In 2002, another paper by the same authors was published. The title is "Criteria for Assessing Classification in Psychiatry." The same arguments have been utilized in both papers.

What are the key ideas that Kendell and Jablensky present in these papers?[19] The application of any test or measure of validity of a psy-chiatric syndrome presupposes that psychiatric syndromes are clearly delineated entities. After all, Robins and Guze wrote in 1970 that "ho-mogeneous diagnostic grouping provides the soundest base for studies of etiology, pathogenesis, and treatment." For example, when talking about "schizophrenia with good prognosis" and "paranoia," it is believed that two distinct entities are involved. (Why would there be two different notions, if there were not two pathological entities?).

However, this is only an assumption, not a fact. The fact is that there is no evidence that individual psychiatric syndromes or disorders are clearly separated, that is, that a natural boundary separates them. Psychiatric syndromes cannot be clearly distinguished on the level of symptoms.[20]

Psychiatric researchers—for example, Kendell and Gourlay (1970), Kendell and Brockington (1980), Kendler and Gardner (1998), as cited by Kendel and Jablensky (2003)—using factor analysis did not manage to show that there is a natural boundary between individual psychiatric syndromes: between psychotic and neurotic depression, affective psychosis and schizophrenia, even between major depression and mental normality.

Also Robert C. Cloninger, one of the most distinguished scholars in the field of personality disorders, maintains that "there is no empirical evidence" for "natural boundaries between major syndromes," and adds that "no one has ever found a set of symptoms, signs, or test that separates mental disorders fully into non-overlapping categories" (1999).

If a clear distinction on the level of symptoms cannot be made between individual psychiatric syndromes or mental disorders, the question arises as to how it is possible to assess the validity of these syndromes or disorders. Namely, the discreteness and distinctiveness of individual syndromes on the level of their defining clinical characteristics (symptoms) is the prerequisite for assessing the validity of that syndrome or disorder by means of a validator.

It is impossible to identify the biological substrate, or any other etiological factor, of a syndrome or disorder if there is no discontinuity (so-called zone of rarity or points of rarity) between it and other syndromes. To put it another way, how would it be possible to detect the etiology of a syndrome if that syndrome has no clear boundaries? If we do not know the object as a clinically clearly delineated entity, how could its etiology be investigated? As I pointed out in the text "Towards a Definition of Mental Disorder," the basic requirement for researching the etiology of a mental syndrome is not met until that syndrome is clinically defined, and the natural boundary (if any) between it and other syndromes is identified.[21]

And that is a Catch-22. The etiological definition of a syndrome is its only validation. An etiological diagnosis is the only valid diagnosis. But in order to find the etiology of a syndrome or mental disorder you have to have clearly defined its borders, that is, a group of subjects the symptoms of which do not overlap with the symptoms of people having other mental disorders. Otherwise you can identify some putative cause (gene, biochemical anomaly, structural anomaly, whatever), but cannot know whether it is the cause of that particular syndrome whose etiology you would like to discover, or of some other syndrome. And clear-cut boundaries between syndromes at the clinical level, to repeat it once more, have not been identified, so far.

Now, the question arises: what should be done if there is no such thing as natural boundaries between supposed clinical entities? What should be done if natural boundaries between supposed clinical entities, or syndromes, cannot be established because they simply do not exist. Groups were formed from people having similar symptoms, similar courses and outcomes of illness, but these similarities turned out to be insufficient for declaring the people in those groups as suffering from a specific, discrete and distinct mental disorder.

Kendell and Jablensky give the only possible answer to this tricky question. "If no detectable discontinuities in symptoms are found in large tracts of the territory of psychiatric disorder, it is likely that, sooner or later, our existing typology will be abandoned and replaced by a dimensional classification" (2003).

There are hints that DSM-V, expected to come out in 2013, will comprise a combination of categorial and dimensional diagnoses.

Norman Sartorius writes that "the questions that will undoubtedly be on the agenda of the working groups seem obvious, easier to pose than to answer" (2006). And one of the first questions will be whether categorial diagnoses should be replaced by dimensional ones.

Would the introduction of dimensional diagnoses pave the way to establish the validity of psychiatric diagnoses and psychiatric classification? (""In medicine, and hence in psychiatry, classification is diagnosis" (Robins and Guze, 1970). No, it would not. The introduction of dimensional diagnoses would probably take us even farther away from the goal of the validation of psychiatrists' diagnoses. Besides, it would create, says Sartorius, new methodological difficulties. "The problem with a dimensional classification is that the making of a diagnosis—the profile of a patient on a fixed number of dimensions—might take a long time and would require the application of a number of psychometric instruments which the psychiatrists and other medical staff are unlikely to use" (2006).[22]

In concluding, due to the mentioned, very serious, conceptual and methodological, hard to resolve difficulties, it seems that the validation of diagnoses of mental disorders is as far away as ever. And to recall, the validity of a diagnosis indicates that the diagnosis is in accord with reality or nature.

Thus the question remains open, is any current classification of mental disorders "a natural classification, a classifications that tracks real, objective underlying similarities, or is it, instead, an imposed classifications that may or may not be useful for us, but expresses our interests, rather than the shape of the world" (Thornton, 2007: 168). It is said that a classification is valid if it "carves nature at its joints." The problem is, however, that it is hard to formulate a claim that a given classification of mental disorders is or is not valid. Why? Because to make such a claim "seems to require stepping outside our classifications to say of them that they line up with real divisions in nature" (2007: 174). Thornton contends that it is questionable whether that is "even notionally possible. How are the 'real divisions' specified without using another classification whose own naturalness will then be open to question." Hence, Thornton infers: "The difficulty of finding a way to *express* the claim threatens to undermine the idea that there is a genuine claim to be made" (2007: 174, emphasis in original).

On the other hand, the comparatively easier identification of the boundary between syndromes in physical medicine and the increasingly sophisticated methods of establishing the etiology of these syndromes has enabled researchers to increase the validity of diagnoses of physical diseases, and correspondingly the validity of the classifications of particular somatic diseases.

As stated, diagnoses of most physical diseases are valid because they are etiological. But the validity of most psychiatrists' diagnoses is very low or nonexistent.

Hence the role or function of symptoms is quite different in physical medicine and in psychological medicine. "'Psychiatric diagnosis," writes José Guimon, "tests the hypothesis that particular signs and symptoms, when regularly found together, belong to a particular class.... In medical nosology, class membership can often predict aspects of aetiology, pathogenesis, therapy, and prognosis, but this is not the case in psychiatry, where diagnostic labels usually provide information only on correlations between symptoms" (1989).

Social Meaning of Physical Diseases and Mental Disorders

The social meaning of physical diseases and mental disorders is quite different, too. The discrepancy between their social meaning is the result of various effects or consequences of each one.

Physical Diseases Biologically Imperil
Humans and the Human Species

The goal of medicine is not only to assist ill people and/or prevent them from falling ill. In a broader perspective, the goal of medicine is to prevent the decline of humankind and secure its survival.

Apart from accidental death as well as death caused by violence, suicide or murder, death enters life through the door of disease. In life, death is closest to us when we are old and when we are physically ill; and these two occurrences are frequently associated. Those who deal with preventing diseases and their treatment shun death, most often caused by disease.

The common denominator of every form of medical practice is found in the goal of medicine. The medical approach serves the purpose of sustaining human life and the survival of the human species.

Even when medical treatment does not result in curing disease and postponing death, by its basic intention and determination it is in the service of sustaining the life of the individual and of groups. In other words, the meaning of medicine is not in its efficacy but rather in its goal, in what the application of the medical approach is intended to achieve.

Since life that is not impaired by disease is one of the preconditions for the development of an individual's and the collective's potentials, and thereby for the survival of the community, medical care to preserve life constitutes a vital or basic human need. This need could be put on the same footing as self-defense and the instinct to procreate which are usually regarded as the paradigm of vital instincts.

In his book *Scientific Theory of Culture* (1944), anthropologist Bronislaw Malinowski names the need for health as one of the fundamental human needs. Medicine is a cultural response to the need for health.

Due to this primary, vital, imperative character of the need for health, this need has been acknowledged and respected in all societies, in all epochs.

The social meaning of disease is in tune with its biological meaning. The sick role defined by Talcott Parson (1951) evidences the accord between the social and biological meaning of sickness. The sick role comprises rights and obligations. There are two rights: the sick person is exempted from "normal" social roles, and the sick person is not responsible for their condition. Also there are two obligations: the sick person should try to get well, and the sick person should seek competent help and cooperate with the physician. The rights and obligations included in the sick role mirror the congruence between the biological and social meaning of health and sickness, respectively. Sickness (health) is so significant both for the individual and society, that society has created the sick role. The sick role is mandatory. It is imposed on the individual. If someone, while ill, does not want to assume the sick role, they risk their life (or incapacity) and thereby do harm not only to themselves but to society as well.

Mental Disorders Menace Sociality

All I have said about the threat to life caused by disease and the need to protect life refers to physical disease. And how are things with mental disorder? Do physical disease and mental disorder share the same meaning?

Even though the mortality rate of mental patients is higher than that of physically healthy people (Felker and Yazel, 1996), mental disorders are not a biological but rather a social menace to humans and the respective community.

As stated in the chapter "Towards a Definition of Mental Disorder," deviation from the behavior and belief standard of a given community is one of the four main characteristics of people with mental illness. Since they do not behave in a socially expected way, mentally ill people endanger sociality. By the notion of sociality I mean an individual's compliance with socially defined meaning of things, events, situations, people. So long as they are social people can exchange messages. At the same time, sociality makes and keeps a society functional: in an universal and in a particular way, that is, relating to a particular society or community.

The acknowledgment of a common social code makes interpersonal communication possible. The communication code consists of a huge number of rules and communication symbols, both verbal and nonverbal. The code is stable, although not fixed once and for all. Over time, people change it slightly. The point is that a system of signals and rules is commonly used by all community members. People use it without thinking about it. Those who make use of the existing communication code—and the greatest majority do it—reaffirm it in meeting their needs and exercising their rights, in exhibiting their sorrows and their joyfulness. They stay within the borders of the real and symbolic order of the community. They are honored as community members.

Hence sociality is both an assumption and an instrument of life in a community and the life of the community.

The appearance of an individual who by their verbal and non-verbal behavior partly or fully ignores or misinterprets the socially fixed meaning of symbols, who with no apparent reason deviates from the widely accepted behavior and belief standard, has an unsettling and even threatening effect on community members. That is why people with mental illness are regarded as a threat. As Derek Bolton put it: "'Normal' mental functioning signifies belonging to a community of shared practices, emotions and beliefs, in which one person makes sense to another and is included in 'we'." Then he adds: "By contrast, 'abnormal' mental functioning signifies a break in perceived sense, a form of practice, emotion or belief which does not make sense and which so far excludes the person from his position as an agent among us" (2008: XIV).

The appearance of a mentally ill individual symbolically or realistically constitutes "a disruption in or threat to organized social life." Horacio Fabrega Jr., Professor of Psychiatry and Anthropology at the University of Pittsburgh, has coined the term "human behavioral breakdown (HBB)" (1993) that bears resemblance to mental disorder, if it is not identical to it. Fabrega indicates that in the syntagma "human behavioral breakdown" "the term breakdown means that the behaviors are defined as constituting a disruption in or threat to organized social life and hence are generally disvalued." I would add that not only the behaviors of those with HBB but also their experiences and talk have a disruptive effect on the fabric of social life, and therefore are perceived as threat.

What Fulfills Basic Needs and Derivative Needs?

Different forces secure the acknowledgment and fulfillment of basic (primary) needs and derivative (secondary, instrumental) needs.

There is no need to coerce people to procure and regularly eat food, to protect themselves from extremely high and low temperatures of the environment, to keep away from predators, to secure premises to live and work, to have children and provide them assistance. All these activities are aimed at fulfilling primary, vital needs.

Biological, instinctual forces urge people to care about their biological existence and the existence of their kith and kin. People need to be taught *how* to better protect their lives, what they should do to stay healthy. But there is no need to teach people the need to care about their own biological existence, their survival, and the survival of their progeny.

Things are quite different with regard to derivative (secondary) needs and their fulfillment.

People incorporate the dominant behavior and belief standard of their milieu through socialization. The process of social learning comprises rewarding those who learn well and quickly, and punishing those who for whatever reason are slow to accept the dominant code or are reluctant to do so.

People feel secure communicating with other people and meeting them, if they know that other people abide by the same social rules as they themselves do.

But when they are confronted with a mentally ill person, people feel insecure. The sociality of people with mental illness is disturbed, and therefore they are unpredictable and irrational; that is the social perception of them, at the very least. Both the unpredictable and irrational are things that people abhor and want to keep far off, to get protected from.

In the context of differentiating the social meaning of physical diseases and mental disorders, it is important to note that socialization and socialized behavior cannot be performed without *surveillance* and *control*. The fulfillment of derivative, secondary needs requires surveillance, control, and even coercion.

Talking about syncretic nature of psychiatry David Pilgrim and Anne E. Rogers assert that "although psychiatry is a medical specialty, its activities are not purely scientific. They are clearly syncretic ... because there is a strong normative aspect to the profession's role." Then they add: "This normative role is one major reason why it has been so controversial especially as it has been regularly characterized by coercion" (2005).

Indeed, any discipline that has a normative role has a regulatory role as well. And the regulatory function is performed by both "soft" methods such as education and "hard" methods such as surveillance, control, and coercion.

On the other hand, surveillance and control are not needed when fulfilling primary, vital, biological needs. Indeed, quarantine in the case of a specific infective disease, mandatory vaccination of children, or when visiting some regions, comprise elements of surveillance and control. Yet, even in these cases society both assists people in the fulfillment of their vital, basic needs, and keeps watch over that process. After all, the fact that people rarely protest against the cited measures, or refuse to comply with them, indirectly indicates that they do not see them as something that is totally imposed upon them.

However, as stated, the fulfillment of secondary needs implies surveillance and control. No matter how reluctant psychiatrists are to see themselves in such a light, they are, among other things, agents of social control. They by their own methods keep watch over and control those who deviate from the behavior and belief standard of the given community due to their mental disturbance.

Since they have an unsettling effect on existing social meanings, since they are regarded as unpredictable and irrational, and due to the fact that the application of repressive measures has no impact on them, people with mental illness are the target of marginalization and stigmatization. (Marginalization is one of the effects of stigmatization.) The marginalization and stigmatization of people with mental illness keeps them at a safe distance from those who are mentally sound. That is how fear of the mentally ill is somewhat calmed down, and/or kept under control.[23]

Unlike people with mental illness, those who have some physical disease do not disrupt the extant social order, their behavior and way of thinking is regarded as predictable. And unlike the perception of mentally ill they are not perceived as people who are likely to harm us as opposed to people suffering from infectious diseases who can harm us by transferring disease towards us. Yet they themselves are not regarded as the agents of violence.

Briefly, people with mental disorder threat those who are mentally non-disordered. Threats are twofold: intangible and unrealistic, and tangible and realistic (Stangor and Crandall, 2000: 74; Alboreda-Florez, 2003). Both produce stigma of mental illness.

On the other hand, physical diseases, except for TB in the nineteeth, and cancer and AIDS in the twentieth century (Sontag, 1991), have not been stigmatized. That is one further difference between mental disorders and physical diseases.

Stigma of Mental Disorder

The importance of stigma of mental disorder cannot be overestimated. "The stigma attached to mental illness and all that is related to it ... is the main obstacle to better mental health care and better quality of life of people who have the illness, of their families, of their communities and of health service staff that deals with psychiatric disorders" (Sartorius and Schulze, 2005: XIII).

One may even say that the impact of stigma on a person's life can be as pernicious as immediate effects of mental disorder on their life

(Corrigan and Penn, 1999). Thus, a mentally ill person, in fact, suffers from mental disorder and stigma of mental disorder as well.

Stigma of mental illness is *universal* and *global* (Thornicroft, 2006: 180; Hinshaw, 2007: 142). Moreover, the results of a great number of studies have shown that the negative attitudes towards mentally ill people worsened in recent times (for example, Link, Ohelan, Bresnaham, *et al.*, 1999; Chou and Mak, 1998; Crisp, 1999).[24]

The assertion made by Gerhard Falk that stigma attached to mental illness is confined to those societies in which the spirit of rationality reigns is unfounded. Falk writes: "The stigma attached to mental illness is severe because we live in a world in which the ability to think and act rationally and in a meaningful fashion has been declared mandatory by public opinion since the Age of Reason began in the early 18th century" (2001: 339). My view is that it is hard to imagine a society that would survive if their members did not follow the principles of rationality and meaningfulness; in other words, if they behaved irrationally. Indeed, there are societies that are more tolerant towards the manifestations of mental disorders—that is the case mostly in developing countries, like, for example, India (WHO: 1979). However, this does not mean that there is no stigma of mental disorder in such societies.[25]

Where does stigma of mental illness come from? What is its origin?

Stigma develops out of a universally held motivation to avoid danger, "followed by (often exaggerated) perception of characteristics that promote threat..." (Stangor and Crandal, 2000: 62-3). Stigma is a way of defense, a defense tactics. "Stigmatizing someone is a highly pragmatic, even tactical response to perceived threats, real dangers, and fear of the unknown.... For the stigmatizer stigma seems to be an effective and natural response emergent not only as an act of self-preservation or psychological defense, but also in the existential and moral experience that one is being threatened" (Yang, Kleinman, Link *et al.*, 2007).

I already explained why and how the mentally ill people endanger *sociality*. But what are the specific characteristics of people with mental illness that discredit sociality? What are the discrediting features of people with mental illness? Virtually all scholars (e. g., Gray, 2001; Wilson, Nairn, Coverdale *et al.*, 1999; Angermeyer, Dietrich, 2006; Fuller, 1994; Magliano, de Rosa, Fiorello, 2004; Littlewood, 1998; Thompson, Stuart, Bland *et al.*, 2002; Byrne, 2001; Jorm, 2000; Heyward, Bright, 1997; Major and Eccleston, 2005) who have dealt with the origin of mental illness stigma agree that there are three key characteristics of people with mental illness that make them subject to stigmatization: the mentally disordered persons are perceived as *unpredictable, unreasonable,* and *unintelligible.* Due to these features people with mental illness are considered as a threat, as a danger. Moreover, these features differentiate mentally disordered from mentally non-disordered as well as from those who suffer from physical diseases.

To stigmatize means to draw a clear dividing line between "them" and "us." Stigmatization emerges when there is a consensual view of one or more characteristics of those who belong to a particular category, and when these characteristics are seen as a reason for keeping them at distance, for avoiding them, from excluding them, and for reducing to minimum activities with those persons who are perceived as the members of that particular category (Leary and Schreidendorfer, 1998).

Stereotype is one of the substantial instruments of stigmatizing. To stigmatize means to categorize. And there are no stereotypes without categorization. When we stigmatize someone we put them in a category. Those who have been categorized or stigmatized are believed to share the same features, that is, to be the same, and, in addition, to be different from members of all other categories (groups).

Prejudice goes with stereotype because prejudice expresses compliance with the content of stereotype. And discrimination goes with prejudice because discrimination implies activities which are in accordance with a particular prejudice. Discrimination targets those who have been stereotyped and against which we nurture prejudice.

All those who deal with people with mental illness know very well how much and how often the latter have been discriminated against, and how many vicious prejudices are there about psychiatric patients.

Conditioning is another important instrument of stigmatization. People are conditioned to connect mental illness with violence, that is, with danger. In the news, in the prime-time television programs, in movies and television shows psychiatric patients are depicted as violent characters. Secondary to such presentation of those with mental illness people are conditioned to believe that psychiatric patients are dangerous. "Not surprisingly, surveys reveal that the close link between mental illness and violence in the popular media is paralleled in the minds of the general public" (Lilienfield, Lynn, Ruscio *et al.*, 2010: 211) And what is most important children as young as 11 to 13 years of age believe that most mentally ill people are dangerous (Watson, Otey, Westbrook *et al.*, 2004).

To stigmatize people with mental illness, that is, to keep distance from them, to excommunicate them, is one of the most efficacious ways to protect ourselves against them.

Do Those with Mental Illness Commit Violent Acts More Often than Mentally Sound People?

The findings related to the connection between mental illness and violence are contradictory. For example, after reviewing the nine epidemiological studies of violence and mental illness published since 1990 Angermeyer (2000) concluded that there is a moderate but significant relationship between schizophrenia and violence. On the other hand, the findings from a variety of studies carried out by the National Institute for Mental Health indicate that "the vast majority of individuals with serious mental illness are not more dangerous than members of the general population" (Fuller, 1994).

Julio Arboleda-Florez seems to be closest to the mark when he writes: "The association between mental illness—specifically schizophrenia—and violence, although confirmed epidemiologically, remains unclear. It seems to flow not so much through direct links of causality as through a series of confounders and covariating causes, such as comorbidities with alcohol and substance abuse (not unlike that which drives violence among individuals without mental illness) and psychopathic personality" (2003).

In any case, if there is a slightly greater proneness of mentally ill people to violence than of mentally sound people, it cannot be the reason for the universal and global, on-going and lately even increasing stigmatization of people with mental illness. The reasons—as I argued in the text above—are more intangible and symbolic. The point I want to make is as follows: when people perceive those with mental illness as a threat they do it more for social and symbolic reasons rather than for tangible, material, reasons. Yet they are not able to discern the former from the latter. After all, they are not interested in doing that. The only thing they do know is that persons with mental illness are to be shunned meaning stigmatized because they are dangerous.

And there are some more intangible and symbolic reasons for shunning those with mental illness. Now, I am going to set them out.

Deeper Currents

The perception of mentally ill people as unpredictable, unreasonable, and unintelligible stirs some deeply entrenched mechanisms that play an important role in initiating and shaping stigma of mental illness.

Thus, Stephen P. Hinshaw maintains that "although the very nature of mental illness makes it understandable that empathy is difficult to sustain, the lack of respect and fairness signals *deeper currents*" (2007: IX, my emphasis). Robert E. Kendell writes along the same lines: "The causes of stigmatization are complex and largely derived from *deeply rooted* cultural attitudes to madness, and assumptions about the nature of mental illness" (2004: XXI, my emphasis).

I will focus on two forms of the deep-level symbolic threat posed by mental illness: evolutionary and biocultural origins of stigmatization, and stigmatization as an instrument for fighting chaos and death.

Evolutionary and Bio-Cultural Origins of Stigmatization

Numerous similarities of evolutionary and bio-cultural concept of the origin of stigma permit me to give a combined sketch of them. Robert Kurzban and Mark R. Leary are the most prominent advocates of the evolutionary origin of stigma, and Steven L. Neuberg of its bio-cultural origin.

Sociality is one of those humans' features that have been selected by natural selection. It enables people to survive both biologically and socially. Those who have better developed sociality are in a better position to transfer their genes to fellow group members. Sociality is in the long history of human species became a biologically founded characteristic of humans (Campbell, 1983). Group benefits most from those who nurture prosocial tendencies such as sharing, cooperation and mutual investment. The more group members are committed to group interests the stronger and more effective group is.

Just "because group living is highly adaptive for human survival and gene transmission, people will stigmatize those individuals whose characteristics and actions are seen as threatening or hindering the effective functioning of their groups" (Neuberg, Smith, and Asher, 2000: 34). They will do it for the sake of their group, and thereby for the sake of themselves.

Mentally disordered people are a prototype of those groups and individuals who not only do not reciprocate in social relations, in social life, but even deconstruct sociality, and by the same token threaten group living. That is why they are the target of stigmatization.

Stigma as an Instrument for Fighting Chaos and Death

People are afraid of disorder and instability because among other things it reminds them of chaos and death which are a permanent source of anxiety. When people believe that everything is in order, stable, under control, predictable, and intelligible, they have the impression or illusion that they are in command, that life imperfections do not have the upper hand, and that nothing unexpected could happen.

Due to the fact that people with mental illness are perceived as unpredictable, unreasonable, and unintelligible, they are at the same time regarded as the epitome of frailness, change, instability, of a lack or loss of order, briefly, of all those things that people are so eager to keep far from their minds and their eyes.

Stigmatization of such people may serve and virtually often serves such a function, the function of fighting chaos and death.

In conclusion, the different social treatment of physically diseased and mentally disordered people is conditioned by different social meaning of the former and the latter. Physical disease imperils the biological existence of people, and potentially of the human species. Medicine is a response to the need for protection from disease, to the need for survival. In so far medicine helps the fulfillment of a primary, vital, instinctual need. People are not urged to fulfill their primary needs. They do it under the dictate of instinctual forces. On the other hand, mental illness disturbs the sociality of people, their abiding by the extant behavior and belief standard, their acknowledgment of current communication code, and of current social meanings of events, situations, people, and so on. In so far people with mental illness are deviants meaning de-social and/or de-socialized. In the course of social learning we are instructed to comply by the existing communication code. We are thought social norms, and social meanings. The needs for respecting the existing social order are derivative or secondary needs. These needs are not instinctual. They are social needs, and their acceptance and performance has to be socially scrutinized and controlled. That is what, among other things, do psychiatrists.

By using their own methods they strive to socialize or re-socialize those who are unsocial or de-socialized. In order to do so they have to relieve mental suffering of people with mental illness, to calm down their distress, and repair their impaired mental functions. Secondary to psychiatric treatment psychiatric patient are expected to abide by the existent social norms, to respect sociality, and to use the governing code in communicating with other people, in expressing their needs, their sorrows and their joyfulness.

Stigma is attached to mental illnesses rather than to physical diseases. This is also an important difference between the former and the latter. Stigma of mental illness is so widespread and so resistant to change that it can contravene, and so often does contravene psychiatric treatment; it thwarts mental health workers' endeavors to provide better services to those with mental illness, to improve their quality of life.

There is no parallel in physical medicine to stigma of mental illness.

Conclusion

The architects of DSMs assert that physical diseases and mental disorders are the same. Martin Roth and Robert E. Kendell, both very prominent psychiatrists, share this view. I am of the opinion that a great many differences between physical diseases and mental disorders justify the distinction between the former and the latter.

Dissimilarity of physical diseases and mental disorders pertaining to the etiology, clinical picture, diagnosis, and social meaning has been demonstrated.

Even though physical-biological, psychological, and socioultural agents and circumstances concurrently partake in the genesis of physical diseases, psychological and sociocultural agents play a comparatively greater role in the engenderment of mental disorders than physical diseases.

We are still in the dark as far as the physical-biological foundation of mental disorders is concerned. The same holds for biological markers of mental disorders. On the other hand, the causes of the majority of physical diseases have been detected. And they are primarily of physical-biological origin.

There is no doubt that mental phenomena are not ghosts, as Karl Jaspers (1997: 459) put it. The brain is the basis of them. However, we do not apprehend the transformation of the physical-biological into the mental. And that kind of transformation is the substantial event in the formation of mental disorders. As for physical diseases things are quite different. Most physical diseases are primarily caused by physical-biological agents, and it is not difficult to apprehend how these kinds of agents cause physical-biological changes. Also we can comprehend the transformation of the mental into the physical-biological if respective mental manifestations are accompanied by physiological changes, as is the case with for example emotions.

In addition, the existence of several psychiatric models hampers research of the etiology of mental disorders. The etiology of mental disorders is differently conceptualized in each psychiatric model. That is not the case in somatic medicine. If there are different concepts about the formation of some physical diseases these concepts are more often complimentary than mutually excluding.

Physical diseases and mental disorders differ in regard to clinical picture, too. The dominance of either mental symptoms or physical signs is the distinguishing feature between the two. Prevailing of mental symptoms in the clinical picture characterize mental disorders, whereas the dominance of physical signs is typical for physical diseases.

Moreover, the personality plays a greater role in shaping the clinical picture of mental disorders rather than physical diseases.

Finally, diagnostic procedure is quite different in psychological and somatic medicine. Numerous aspects of the difference between the two originate from diagnoses in medical disciplines other than psychiatry being mostly etiological whereas in psychiatry they are not etiological. This gives rise to complex problems associated with the assessment of reliability and validity of mental disorders. On the other hand, in somatic medicine the reliability and validity of physical diseases is far from being as serious problem as it is in psychiatry.

If different social meaning of physical diseases and mental disorders were not grasped it would not be possible to form a complete picture of how dissimilar the former and the latter are. Physical diseases, directly or indirectly, imperil the biological foundation of humans, and broader of the human species. Somatic medicine is the response to this danger. On the other hand, mental disorders primarily endanger the sociality of humans. The sociality is the assumption and guarantee of the existence of life in the community and the life of the community. The sociality is threatened by various kinds of deviants and social occurrences. Psychiatry is the response to the threat to the sociality coming from the mentally ill people. So is stigma of mental illness.

Different social meaning of physical diseases and mental disorders determine different social meaning of, on the one hand, medical disciplines other than psychiatry and of psychiatry, on the other.

The cited differences between physical diseases and mental disorders are more than sufficient to oblige us not to consider them as the same.

Notes

1. Frederick C. Redlich, Professor of Psychiatry at Yale University, points out differences between physical diseases and mental disorders. Redlich writes: "I propose to distinguish between the concepts of physical disease and psychological, mental, or behavioral disorders. Some of these psychological disorders are the result of cerebral disease, or sooner or later may be recognized to be the consequences of such disease. Others fall into a somewhat vaguely defined in-between class of psychophysical diseases. However, the bulk of what we call behavior disorders are sufficiently different in their observable manifestations, etiology, methods of detection, and methods of treatment to deserve separate discussion, even though close and practically important relationships between the two categories exist" (1976).

     Norman Sartorius, on his part, stresses out the difference between physical diseases and mental disorders as follows: "A condition can be considered to have the status of a disease when its causes and pathogenesis are known, its clinical picture well described, its natural history known and its reaction to treatment and other interventions predictable. None of the mental and behavioral disorders satisfies these requirements" (2002: 202).

2. It is of note that R.L. Spitzer and J.B. Williams (1982) were no happy with the term "psychiatric disorder" because it suggests that no mental health workers other than psychiatrists are qualified to deal with such kind of disorders.

3. Dan J. Stein, Katharine A. Phillips, Derek Bolton *et al.* (2010) address the question of whether the term "mental" is optimal in a paper dealing with a potential definition of mental disorder in DSM-V. After ascertaining there is no optimal term they propose two options: either "the awkward term 'mental/psychiatric,'" or "a more conservative approach" that would be "to retain the term 'mental disorder.'" In may view, the term "mental/psychiatric" is awkward, indeed.

4. Dusan Kecmanovic (2009b) criticized Bulmore, Fletcher, and Jones's "Proposal for strategic action" (2009) aimed at supporting "the future growth of a brain-based medicine of the mind and its psychiatric practitioners." The goal of the fifth of the five proposed actions is to enhance psychiatrists' efforts to communicate the neuroscientific basis of mental disorders to patients, their families and the general public since "greater knowledge of the physical basis of mental illness should have," as the authors put it, "a destigmatizing benefit for our patients." However, as stated, to communicate a brain-based medicine of the mind to the public is not conducive to the attenuation of negative attitude towards mental illness.

5. There are many ways in which the difference between the hypothetic-deductive and hermeneutic-interpretive approach can be described. For example, Paul Verhaeghe, Professor of Psychoanalysis at the University of Ghent in Belgium, who fosters a Freudo-Lacanian perspective, dubs the hypothetic-deductive approach *medical diagnostics*, and the hermeneutic-interpretative approach *psychodiagnostics*. He argues that medical diagnostics is restricted to the individual while psychodiagnostics cannot be restricted to the individual. "Psychic identity, with its potential psychopathology and aberrant behaviors, must be conceived in such a way that it grants the other a place equally important as the individual's." The second difference between the cited approaches is as follows. "Unlike what takes place in medical diagnostics, here one cannot similarly bind a number of isolated symptoms into an objective, universalizable syndrome that holds for just about every case. To the contrary, the more information the diagnostician acquires, the more specific the situation becomes, to the effect that generalization becomes all the more difficult. In medical diagnostics the symptoms are interpreted as *signs* pointing to

an underlying disturbance that can be both isolated and generalized. In clinical psychodiagnostics we are confronted with *signifiers* that carry endlessly shifting meanings in any given interaction between the patient and the Other" (2008: 5, emphasis in the original). In concluding the comparison Verhaeghe maintains that "central to medical diagnostics is the gaze, whose focus is on detecting signs that point toward objective, measurable parameters. In contrast, in clinical psychological psychodiagnostics the focus is laid primarily on listening to signifiers that remain open to interpretation. Medical signs pertain to an illness scenario; signifiers, on the other hand, derive their meaning and function from a specific relation with Other" (2008: 17-8).

6.   It is debatable whether different methods describe from various angles one and the same phenomenon, one and the same world, or, as contended by John Law and John Urry (2004), various methods create different worlds, which are equally valid, equally true, but are not similar. Thus the question is whether various methods from various angles describe the same reality, or create different realities. (The implication of the second possibility is that there is no one world, one reality but rather more different parallel worlds, or realities.) The claim is that a particular method does less to describe an occurrence and help to learn about it; rather, it creates a new occurrence, shifts the consideration of the nature and reach of methods from the epistemological to ontological level.

It would be worth thinking about whether psychiatric models, in fact, create different mental disorders, i.e., different sorts of mental disorder.

7.   In an attempt to find out why there is a decline in the numbers of medical graduate who opt for training in psychiatry Assen Jablensky compares the state of affairs in general medicine and psychiatry. "General medicine is becoming increasingly 'molecular', hence more attractive and intellectually challenging to young minds. This kind of transformation has not occurred in psychiatry. Hardly any of the recent advances in neuroscience, molecular genetics and genomics has translated into practical clinical tools, disease markers, treatment or novel conceptual paradigms in out understanding of the nature of mental disorders. Notwithstanding hyperbole and periodically appearing false promises of imminent breakthroughs, the gains in real knowledge of the genetic and neural basis of the major mental disorders have been modest, while the looming complexity of the task has become obvious" (2010).

8.   Erik R. Kandel, an eminent scholar in the field of the relationship between brain functions and mental processes, writes: "The details of the relationship between the brain and mental processes—precisely how the brain gives rise to various mental processes—is understood poorly, and only in outline" (1998).

9.   The fragmentation of neuropsychiatry into neurology and psychiatry began in the fifties and sixties. Journals like *Acta Neurologica and Psychiatrica Scandinavica* were splintered into *Acta Neurologica Scandinavica* and *Acta Psychiatrica Scandinavica*, and *Acta Neurologica and Psychiatrica Belgica* into *Acta Neurologica Belgica* and *Acta Psychiatrica Belgica*.

There has been a resurrection of interest in neuropsychiatry over the last decades (for example, Price, Adams, Coyle, 2000; Martin, 2002). The recent progress in neurosciences probably gave rise to the revival of interest in neuropsychiatry.

I am of the opinion that the re-integration of neurology and psychiatry will not occur. In that sense I agree with David H. Brendel (2006: 114), who writes that any advocating of reunification of neurology and psychiatry either undervalues or ignores the role played by psychosocial factors in the genesis of mental disorders, as well as adaptation, intention and meaning which are key elements of psychiatric symptoms. After all, all arguments for differentiating physical diseases and mental disorders justify the separation of neuropsychiatry into neurology and psychiatry.

Joseph B. Martin in the paper "The integration of neurology, psychiatry, and neurosciences in the 21st century" (2002) argues for the break down of the barriers separating neurology and psychiatry. He writes: "Neurology and psychiatry have, for much of the past century, been separated by an artificial wall created by the divergence of their philosophical approaches and research and treatment methods."

Does Martin want to say that the divergence should not have happened? If he thinks so he should have explained why there are nowadays, as has been for much of the past century, divergent epistemological perspectives, different research and diagnostic and treatment methods, in neurology and psychiatry. In other words, he should have elucidated what has conditioned the cited divergence. If the reasons for the divergence have been artificial how could they caused so persistent, long-term divergence of neurology and psychiatry? Martin is right: neuroscience is a meeting point of these two disciplines, but they differ as far as their etiology, clinical picture, diagnostics and social meaning is concerned.

Perminder S. Sachdev (2007), in the text titled "An agenda for neuropsychiatry as a the 21st century discipline," published in *Acta Neuropsychiatrica*, contends that "despite calls for the amalgamation of neurology and psychiatry into a supersized specialty of neuropsychiatry, it is likely that the two disciplines will retain their independent identities, and neuropsychiatry will only have a future as a third discipline."

10. Kay R. Jamison, a psychologist suffering from bipolar disorder, describes her husband's battle with lung cancer in her book *Nothing was the Same* (2009). Her husband, Richard Wyatt, a renowned psychiatrist and scientist, was first diagnosed with Hodgkin's disease. He underwent "an aggressive combination of radiotherapy and chemotherapy that cured him from his disease but at considerable cost." Years later he was diagnosed with lung cancer. He wrote the following lines in a letter to his wife: "The disease and the magic bullets have left their traces or scars but they are not a part of me in the way yours are. All the more so because yours are integral to your personality. Because of this I am luckier than you; I can love a manic-depressive in a way you cannot love a Hodgkin's disease" (2009: 25-26). This is a subtle depiction of the notion that mental illness is an integral part of the personality, unlike physical disease that is viewed as external, as alien.

11. One year later, i.e., in 1972, a monograph entitled *Psychiatric Diagnosis in New York and London* by John E. Cooper, Robert E. Kendell and others was published.

12. Joan Bushfield also pays attention to the distinction between research and clinical practice in regard to psychiatrists' observing the diagnostic rules formulated in DSMs. "While the need for standardization is clearly recognized in research contexts, it seems likely that in clinical practice psychiatrists will not only want to retain some element of discretion in their use of diagnostic categories (they will continue to argue that particular categorizations should be abandoned and new ones introduced), but they will also want to retain an element of clinical judgment in making their diagnosis. Overall the pressure for consensus and the commitment and the need for standardization is far weaker in the clinical context, given the commitment to the needs and interests of the individual patient. Consequently, it seems likely that although reliability in clinical contexts may increase, it will never reach the high levels shown in research contexts"(1986: 69).

Peter Joce, Professor of Psychiatry in Christchurch, New Zealand, is one of many prominent psychiatrists who share Spiegel's view that in day-to-day diagnostic practice psychiatrists do not keep to the operational definitions of mental disorders set out in the American classification of mental disorders. "In principle the introduction of diagnostic criteria should enhance reliability, although it is surprising the number of clinicians who, despite saying that they are using DSM-IV criteria, cannot actually recall what the diagnostic criteria are" (2008).

Patrick D. McGorry, Ian B. Hickie, Alison R. Yung *et al.* (2006) join the club of those who are skeptical about how much psychiatrists in day-to-day clinical practice follow the DSMs' diagnostic prescriptions: "Despite efforts to shore up reliability, the later remains a problem outside of research setting...."

13. Here is the comment by Frederick K. Goodwin and Kay R. Jamison on disregard of personal experience induced by DSMs' operational definitions. "The requirements of sound research have produced operational criteria for selecting homogenous groups of clinical subjects. Extended into clinical diagnostic systems, the criteria as noted have made diagnoses more objective and reliable. Commendable as they are, these achievements have been purchased at a price. Rarely does one encounter discussion of mental illness in current journal articles that fully represent the *varieties and texture of experience*." (1990: 4, my emphasis)

14. Theodore Millon (1991) writes: "The current state of psychopathologic nosology and diagnosis resembles that of medicine a century ago. Concepts remain overwhelmingly descriptive. To illustrate, the third edition of the *Diagnostic and Statistical Manual of Mental Disorders* (*DSM-III*; American Psychiatric Association, 1980) was not only formulated to be atheoretical but addressed itself *exclusively to observable phenomena*." (1991, my emphasis) Robert L. Spitzer, in the same issue of *Journal of Abnormal Psychology*, protested against the claim that DSM-III diagnoses are made on the basis of only those phenomena which are accessible to sensory inspection. Thus, he asserts: "The Task Force (of the DSM-III) always recognized that making clinical judgment about psychopathology involved more than 'direct sensory inspection'. It never believed that it was possible or desirable to limit diagnostic criteria to 'attributes that could be readily observed' " (1991).

15. It is of note that Michael Grube (2006) empirically validated the intuitive diagnosis of schizophrenia by means of "praecox feeling." Compared to the standardized diagnostic classification, the precision of intuitive reasoning was remarkably high with a sensitivity of 0.85, a specificity of about 0.80, a positive predictive power of about 0.90.

16. Maj (2005) mentions three other possible reasons for an increase in 'psychiatric comorbidity' as a by-product of recent diagnostic systems. First, the rule that those who constructed DSMs did not proclaim but still respected that "the same symptom could not appear in more than one disorder" (Robins, 1994). For example, "DSM-IV does not allow the presence of anxiety in a patient with major depression to be recorded either as a symptom or ... as a specifier for the diagnosis. The concomitant diagnosis of major depression and panic disorder is encouraged (being one of the most common form of 'psychiatric comorbidity'), whereas the concomitant diagnosis of major depression and generalized anxiety disorder is not allowed (unless generalized anxiety occurs also when the patient is not depressed)." Second, the proliferation of diagnostic categories carries the risk that demarcations "are made where they do no exist in nature." And if that is the case, "the probability that several diagnoses have to be made in an individual case will obviously increase." Third, in pre-DSM's era, if a psychotic patient had neurotic symptoms, "the pos-

sibly concomitant neurotic disorders would not be diagnosed because they would be regarded as part of the clinical picture of the psychotic condition." Today, those who stick with the DSM's diagnostic rules diagnose that patient as suffering from both Schizophrenic Disorder and Panic Disorder.

17. Allen J. Frances points at the discrepancy between experts' and clinicians' activities in relations to field trials: "All diagnoses have the inherent problem of having been created by experts who have highly specialized research and clinical experiences for use by clinicians who treat a much less selected, heterogeneous population. Experts worry most about missed cases and distinguishing between similar disorders, while the risk in general use is more likely to be false positives" (2009b).

18. A World Psychiatric Association workgroup has formulated a comprehensive model of psychiatric diagnosis which is designed to correct desubjectivization and decontextualization of psychiatric diagnosis introduced by current diagnostic and classificatory systems. Thus, "International Guidelines for Diagnostic Assessment" (IGDA) have been defined. The new diagnostic model has been dubbed "Ideographic (personalized) diagnostic formulation" or "Comprehensive diagnostic model". "It integrates a standardized multiaxial formulation (illness, disabilities, contextual factors and of life) and an ideographic personalized formulation (culturally informed and contextualized clinical problems, patient's assets pertinent to care, and expectations of health restoration and promotions as jointly understood by clinician, patient and family" (Mezzich, 2002). According to IGDA, the comprehensive diagnostic process "involves more than simply identifying a disorder or distinguishing one disorder from another. It should lead to a thorough, contextualized and interactive understanding of a clinical condition and of the wholeness of the person who presents for evaluation and care" (IGDAWorkgroup, WPA, 2003).

I would say that, if introduced, "comprehensive psychiatric diagnosis" as conceptualized by IGDA will throw overboard even traces of the reliability of psychiatric diagnoses. By the same token, it will stand in the way of establishing the validity of psychiatric diagnoses.

Tim Thornton, Professor of Philosophy and Mental Health at the University of Central Lancashire (UK), argues that idiographic judgment as a kind of individualized judgment "has no place in psychiatry" (2008). It "threatens psychiatric validity." Also, Thornton maintains that "narrative judgment does seem to provide a genuine addition to a narrow model of psychiatric criteriological diagnosis. Narratives are essentially normatively structured, reason-based accounts of individual thought and action. There are the perspectives from which a subject, as a person, comes into view. But, unlike supposed individualized judgments, they are essentially general and thus there is no a priori argument against their validity" (2008).

19. It is noteworthy that Robert E. Kendell in a paper entitled "Five criteria for an improved taxonomy of mental disorders," published in the book *Defining Psychopathology in the 21st Century* (2002), and edited by John E. Helzer and James J. Hudziak, presented the key ideas which he and Jablensky elaborated in the paper "Distinguishing between the validity and utility of psychiatric diagnoses" (2003).

20. The authors of DSM-IV concede that there are no clear boundaries between categories of mental disorder. "In DSM-IV, there is no assumption that each category of mental disorder is a completely discrete entity with absolute boundaries dividing it from other mental disorders or from no mental disorder... The clinician using DSM-IV should therefore consider that individuals sharing a diagnosis are likely to be heterogeneous even in regard to the defining features of the diagnosis" (1994:

XXII). The same view has been expressed by Allen J. Frances. He writes: "It has long been realized that the mental disorders described in our diagnostic system are fuzzy sets that lack clear boundaries between themselves and with normality" (2009a).

21. Every new edition of DSM has more mental disorders than the previous one. There is a tendency to pathologize problems in living, that is, to label them as mental disorders. This kind of expansion of psychiatry will make the search for causes of mental disorders even more difficult. This is particularly true when searching for the cause of mental disorders in brain pathology that is a specific feature of the medical psychiatric model. This is one of paradoxes in contemporary psychiatry: the dominance of the medical model, on the one hand, and expanding mental disorders to include problems in living with a very dubious pathological character, on the other. Needless to say that detecting brain origin of the latter is extremely difficult, if at all possible. And brain origin of mental disorders is one of the key postulates of the medical model. Stuart A. Kirk pointed out this paradox in the text "Introduction: clinical perspectives." The text was published in the book *Mental Disorders in the Social Environment. Critical Perspectives* (2005), edited by S. A. Kirk.

22. It is of note that there are scholars who maintain that "the concomitant use of both approaches (the categorical and the dimensional one, D.K.) may best conceptualize the richness of psychopathology and provide the most useful description of psychotic patients" (Demjaha, Morgan, Morgan *et al.* 2009).

23. In addition to feeling the mentally ill as unpredictable and irrational, people are afraid of them because at times they see in their verbal and nonverbal behaviour indication of an unknown order of things the meaning of which they cannot detect. "Psychological dysfunction is marked by breakdown of meaningful connections in psychic life: between perception and reality, between beliefs and evidence, between emotion and its object (its cause), between reasons and action... The question is whether the apparent disruption of meaning and reason is a pure deficit, or is rather on the surface, beneath which there is—after all—order..." (Bolton, 2008: XVI-XVII).

I am not referring to the order (meaning) that more or less all psychological conceptions read into dis-order of mental illness. Nor am I pointing at the hidden meaning of things which madness sometimes reveals. I have in mind the possibility that verbal and non-verbal behavior of people with mental illness foreshadows a different framework of meanings, of "functioning below the level of an appropriate 'normal' group" (Bolton, 2008: XVII). Those who have no idea of any other order of things which would be different from the existing one—and that is the case with the majority of people—feel threatened by the possibility itself, suggested by people with mental illness, of a radically different "state of affairs." This is one of the reasons for fear of disorder of the mentally ill.

24. Stephen H. Hinshaw (2007: 151-2) provides an explanation for the finding that stigmatization is increasing despite greater public knowledge related to mental illness. First, increased urbanization and the closing of mental hospitals have made greater proportions of the public exposed to larger numbers of individuals with serious mental illness, and rendered them less tolerant towards the manifestations of mental disorder. Second, today's competitive labor market made more visible reduced functional capacity of the mentally ill people, and thus increased stigma of mental illness. Third, "the extensive growth of a middle-class may have caused a tendency towards standardization of behavior." Nonconforming behavior of people with mental illness cannot fit in a conformity-prone environment, and thereby is subject to stigmatization. Fourth, due to enormous technical innovations a stereo-

typed image of the mentally disturbed person is more easily spread today than it was in the past.

25. Asmus Finzen and Ulrike Hoffmann-Richter (1999: 13-19) claim that in recent times schizophrenia has taken up the role of the most terrifying illness. Susan Sontag (1991) argued that first TB and then cancer and AIDS were regarded as the most frightening diseases in the nineteenth and twentieth century respectively. And she provided convincing evidence that supports such a claim. Unlike Sontag, Finzen and Hoffmann-Richter did not substantiate their claim. The truth is that nothing indicates that schizophrenia has become the most terrifying illness in recent times. As a metaphor for all serious mental disorders schizophrenia has always been regarded as a very terrifying disorder, indeed.

4

Conceptual Cacophony in Psychiatry

> *Because no particular orientation or limited*
> *subgroup of schools has established its creden-*
> *tials as the sole scientific approach, there remains*
> *no scientific criterion for officially adopting one*
> *orientation over others.*
>
> Michael A. Schwartz
> and Osborne P. Wiggins, 1988

Psychiatry abounds in models.[1]

These models have been dubbed "prominent emphases within psychiatry" (Sabshin, 1990), "predominant theoretical representations of psychiatry" (Beigel, 1995), "approaches to the mind" (Havens, 1973, 2005), and "systems of explanation" (Moncrieff and Crawford, 2001).

A great many psychiatrists are mostly unaware of how much the particular model they endorse influences their way of thinking about mental illness and their clinical practice. They usually take their chosen model for granted. They do not question its assumptions, and they do not discuss its weak points. They are not very interested in other models, in what is going on beyond the model they consider as the best among all the possible models.

They are so engrossed in their model that they never think about making it explicit except when they oppose it to other models.[2]

To date, critically assessing one model from the vantage point of another has not borne fruit. In most cases it was followed by a stronger embrace of one's own model. Partisan psychiatrists are so little amenable to criticism coming from the other side of the fence.

From the first days of psychiatry until today there has always been the dominance of one, and rarely two, conceptual models. Seemingly, never in the same period have three or four models had the same relevance in the psychiatric community and society at large.

The proponents of one model rarely change sides.[3] If they do, they do it most often so as to benefit from the popularity of one particular model in a certain epoch. When one model takes center stage, not only in psychiatry, but also in the broader community's perception of what is a proper model (and these two processes usually coincide), it is much easier for the advocates of that particular model to get research funds and public approval; they are held in higher esteem and are consequently more praised than those psychiatrists who stay committed to one of the "shadow models."

The influence of the dominant psychiatric model can be traced in various aspects of psychiatric activity. For example, it is mirrored in the content of psychiatric journals (Kecmanovic and Hadzi-Pavlovic, 2010). Also, "with each dialectical shift in the prevailing theoretical paradigm, the vantage point for the retrospective construction of the history of the discipline has changed." Mark S. Micale dubs this phenomenon "the paradigmatic structuring of psychiatric historiographies" (1996).

The large number of models in psychiatry and the fact that models do not exist in other medical disciplines, or if they do they do not produce a conceptual cacophony in them,[4] requires an answer to the question as to why psychiatry abounds in models. Given the degree of discord among individual models, the question is even more seemly.

The epistemological premises of various general concepts about the basic nature, causes and treatments of mental disorders are discordant. "They tend to be more than simply differences in perspective; each is an encompassing view resting on certain assumptions of legitimacy and importance; and each develops in part in opposition to the other" (McHugh and Slavney, 1983).

The same view is echoed by Normal Sartorius who has written the following lines: "No other branch of medicine has developed such different orientations nor as much animosity between the defenders of different theoretical and practical orientations. Like Gods in anger, the sects in psychiatry seem to be ready to reject all the knowledge or insights that sects other than their own held: the good and the bad in others have been equally viciously attacked.... A vital step in the development of psychiatry is its unification.... War and anger within psychiatry is wasteful and diminishes the probability that we shall make progress in knowledge and in its useful application" (2002: 194).[5]

Why are There Many Models in Psychiatry?

There are several reasons for the existence of many models in psychiatry.

First, there is no a widely accepted theory of the mind-body relationship in the mentally sound and mentally disordered. It is missing in psychiatry because it is missing in philosophy.[6] The existence of different philosophical conceptions of the mind-body relationship—for example, Cartesian dualism, parallelism, epiphenomenalism, theory of double aspect—provides a fertile ground for the articulation of different psychiatric models. Neither psychiatrists nor clinical psychologists will be able to reach a consensus in regard to the fundamental issue of the relation between the physical and the mental until a general accord is attained in philosophy or at least until one view of the cited relation prevails in philosophy.

It is easy to identify the philosophical background of some psychiatric models; for example, epiphenomenalism underlies the medical model. The leading figures of some other models refer to the philosophers in the writings of which they find inspiration and foundation for their concepts and practical activities; for example, the advocates of the phenomenological-existential model (Ludwig Binswanger, Eugène Minkowski, V.E. Freiherr von Gebsattel, Ronald D. Laing, and others) quite often make references to the writings of Martin Heidegger, Edmund Husserl, Jean-Paul Sartre.

Second, biological, psychological and sociocultural factors co-determine the genesis and shape of mental disorders. As there is no unifying perception of these factors, of how they are intermingled in each individual, be they a mentally healthy or mentally sound individual, each psychiatric model addresses only one of the cited factors. "We must apply different sets of concepts to these factors, and we must employ different logics in our reasoning about them" (Schwartz and Wiggins, 1988).

By addressing only one side of mental disorders, each psychiatric concept or model ignores all other sides. By focusing on only one aspect of mental disorder it affirms its specificity. As the advocates of each individual perspective or model do not take into account other possible perspectives on the same phenomena, they do not see, or more accurately, they cannot see the deficiencies of their own vantage point. Thus each model follows its own presumptions, and thereby prevents a possible conversion of different models.

Third, the truth is that the same psychopathological occurrence can be explained and interpreted, that is, can be conceived as the result of causation and intention. For example, depression and associated suicidal ideation may be understood as the consequence of distorted neuron-chemical processes, or a person's intent to punish someone who will feel hurt by that person's death. And what is most important, there is no way to confirm or dismiss either view. In reply to possible remarks that the efficacy of antidepressant drugs in alleviating or eliminating depression does testify to its biological origin, I would refer to Parker's view that "evidence of any 'treatment specificity effects' is hard to find despite enormous database" (Parker, 2009). Moreover, "studies have shown that cognitive therapy is as efficacious as antidepressant medication at treating depression," and it seems "to reduce the risk of relapse even after its discontinuation" (DeRubeis, Siegle, and Hollon, 2008).

Thus there is no convincing evidence that any approach (model, perspective) is superior to other(s), that is, that any model should be discarded altogether. Secondary to such a state of affairs, however strong is the dominance of a particular model at a particular time, other models do not disappear without a trace. They keep on existing as shadow models.[7]

Fourth, the dominance of one, and rarely two, conceptual models is conditioned by social, financial, and ideological reasons (Kendler, 2005). As these reasons change so do the dominant models; thus if not dominant at the moment, a particular model is a model in waiting. Its time will come.

Fifth, there is an epistemological seductiveness in single perspectives. Schwartz and Wiggins (1988) draw attention to this phenomenon originally described by Karl Jaspers in his work *Psychology of Weltan-schaungen*. However paradoxical it may sound, each single perspective is universal in spite of not being able to be universal. It is not able to say everything about all aspects of reality, but it can say something regarding everything. For example, the medical model can say something about any psychopathological phenomenon. It provides an explanation for such different occurrences as lack of concentration, depression, high mood, delusions, hallucinations and aggressiveness. "Because one can assert something about everything, one can mistakenly suppose that one can assert everything 'worth saying' about everything." This epistemological seductiveness may be one of the subjective reasons for the sustainability of different psychiatric models.

Sixth, Peter Tyrer and Derek Steinberg, British psychiatrists, the former from Nothingam, and the latter from Kent, have a fair answer to the question of why are there so many different models in psychiatry. "Knowledge in psychiatry," they write, "is far outstripped by theories and opinions and these are allowed to flourish because the evidence needed to contradict them is not available" (1987: 2).

How Do Psychiatrists Choose Their Preferred Model?

In writings about models in psychiatry, due attention has not been accorded to the important question of the choice of the preferred model. If one bears in mind that it is a rather significant decision in the professional life of a psychiatrist, it is even more astonishing that this question has not been fully addressed to date. Such a decision tailors how psychiatrists look at their patients, how they conceptualize their distress; such a decision determines the kind of services they will provide to their patients; whether they will spend more working hours in emergency psychiatric departments, state hospitals, public or private facilities; which conferences they will be attending; which colleagues they will preferably associate with; where a significant portion of their earnings will come from, and so on.

I will list some of the most common reasons for psychiatrists' decision to pick one particular model rather than another one.

The conceptual orientation of the leading figures in the institution where one starts a professional career. During residency, psychiatrists work at different departments, at different facilities, whose staff prefer this or that psychiatric model. Thus residents have the opportunity to get acquainted with different models. A number of them express their preferences for a specific psychiatric model under the influence of one or more leading figures in the institution where they start working as psychiatrists. At times, such a decision is made, consciously or unconsciously, through identification with one's superiors; at other times it is a matter of opportunism, the manifestation of one's compliance with the dominant orientation of the given institution or department.

Biological or psychological mindedness. Some psychiatrists are more biologically than psychologically minded even before they start studying medicine. The inclination towards biological sciences somewhat predisposes them to adopt the medical model once they become psychiatrists. Those who are more psychologically minded are likely to prefer the psychological model. Those who are mostly interested in social and cultural issues will probably give priority to the social-cultural model. There are people who have the image of psychiatry as a more psychological, even spiritual rather than biological, discipline. And that is what makes psychiatry attractive in their eyes. They complete medical studies because there is no psychiatry without medicine, but all the time, that is, from the first years of medical studies they keep an eye on psychiatry. They are more likely to endorse the psychological or maybe the social-cultural rather than the medical model.

The dominance of a particular model. The psychiatric model that prevails at a particular time has high recruiting potential. It is hard and usually not very rewarding to swim against the tide. On the other hand, there are many advantages to being in tune with the model governing most psychiatrists' practice. Those who are part of mainstream psychiatry get employment comparatively easily; they are more sought after than those who are not; there are more conferences dealing with various aspects of the prevailing model; information related to this model is more frequently presented in the mass media and general psychiatric journals, and so on. Thus the popularity of a particular model motivates a number of psychiatrists to espouse it.

It is truism to say that the dominant culture cannot help but to favor a particular psychiatric model. Thus Paul R. McHugh writes: "During the thirty years of my professional experience, I have witnessed the power of cultural fashion to leave psychiatric thought and practice off in false, evens disastrous directions." And then he adds: "I have become familiar with how these fashions and their consequences cause psychiatry to loose its moorings" (2006: 3).

The financial interests. Of course, no one talks about them when discussing the benefits of preferring a particular model. But the financial rewards may play a role in prioritizing one particular model over others. This does not mean that the expectations of better financial remuneration when practicing one particular model are always real, that they are realized in most cases. What is important is that some psychiatrists do believe that they will earn more money if they provide services according to the principles of the medical model, or of the psychological model. I did not mention the social-cultural model because this model is believed to be the least financially rewarding.

What matters is a psychiatrist's conviction that a particular model he or she has chosen suits the reality of mental disorders better than other models. Such a belief certainly has a motivating force. The question is, however, whether it precedes the decision to endorse a particular model, or is the result of rationalizations, i.e., post hoc justifications, or results from the practice of a model that generates the certainty that there is no other model worth considering than the chosen one.

Numerous Models in Psychiatry: Advantages or Imperfections?

The existence of many models in psychiatry might be perceived both as psychiatry's advantage and as its disadvantage.

A general favorable remark about having many models is that it indicates how dynamic and vital psychiatry is. One could also say that it is good to have several perspectives in psychiatry because reality is heterogeneous. So every aspect of reality is to be approached in a different way, and that is why multiple concepts are needed.

There are arguments that different approaches are necessary because to claim that "the meaning of any psychiatric fact depends upon the particular perspective employed is to say that apart from all perspectives, facts make no sense" (Schwartz and Wiggins, 1988). The idea, originated by Karl Jaspers, is that "perspectives arrange the mass of data in an intelligible order. They tell us what regarding the patient is relevant to his or her disorder and what is irrelevant."

Two critical remarks can be leveled at this idea which somewhat defends the existence of many models in psychiatry. First, a unified theory about different aspects of reality could perform the same function of organizing reality, of making it intelligible. Such a theory or concept would be of greater help in understanding reality because it would not provide different perspectives on different aspects of reality. Second, by introducing order into chaos, different approaches or concepts parcel reality and thereby create different sections of reality. Briefly said, they make sense of reality but at the price of fragmenting it; thereby they sow seeds of new misunderstandings, and conflicting opinions about one and the same reality. With a bit of exaggeration one might say that the formation of many concepts about reality has replaced a big chaos by a not so big chaos.

In my view, the downsides of having many legitimate models in psychiatry far outweigh the possible advantages. Indeed, the existence of many models in psychiatry nurtures "a continuing view that psychiatry is a discipline without a clear sense of identity or focus" (Beigel, 1995) However, this is not the most negative fall-out of the legitimacy of more than one psychiatric model. There are far more serious effects such as alternative explanations of the same psychopathological phenomenon; confusion in patients caused by different messages coming from the advocates of different models; dilemmas about the "right" treatment;

latent or open antagonism among psychiatrists favoring different perspectives, and so on.

Sidney Bloch, Professor of Psychiatry at the University of Melbourne, is of the opinion that "psychiatry's continuing failure or mere lip service to address both biomedical and psychosocial dimensions of professional knowledge in an integrated fashion has been a major hindrance to its progress." Competing explanations, "not uncommonly contradictory," are dividing psychiatry from within. In my view, Bloch is very realistic when he writes that "an integrating paradigm to counter fragmenting forces seems elusive." Hence his conclusion: "the unfortunate outcome is a profession working without a sense of unity seemingly oblivious of the peril it faces" (1997).

Heinz Katschnig, Professor of Psychiatry at the University of Vienna, shares the same view. After pointing out that our discipline is threatened by the existence of *de facto* ideological subgroups, he states that "if psychiatry is to persist as a profession, it needs to have a conceptual centre." And he adds: "What this might be in the future is not clear." It is not clear, indeed.

Psychiatry: Multi-Paradigmatic or Pre-Paradigmatic

Are conceptual models in psychiatry the same as *paradigms*? Do they fit with the meaning that Thomas Kuhn gave to the notion of paradigm in his classical work *The Structure of Scientific Revolutions* (1962)?

Psychiatric conceptual models and paradigms in Kuhn's terms could not be considered as being the same. Kuhn called *paradigm shift* a radical change in key epistemological assumptions, not only within science, but also in relation to the dominant world-view. According to this author, a new paradigm, i.e., a new world-concept, excludes the fundamentals of the old one. In other words, two different paradigms never co-exist; one always replaces the other. That is not the case in psychiatry. As stated, different models co-exist in psychiatry. The dominance of one model never makes all other models totally obsolete. As I said in the text above, when one model loses its dominant position, this does not mean that it will not be resurrected, that it will not resurface years later, and retake center stage.

Yet, Kuhn's paradigm and psychiatric paradigm—if for the moment we call psychiatric models paradigms—appear to have two common characteristics. According to Kuhn, the new paradigm is acknowledged as dominant not so much due to its capacity to explain reality in a more accurate, or more sophisticated way, as "because it is better able to justify the social practices of the relevant discipline" (Horwitz, 2002a: 57). The same holds for psychiatry. No psychiatric model becomes prevailing because it more accurately explains mental illness and is more useful when its principles are implemented in clinical practice, but because it is in tune with the current social circumstances.

Moreover, according to Kuhn, paradigms are matchless. Paradigms are so different that one paradigm cannot be translated into another. It is the same with psychiatric models. Although a few attempts have been made to identify the common features of two models—for example, Eric R. Kandel (1999, 2005) did it when he strived to explain that psychological (psychodynamic) and biological models have some common points, and Jules V. Coleman (1971) did it when he contended that the psychoanalytic approach to symptom formation can be understood as a social process—individual psychiatric models are incommensurable, to use Kuhn's phrase.

Kuhn asserts that paradigms are incommensurable for three reasons. First, the dominant paradigm determines the perception of reality, which means that the perception of reality differs from one paradigm to another. Second, the meaning of individual topics within a paradigm also differs from the meaning of individual topics within another paradigm. Third, each single paradigm gives different importance to individual phenomena.

Could the same reasons for incommensurability be identified as far as the incommensurability of psychiatric conceptual models is concerned? Let us consider two psychiatric models: the medical and the psychological (the psychodynamic variant of the psychological model). Biologically oriented psychiatrists are primarily interested in the symptoms an individual presents; on the other hand, psychodynamically orientated psychiatrists focus on how the client experiences the therapist, how they relate to the therapist. Those who favor the medical model believe that brain pathology causes the appearance of the symptoms, whereas those who stick to the psychodynamic model search for the meaning of symptoms in the personal history of the client, in their emotional past and in how they relate to the therapist. The biologically oriented psychiatrist has no doubt whatsoever that brain structural and biochemical anomalies have caused the patent's symptoms. On the other hand, the psyhodynamically oriented psychiatrist focuses on how the client has gone through the phases of psychosexual development. There is the clue to the client's current mental suffering.

I will list a number of other differences between a psychiatrist biologist and a psychiatrist psychodynamist. The former deals with psychotic and non-psychotic patients and the latter deals mostly with non-psychotic patients. The former strives to attenuate or eliminate the patient's symptoms. The latter's ambition is to assist the client in gaining insight into the dynamics of the formation of their mental problems. The former wants to rid the patient of the symptoms or make the symptoms less disturbing, so as to enable the patient to properly function in the community. The therapeutic ideal of the latter is to produce a change in the client's personality

For several years Tanya M. Luhrmann, anthropologist, observed how American psychiatrists in various psychiatric facilities diagnose and treat patients. She came to the conclusion that American psychiatry is deeply divided. That is why she called her widely cited book *Of Two Minds*. Luhrmann writes: "Psychiatrists are taught to listen to people in particular ways: they listen for signals most of us cannot hear, and they look for patterns most of us cannot see. Their two primary tasks, however—diagnosis and psychopharmacology, on the one hand, and psychodynamic therapy, on the other—teach them to listen and look in *different ways*" (2000: 22, my emphasis).

Luhmann's conclusion about the deep divide in American psychiatry is valid for psychiatry in any country where psychiatrists do not espouse the same conceptual model. And that is the case with most countries across the world.

Rachel Cooper (2007: 88) points out that the concurrent legitimacy of several models is not specific to psychiatry. Reportedly it is valid in psychology and allied disciplines alike. Cooper dubs all these disciplines "psy-sciences." If we talk about the medical, the psychological, and the social model, it is fair to say that the psychological model is by far the most popular model among psychologists, in particular among practicing psychologists. In so far Cooper's assertion is flawed. However, if Cooper meant that there are several rather different concepts within the psychological model, she is right.[8]

In conclusion, psychiatry could be considered as multi-paradigmatic in view of the fact that there is no such thing in psychiatry as a dominant psychiatry model endorsed by all psychiatrists without exception, in a particular region, in a particular era. At the same time, psychiatry could be pronounced pre-paradigmatic because at any given time, different models exist in psychiatry (a pre-scientific battle of paradigms, Kendler, 2005).

Main Models in Psychiatry

As stated, there are different models in psychiatry. Roughly, all of them can be reduced to three main models: *the medical model, the psychological model, and the social-cultural model.*

The Medical Model

Advocates of the medical model[9] maintain that the only thing that matters is occurrences at the level of structures and functions of individual organs, of the brain in the case of mental disorder.

Psychic manifestations are epiphenomena of what is going on at deeper levels, primarily at the levels of synapses. Therefore, proper treatment aims to produce changes in the brain structure and functions.

Subjective experience, the specific way a person relates to themselves and others, is beyond the scope of interest of the advocates of the medical model; in any case it is something that is of secondary importance.

As for the therapist's skills such as empathy and intuition, which significantly differ from one therapist to another, they are not held in esteem within the medical model; they are low on this model's agenda.

Advocates of the medical model ignore the differences, no matter how big they are, between the subjective worlds of different individuals. They endorse the principle that the brain's structure and neurochemistry are the same in different individuals. And they are disordered in the same way in those who suffer from the same kind of mental disorder. What is going in an individual's brain is relevant rather than what is going between them and other people.

Notions such as the patient's viewpoint, their specific experience of themselves and other people, their hopes and disappointments, simply do not exist in the vocabulary of those favoring the medical model (Dewhurst and Watson, 1996). Hence it is with good reason that the medical model is considered apersonal.

Within this model there is a clear distinction between disorder and non-disorder. Correspondingly the advocates of the medical model prefer categorial diagnoses to dimensional diagnoses.

The Psychological Model

Within the psychological model—in particular that of the psychodynamic kind—symptoms are seen as external manifestations of deeper currents that comprise recent and remote experiences as well as internal conflicts. Some times the latter are close to consciousness, at other times they are not.

Therapeutic alliance, everything that occurs in the relation between the therapist and client, is of utmost importance, both in terms of diagnostics and therapy.

Since the therapist's personality is the key vehicle and instrument of the treatment, the therapist is required to undergo special training (or analysis) aimed at reducing their own internal conflicts that might prevent them from properly treating those in need.

A psychodynamic orientation is one among many orientations within psychological model. Behavioral and cognitive therapy are other orientations that deserve attention, because they are most frequently used today.

Behavioral therapists draw on behaviorism. By using various techniques such as classical or operant conditioning they strive to eliminate the patient's "bad habits," that is, their ill-adaptive behavioral patterns.

But the basic premise of cognitive therapists is that cognitive processes play a key role in the genesis of mental disorders. Hence it is by modifying a person's habitual way of thinking that it is possible to improve their mental condition. The royal road to recovery is a new, balanced view of ourselves, of other people and of events that are related or non-related to us.

Those who use the psychological model do not need medical knowledge. Notions such as neurotransmitters, sub-cortical regions, synapses and the like cannot be found in the vocabulary of the advocates of the psychological model.

Unlike the medical model that is apersonal, the psychological model is personal. It deals with emphatically personal rather than universal data.

Within the psychological model there is no clear-cut distinction between the normal and the pathological. The dividing line between them is blurred or nonexistent.

Since disorder and non-disorder are relational notions according to the psychological model, it is no wonder that the advocates of this model consider dimensional diagnoses as superior to categorial ones.

The Sociocultural Model

In the view of those who prefer the sociocultural model to other models, the sociocultural environment plays a major role in the engenderment, course and outcome of mental disorders.

Sociocultural occurrences that comprise a sudden change, and this most often means a loss, for example, social disorganization, death of loved ones, emigration, have the greatest disturbing potential in terms of preventing people from meeting their needs, and thereby the greatest potential to upset their mental balance.

The therapeutic arsenal of the sociocultural model is large. It encloses various methods and measures from group therapy, therapeutic community, occupational therapy, to providing support to the family, and making efforts to change the existing social and even political environment.

From the foregoing it is obvious that cognizance of the social rather than the medical sciences is instrumental in enabling people to gain (better) insight into social occurrences that might have played a role in generating and shaping mental disorders, and determining their course and outcome.

Medical knowledge cannot be of much use to advocates of the sociocultural model.

Within this model an individual is viewed through the lenses of their group membership, their relation to their referring group and other groups, and the relation of them as a group member towards members of other collectivities.

Notions such as role conflict, lawlessness, alienation, dehumanization, labeling, specific social normative system, are frequently used by culturalists. These notions can rarely be found in the vocabulary of the psychological model, and never in the vocabulary of the medical model.

The border between the normal and the pathological is not stable within the sociocultural model; it is not clearly visible in any case. The pathological is located more in the social-political environment, in the relationship of an individual to their referring group(s) rather than in the individual themselves.

What are the Effects of the Existence of Several Models?

An individual would be very confused, or even additionally deranged, if told by a psychiatrist that their mental suffering was most probably caused (or precipitated or triggered) at the same time by their brain chemistry, their psycho-social (including sexual) upbringing or development, by their cognitive or behavioral patterns (bad habits and wrong explication schemata), and the sociocultural milieu they live in (anomic social situation).

Is it possible that all the cited circumstances and factors truly co-determine a particular disorder? Yes, this could be the case. But the same could be said for any mental disorder because none of the arguments of any model can be easily and totally refuted, or confirmed, in any particular case, except perhaps for an anomic social situation. Yet, if the notion of social situation primarily refers to family situation, psychiatrists and clinical psychologists will not be at great pains to show that the family of a particular patient was "in fact" dysfunctional. And if someone contacts several psychiatrists, and each one of them says the same thing, i.e., that all the cited factors may have caused their mental problems, the person will easily jump to the conclusion that psychiatrists do not know very much or do not know anything about where their patients' problems come from, and will consequently infer that psychiatrists are not be trusted.

With a bit of cynicism one might assume that in a good number of cases psychiatrists stick with only one model in order to present themselves as competent. Namely, in the public's eyes, and not only in the public's, the more a doctor pinpoints a specific reason as the very reason for someone's problems the more they are to be trusted. Those who state that nearly everything could have caused, or could have contributed to someone's either physical or mental suffering, are held in much lesser esteem than those who are confident they know the very reason for someone's health problems; not a reason but *the* reason.

Since each psychiatric model has its own epistemological foundation, it is hard to compare them and say which one is better in the absolute and in the relative sense, as we will see when discussing methodological pluralism. This is all the more so as the outcome, as one of the key categories in medicine, is differently conceived in each model. In other words, the meaning of a good outcome differs from one model to the other.

It is worth noting that the existence of various models has a negative impact on team work in psychiatry as well. For example, since psychiatrists more sign up with the medical model than other team members, and since psychiatric social workers are inclined to overvalue psychosocial intervention, covert or open frictions and misunderstanding among team members are no rare, especially in regard to patients who are "somewhere on the road between distress and illness" (Colombo, Bendelow, Fulford *et al.*, 2003).[10]

All the above-mentioned consequences of the conceptual cacophony in psychiatry have prompted psychiatrists—interestingly enough, mainly those psychiatrists who hold a degree in philosophy as well—to try to find a solution to the conceptual, and not only conceptual conundrum in psychiatry. (This does not refer to George Engel, the author of the biopsychosocial model, who is not a psychiatrist.)

Attempts to Overcome the Conceptual Cacophony in Psychiatry

In recent times there has been talk that the empirical approach will resolve the sectarianism in psychiatry. The mantra of this move is that only empirical evidence can disperse the clouds of the theoretical confusion caused by different perspectives.[11]

Michael A. Schwartz and Osborne P. Wiggins (1988) elaborated upon this issue, and I will rely on them in depicting the true character of this determination to put things in order with regard to psychiatrists' confronting views of the same phenomena.

Speaking in more concrete terms, the aim of those who are determined to give priority to the facts is to "link specific kinds of therapies and techniques with specific kinds of disorders." The idea is that once "diligent and systematic empirical investigations have finally established the most effective approaches to the different kinds of disorders," there will no longer be room for claims coming from the practitioners of different models that their approach is the most successful one. The relocation of psychiatry back into medicine is supposed to be a collateral and worthy effect of such new state of affairs.

Schwartz and Wiggins grasped the danger of this tendency "to install positivistic methods of inquiry as the only acceptable ones." And promoting the positivist approach as the only right approach is nothing less than reaffirming the medical model as the only valid model. "If one wished to discuss forms of treatment, for example, one could do so only by offering statistical analyses of clinical trials of groups of patients. These clinical trials would see highly specified techniques and procedures, careful definitions, standardization, treatment manuals, and the like. For the new psychiatry, evaluations and procedures should be as mathematical as possible."

This is a new form of sectarianism under the guise of the medical model, as Schwartz and Wiggins rightly noted. Mathematical and statistical methods are welcome and useful in psychiatry. However, psychiatrists must be aware of the limitations of the application of these methods to understanding psychiatric phenomena. Regardless of the claims of the advocates of these methods, they cannot be accepted as universally valid in psychiatry.

Such claims enunciated in the eighties seem to have heralded today's claims that there is no psychiatry unless it is evidence-based psychiatry. And the same criticisms that have been leveled at evidence-based psychiatry apply to this kind of new sectarianism.

There have been still other attempts to resolve the conceptual conundrum (conceptual "trichotomy") in psychiatry. As the mind-body dualism underpins the majority of conceptual hard-to-resolve questions in psychiatry, David Dewhurst and I. Patrick Burges Watson (1996) have resorted to the notion of a person, which is supposed to bridge the divide caused by the mind-body dualism. The cited authors are of the opinion that the concept of a person could provide psychiatrists with a powerful instrument in overcoming the various dualistic and materialistic perspectives. Why? Because "a person is a psychobiological being whose psychical and physical aspects are integrated, with psychological and physical qualities being ascribed to the very same subject." In addition, as a member of the community "a person is involved in various interpersonal and social relationships." Thus the notion of a person would connect all three aspects or sides (biological, psychological, and social-cultural) dealt with by individual psychiatric models.

I do not find using the notion of a person very heuristic in resolving the psychiatric conceptual puzzle.

So far I have made a brief reference to some not fully developed ideas about how to overcome conceptual cacophony in psychiatry. Now I will pay attention to several more elaborated endeavors to achieve the same goal.

There have been several attempts to solve conceptual heterogeneity in psychiatry. I will focus on *eclecticism, the biopsychosocial model, methodic pluralism* and *pragmatic psychiatry*. Eclecticism is not an authorized attempt. The rest are.

I will sketch each one of them and show that none of them have proved successful.

Eclectic Psychiatry

Eclectic psychiatry is not a particular psychiatric model. "Given the countless tributaries that flow into clinical psychiatry, it goes without saying that psychiatry is an eclectic discipline" (Knight, 1995).

The term *eclecticism* has two meanings: first, eclecticism is the reluctance to accept a particular concept, and only taking some bits or fragments of individual conceptions or models; second, eclecticism is choosing the best one, and that is the original meaning of the ancient Greek notion *"eklektikos"* from which the word eclecticism is derived.[12]

Both these meaning of the notion of eclecticism can easily be found in the practice of eclectic psychiatry.

Eclecticism is not legitimate in medical disciplines other than psychiatry. There is no mention of something called, e.g., eclectic ophthalmology, eclectic anesthesiology, or eclectic otolaryngology. The fact that not only has eclecticism the right to exist in psychiatry, but is also welcomed by a number of psychiatrists, is one indication more of how specific psychiatry is compared to other medical disciplines.

There would be no psychiatric eclecticism if there were not many (legitimate) psychiatric models. At the same time, there would be no psychiatric eclecticism if all psychiatrists were happy to stay with only one model.

There are many reasons for the attractiveness of eclecticism. Talking about the perils of eclecticism in psychology Brent D. Slife (1987) mentions three main ways in which eclecticism attracts psychologists. It seems to me that eclecticism attracts psychiatrists in the same ways in which it attracts psychologists.

First, those psychiatrists who are for whatever reason reluctant to follow any one theory find eclecticism helpful in escaping any particular conceptual orientation.

Second, eclectics "look around at existing orientations and see no clear winner from either the basic or applied literatures, and thus assume that each orientation has something to offer." So they select those elements of all systems that they consider the best.

Third, to be eclectic bears resemblance to be open-minded, flexible, non-dogmatic. Since those who sign up to a particular conceptual model are considered dogmatic and inflexible, it is alluring not to be like that.

If there are good reasons for the existence of psychiatric eclecticism, and it seems there are, and if a number of psychiatrists find psychiatric eclecticism convenient, i.e., the best possible option to overcome the models' one-sidedness, the question arises why eclecticism is not more talked about and discussed. Why are there no professors of eclectic psychiatry, as there are professors of biological and social psychiatry; why are there no textbooks on eclectic psychiatry—with the exception of Rudolph Kaelbling and Ralph Patterson's 1966 book *Eclectic Psychiatry*—as there are textbooks of biological psychiatry and social psychiatry?

Medical students are taught that all sides of the mentally disordered are relevant in the genesis, course and outcome of mental illness. At exams, either at undergraduate, or postgraduate level, or at the end of residency, students are expected to demonstrate knowledge and expertise in biological, psychological and social psychiatry. What they are not taught is eclectic psychiatry, i.e., how to combine methods of the cited three kinds of psychiatric orientations. It is as though psychiatry teachers look down on eclectic psychiatry and do not think it is a topic worth theirs and students' attention.

One of the possible reasons for undervaluing eclectic psychiatry is the fact that eclectic psychiatry has no clear and stable profile and identity, that it is a mixing (not melting) pot. After all—the argument goes—what kind of psychiatry is one whose initiator(s) and leading figures are unknown and whose greatest achievements are unknown.

There are two main forms of eclectic psychiatry.

Eclectic Psychiatry as a Combination of Different Models

Eclectic psychiatry might mean the simultaneous application of the principles of the medical, the psychological, and the social-cultural model. For example, when a depressive patient seeks help, their depression could be interpreted in the following ways: they are depressive because the level of neurotransmitters in their brain, above all serotonin and noradrenalin, is low; because of a genetic predisposition; because of a hormonal deficit (for example, low level of thyroxin); because of some somatic ailment(s); because they took substances that might cause or precipitate depression (for example, corticosteroids); because they took some illegal addictive drugs; because of so-called depressive diathesis meaning a propensity to react by depression to various events either in the environment or within the organism (*biological psychiatry*); because an aggressive response to inhibition was thwarted, and consequently aggression turned inwards (psychodynamic explanation); because of learned helplessness (*cognitive psychology approach*); because of the lack of positive confirmation (*behaviorist approach*); because of some life-event the patient experienced either over the last six months (for example, the loss of one's spouse, or the loss of one's job) or in the distant past (for example, the loss of one parent in childhood); because of life in an anomic social-cultural environment; because of difficulties in adaptation to a new social-cultural milieu (for example, acculturation stress) (*the social-cultural model*), and because of a failed search for meaning (*the existential model*).

From the foregoing it is obvious that the possible explanations for the depression of a particular patient greatly vary. If an eclectic psychiatrist keen on combining the principles of different psychiatric models finds all the cited explanations of the patient's depression fitting, the question arises: how would it be possible to implement them in clinical practice, that is, in the treatment of that particular patient.

Psychiatrists might note that the patient's anamnesis and examination might rule out many circumstances and factors as possible reasons for depression, so there is no need to use therapeutic methods and techniques that are specific to a number of concepts about the origin of depression.

For example, examining the patient's physical and biological state (including measuring specific hormones), ruling out the patient's addiction to illicit drugs and their insufficient exposure to light, the possibility can be rejected that some physical-biological factor might have caused the depression.

In addition, if the patient tells the psychiatrist that they have not experienced any loss in the recent or distant past, and that they have not moved to another country, and the like, the psychiatrist can dismiss the possibility that the patient's depression might have been caused or precipitated by those circumstances.

Yet, how can it be asserted with certainty that the patient's depression does indeed originate from their "learned helplessness," or lack of positive reinforcement, or unsuccessful search for meaning, or aggressiveness turning inward. If a psychiatrist looks for data that might confirm that their assumption about the origin of the patient's depression is right, they will find them. There are a great many elements in the history of any depressive patient, and in particular in their current mental condition and way of thinking and feeling, and relating to themselves and others, that might indicate that they are depressive because of learned helplessness, because of the lack of positive reinforcement, because of turning aggressiveness inward, because they did not manage to find the meaning of their existence, because some of their relatives were prone to depression.

One thing is certain. As stated, it is hard to imagine what the treatment of a patient would be like if their depression was understood as resulting from all the cited factors and circumstances, and corresponding kinds of treatment were applied. Of course, this is assuming that one and the same psychiatrist is able to apply various treatment methods and techniques, which is more the exception than the rule. In practical terms it would mean that a single psychiatrist uses psychodynamic techniques, cognitive as well as behavioral methods and techniques, that they are cognizant of pharmacotherapy, in particular the pharmacotherapy of depressive states, and familiar with various methods aimed at helping the patient find specific meaning not only in their depression but also in their own life (spiritual coaching, life coaching).

Another question is what would be the patient's reaction to the diverse messages coming from such different treatment methods and techniques. If the therapist explains the reason for using such diverse treatment methods and techniques, and the basic principles of the concepts from which they are derived, as a therapist is expected to do, this question is even more appropriate. It goes without saying that people are readier to accept explanations of their health problems that are coherent, logical, and make sense rather than those that are contradictory.

I made a passing reference to the question of how a psychiatrist could be equally well trained in applying different treatment methods and techniques specific to different psychiatric models. The same question is valid with regard to various techniques that are specific to various orientations within one and the same model. For example, there are several hundred psychotherapeutic orientations (concepts, schools). All of them are covered by the same notion of the psychological model. How could a psychiatrist be trained in the treatment techniques of so many more or less different psychotherapeutic orientations? The time that is necessary to complete training in dozens of methods and acquire experience in their use hinders a psychiatrist from properly doing such a job. In that regard Fernando Lolas rightly notes that "the many aspects of a seemingly heterogeneous profession, ranging from Bohemian speculation to hardcore empirical research, do not find a reasonable harmonization within individual practice of psychiatrists." And then he adds: "In order to honor all the heterogeneous discourses constituting the historical knowledge base, they should resemble 'Renaissance men' and this is seldom the case, particularly in an era of state controlled or marked-driven practice" (2010).

Eclectic serialism is the second form of eclectic psychiatry.

Eclectic Psychiatry as Psychiatric Serialism

The notion *psychiatric serialism* was first used by Eugene M. Abroms. Psychiatric serialism is a specific kind of eclectic psychiatry.

Two forms of psychiatric serialism may be differentiated. Let us see what the first form of serialism is like.

According to Abroms, serialism means that after therapeutic alliance has been established, the therapist must determine whether there is an obvious somatic basis to a concrete mental disorder, and where possible, use proper physical-biological treatment methods. "What it means in practice is that, after forming a treatment alliance, the therapist must always assess the evidence for a biological substrate of the disorder and, where feasible, administer the appropriate biological treatments. On a stable biological platform, psychosocial interventions can then be utilized to promote the goals of *lieben* and *arbeiten*, and an existential therapy relationship can be forged to promote personal integrity" (Abroms, 1983).

Why is the search for the biological foundation of a particular disorder prioritized? If it is found that a physical (neurochemical) cause underlies someone's mental symptoms, and if that cause could be eliminated, the symptoms would most likely disappear. Depending on the nature of the somatic cause, its removal—for example in the case of a brain tumor—might save the patient's life. In that sense elimination of the possible somatic causes of mental disorder at the very beginning of a patient's treatment is more than recommended.

The reader should note two circumstances. First, in regard to the number of depressive states, substance use disorders, personality disorders, and anxious states as the most common forms of mental disorders, the number of so-called organic mental disorders, i.e., disorders caused by some identifiable somatic disease or malfunction, is negligible. (This does not refer to some forms of dementia that are more neurological or neuropsychiatric rather than psychiatric disorders.) Second, except for a very small number of cases, it is not possible to establish a cause-effect relationship between the somatic-biological substrate and a particular psychiatric syndrome.

Furthermore, what is meant by "on a stable biological platform, psychosocial interventions can then be utilized?" Does it mean that social-psychological interventions should not be used if the biological substrate of the disorder has not been detected? What happens if the psychiatrist cannot establish the biological underpinning of mental symptoms, which is most often the case? Does this mean that it is senseless to use both biological treatment methods, because the biological cause is unknown, and social-psychological treatment methods?

Strictly following the reasoning of those who favor the second form of psychiatric serialism, it turns out that there is no place for psychiatric therapy where the biological substrate of mental symptoms has not been identified. Such a view is not far from *monotheistic biologism* (Silove, 1990).

Now a few words about the second form of eclectic serialism. Psychotic disorders are quite often said to be more biologically than psychologically or socially conditioned. The opposite case is true with non-psychotic disorders.

Advocates of the second form of psychiatric serialism claim that disorders that are mostly biologically conditioned should be treated by biological treatment methods, and that disorders in the genesis of which social-psychological factors play a more important role should be managed mostly by non-biological treatment methods.

The starting point of such a belief and/or practice is an assumption rather than empirical evidence. For example, the hereditary factors of schizophrenic disorder(s) and bipolar disorders have been more explored than the hereditary factors of anxious disorders, for example. Yet, how is it possible to refute the view that such a disproportion in knowledge about the genetics of psychotic and non-psychotic disorders is due to the more reliable diagnostics of the former compared to the latter rather than to the real difference between psychotic and non-psychotic disorders in regard to their biological underpinning.

The first form of psychiatric serialism is biologism in disguise. The second is based on the premise that biological foundation of psychotic disorder is more certain than the biological underpinning of non-psychotic disorders. This premise is disputable.

In conclusion, I would say that shaky conceptual ground on which a great deal of eclectic psychiatry practice resides is caused by a lack of theory of this kind of psychiatry. Eclecticism takes no stands, as S. Nassir Ghaemi (2003: 82) put it. Eclectic psychiatry begins and ends with the assertion that in dealing with people with mental disorder one has to take into account all aspects (biological, psychological, and social-cultural) of those people. This is commonsensical, but this is not a theory, let alone a model. Least of all, eclectic psychiatry is a way to solve or overcome the conceptual puzzle caused by the legitimacy of many models in psychiatry.

Finally, it is difficult to define psychiatrists who declare themselves as eclectic. Quite often psychiatrists who declare themselves as eclectic or are recognized as such by others differ from each other more than eclectic and non-eclectic psychiatrists do.

In conclusion, I would say that Peter Lambley (1971) was right when he said that eclectic psychiatry in some variants is more like technical maneuvering than a conceptually meaningful activity.

The Biopsychosocial Model

Advocates of the biopsychosocial model claim that it is a corrective of other models, the biological model above all, insofar as it integrates the specificities of all traditional models.

George Engel is the author of the biopsychosocial model. He is an internist (gastroenterologist) who trained in psychoanalysis with Franz Alexander. Engel inaugurated the model in two papers: "The need for a new medical model: a challenge for biomedicine" (1977) and "The clinical application of the biopsychosocial model" (1980). Although the latter was published in *The American Journal of Psychiatry*, it elaborates the implications of the psychological-social model for the study and care of a patient with acute myocardial infarction.

Conceived of as holistic, this model pays equal attention to various explanatory concepts in natural sciences, individual psychology, sociology, economics, politics, and anthropology.

According to the biopsychosocial model, all dimensions of the mentally ill are interrelated, that is, they influence one another.

The model has attracted the attention of and is heeded by those who are interested in how to resolve the conceptual cacophony in psychiatry because it is comprehensive and gives equal weight to all aspects of the mentally ill.

Has the biopsychosocial model achieved the goal of being an alternative to the reductionism of the biological, psychological and social-cultural models? Many critics of Engel's concept (for example, Paul Fink, Michael A. Schwartz and Osborne Wiggins, Laurence Foss, Kenneth Rothenberg) hold that the biopsychosocial model does not address the practical aspects of clinical work.

The major problem with the model is that however good it might be as a concept, it does not provide a recipe for how to implement it. It recommends a diversity-of-sciences approach but provides no guidelines for selecting the science that applies to a particular patient at a particular time (Schwartz and Wiggins, 1985). "Moreover, the biopsychosocial model provides no formal model of anticipating the idiosyncratic problems that every individual patient presents; only the interdependence of the various system levels is emphasized" (Sadler and Hulgus, 1992).

Furthermore, however comprehensive it may be, the biopsychosocial model is not specific.

"With any particular patient ... only a limited number of factors will play a role in treatment, but the biopsychosocial model offers no help in

delimiting and circumscribing them. For one patient the spiritual support afforded by his religion may prove relevant. For another patient the
financial support he lacks may be crucial. For even another patient, the
political support he receives from his constituents may be quite important. The biopsychosocial model provided no guidance in locating and
specifying the relevant variables" (Schwartz and Wiggins, 1985).

Apart from its comparatively small usefulness, the biopsychosocial
model has not provided even at the conceptual level what could be
expected of it, given its name and claims. The biopsychosocial model
has not managed to synthesize the achievements of the traditional individual models in a new concept that would assist psychiatrist in getting
a comprehensive view of the complexity of mental illness. "Engel's
model lists the ingredients but dos not provide a recipe" (Slavney and
McHugh, 1987: 122).[13]

None of traditional conceptual models has lost its identity in the
biopsychosocial model. On the other hand, it is difficult to perceive the
identity of the biopsychosocial model itself.

There is no better way to present Engel's way of thinking, to give
the reader an idea of how much the biopsychosocial model is lacking in
practical guidelines which are precondition for its clinical implementation than to cite Engel himself.

After having mentioned diabetes and schizophrenic disorder as
paradigms of physical diseases and mental disorders, Engel says that
the biomedical model is not of much help in the proper interpretation,
explanation and treatment of these maladies. Then he adds: "To provide
a basis for understanding the determinants of disease and arriving at
rational treatment and patterns of health care, a medical model must
also take into account the patient, the social context in which he lives,
and the complementary system devised by society to deal with the disruptive effects of illness, that is, the physician's role and the health care
system. This requires a biopsychosocial model. Its scope is determined
by the historic function of the physician to establish whether the person
soliciting help is 'sick' or 'well'; and if sick, why sick and in which
ways sick; and then to develop a rational program to treat the illness
and restore and maintain health."

The knowledge provided by individual psychiatric models cannot
be ignored. If we did that we would ignore psychiatric knowledge. The
point is that there is no psychiatric knowledge outside the knowledge
afforded by individual psychiatric models. At this moment, there is no
useful knowledge for psychiatric practice other than the knowledge ac-

quired within individual psychiatric models. The biopsychosocial model which upholds a conceptually, in fact, neutral position does not offer new psychiatric knowledge that could either supplement or replace existing knowledge. It is one thing to say that psychiatric practice and theory should integrate the contributions, no matter how partial, of individual psychiatric models, and another thing to create new knowledge.

In conclusion, while opposing "one-sided knowledge" (Eisenberg, 1977) of the traditional models, the biopsychosocial model did not provide "multisided knowledge." Hence, it is not surprising that the biopsychosocial model has been accepted as a catch phrase but has not been translated into a new form of clinical practice.

Methodic Pluralism

Due to the fact that Karl Jaspers was the first one to assert that psychiatrist should make use of both causal explanation and meaningful understanding, this psychiatrist-turned-philosopher should be considered the forefather of methodic pluralism. S. Nassir Ghaemi holds that, apart from Karl Jaspers and himself, Leston L. Havens, Paul R. McHugh and Phillip R. Slavney are advocates of methodic pluralism. Ghaemi presented his ideas in his seminal work *The Concepts of Psychiatry. A Pluralistic Approach to the Mind and Mental Illness* (2003). More recently he has written on methodic pluralism in the paper titled "Pluralism in psychiatry: Karl Jaspers on science" (2007).

In order to delineate the specificity of methodic pluralism as clearly as possible, Ghaemi, Professor of Psychiatry at Tafts University in Boston, points out the difference between eclecticism and the biopsychosocial approach. As stated, these two approaches might be conceived as a defense against dogmatism, that is, against commitment to only one model. Ghaemi criticizes eclecticism and the biopsychosocial model alike. According to him, the former is "an obstacle to further progress" (2003: VII). As for the latter, he writes that "the problem exists, perhaps, in the failure of the model itself, not failure to implement it" (2009).

Ghaemi's basic assumption is that keeping to only one method is not sufficient in psychiatrists' approach to the mentally ill because every method is partial, and thus suitable for only one aspect of those with mental illness. "Multiple independent methods are necessary in the understanding and treatment of mental illness" (2003: 15).

Eclectics say that since physical-biological and mental factors concurrently determine mental disorders, all methods are welcome in diagnosing and treating people with mental illness. And they should be used simultaneously. On the other hand, according to pluralism, to which Ghaemi signs up, individual methods and techniques should be used separately and purely. Psychiatrists should know the strengths and weaknesses of each individual method and technique. On the basis of such knowledge they should know when it is recommended to use one particular method (somatic, medical or psychotherapeutic), and when some other method or technique (medical, somatic or psychotherapeutic) is preferable.

Eclectics, Ghaemi adds, do not assess the perfections and imperfections of individual methods and techniques. "Little work is done on specifying when and why medications work or do not work, when and why psychotherapy is effective or not, and when they might (or might not) work best together" (2003: 82).

Thus the key difference between eclecticism and the biopsychosocial approach, one the one hand, and methodic pluralism, on the other, is that the practitioner of methodic pluralism is cognizant of what might be achieved by using a particular method, and therefore selectively applies this or that different method. They use one or more particular methods only in those cases where research results have shown that this is likely to give the best results.

In line with his pluralistic approach, Ghaemi is a fervent advocate of the two-person model. He devotes the concluding pages of his book to this model.

The two-person model, as its name indicates, comprises two therapists: a psychiatrist who prescribes drugs, and a psychologist and/or social worker who provides psychotherapeutic services.[14] This model is gaining popularity particularly in the United States.

What are the advantages and downsides of the two-person model? There are two putative advantages of this model. The first one pertains to cost-effectiveness. As psychiatric services are more expensive than the services provided by psychologists and social workers, the economic rationale says that a psychiatrist sees a patient for medication management a few times yearly, and that non-medical therapists see them on a weekly or fort-nightly basis. (There is, however, no convincing evidence that the two-person model has a fundamental advantage.) The other putative advantage of this model is that it is vehicle of the pluralistic approach, its organizing basis.

And what are the downsides of this model? They have been elaborated in the paper "The fate of integrated treatment: whatever happened to the biopsychosocial psychiatrist" (2001) by Glen O. Gabbard and Jerald Kay.

I will mention only a few of them. First, two therapists, one in charge of the brain, the other in charge of the mind, suggests tacit acknowledgement of the appropriateness of Cartesian dualism. On the other hand, the one-person treatment model implicitly endorses an integration of mind and brain in both the psychiatrist's and the patient's perspective. Second, the therapeutic alliance between one patient and two therapists is less beneficial than the alliance between one patient and one therapist. Third, if the psychiatrist's role is reduced to the role of psychiatrist-prescriber, the patient is likely to experience medication treatment as something that has nothing to do with their mind and mental suffering, with an ensuing negative attitude towards medications in general and low adherence to prescribed medications in particular. Fourth, since health insurance companies are not ready to compensate therapists for the time they spend discussing about the patient, they quite often do not exchange opinions about the patients they treat, about how the treatment is going, what should be done to improve its efficacy, and so on. It is not uncommon for therapists dealing with the same patient to never meet and not know each other. Such a lack of communication between therapists cannot help but to have a negative impact on the treatment of a patient, and in some cases might even be harmful.

As stated, Ghaemi is a strong advocate of the two-person treatment model. His view of this model is rather radical.

Ghaemi writes: "There is absolutely no general reason why one treater would be better than two, three, or four. There is absolutely no general reason why a psychiatrist would provide better psychotherapy treatment than a psychologist or social worker. For that matter, there is no reason to assume that a psychiatrist would provide better psychopharmacology treatment than a highly skilled and experienced nurse practitioner. It all comes down to knowledge, experience, and conceptual clarity" (2003: 306).

I agree with Ghaemi's first assertion. Psychologists and/or psychiatric social workers who are well trained and skilful in providing psychotherapy might be therapeutically more successful than a psychiatrist who does not have additional psychotherapeutic training and/or experience. However, it is highly doubtful that a nurse, no matter how skilled and experienced, could know more about psychopharmacological treatment than a psychiatrist. The knowledge about neurochemistry, physiology, pathophysiology, neuroanatomy and pharmacology that a psychiatrist acquires during medical studies makes them much more knowledgeable about psychopharmacotherapy than a nurse.

Ghaemi points out that "the best treatment is provided by the most expert treater" (2003: 306) and adds that no single clinician can be extremely expert at more than one approach or method in psychiatry. For example, a psychopharmacologist is not equally competent at the psychopharmacological treatment of all kinds of mental disorders. There is no such a thing as a universally competent psychopharmacologist. A psychopharmacologist who is expert in the treatment of bipolar disorder can provide the best psychopharmacological treatment for people suffering from this kind of disorder. The same holds for psychotherapists. A psychotherapist who is highly qualified for the treatment of general anxiety disorder, for example, can provide the best psychotherapeutic services to those with this disorder. "The best outcome will arise from multiple treaters, each of whom is expert in what she or he does" (2003: 307).

In addition, empirical evidence about the kind of psychopharmacological or psychotherapeutic treatment that is the most effective should determine the choice of both the treatment and therapist. In other words, prior to the application of any kind of therapy, a decision is to be made regarding the kind of treatment and therapist. First, a decision is made on the basis of empirical evidence of which kind of treatment has proved the most successful in the management of that particular disorder. Second, a decision is made after searching through a list of therapists (both psychopharmacologists and psychotherapists) where they are classified according to their expertise in the management of particular disorders. If such a list exists at all!

Several questions arise in regard to the cited way of deciding which kind of therapy to administer and which therapist(s) to recruit.

First, there are several hundred types of psychotherapy today. In order to know which one gives the best results in the management of a particular disorder, one has to know how many kinds of psychotherapy have been tested in regard to their efficacy in the treatment of that particular disorder. In addition, bearing in mind that measuring the outcome of psychotherapy is not the best side of the studies dealing with the efficacy of psychotherapy, it is questionable whether a valid conclusion can be reached regarding which kind of psychotherapy is best suited to this or that kind of disorder.

Second, there are several hundred forms of mental disorder in DSMs. We are far from having experts, either psychopharmacologists or psychotherapists, able to manage hundreds of forms of mental disorder. So what should be done in those cases where there are no experts at treating them? Is the two-person model justified in these cases, or is its usefulness confined to people with mental disorder where experts have been confirmed and sanctioned in its management?

Third, if subspecialists in a specific type of treatment of a single mental disorder will be more in demand in years to come, and consequently the ambition of more and more psychiatrists will be to be experts at the management of only one disorder by only one therapeutic measure, we can expect in the not so distant future that there will be psychopharmacologists dealing only with Depression type I, or only Depression type II, or those who are the best in the management of Delusional Disorder, and those who are the most competent in the management of Schizophrenic Disorder? Or, along the same lines of reasoning, will there be psychotherapists who excel in the treatment of Generalized Anxiety Disorder, but are not as good in the management of Panic Disorder. (Given the rather frequent change of the names of psychiatric syndromes or entities, it will not be easy to make out which disorder a psychopharmacologist or psychotherapist excels in managing!)

Fourth, as comorbidity is ever more frequently diagnosed, does this mean that experts in the management of each single disorder should provide services to a patient who suffers simultaneously from more than one disorder? If the answer is in the affirmative, does this mean that the two-person model should, in those cases, be superseded by the four-person or the six-person model? (Two therapists for each disorder.)

Fifth, in how many regions around the world would it be possible to organize the provision of mental health care according to the principle of the two-person model? In how many countries are there experts in the management of particular disorders, and how many of them are available to those suffering from this or that kind of mental disorder? In other words, demanding that the best treatment should be provided by the most expert treater, however sensible it might sound, seems elitist in its assumption and fall-outs.

In addition, by advocating the two-person model, Ghaemi acknowledges that a psychiatrist is not able to skillfully master different methods originating from different psychiatric models. By the same token he affirms a division within psychiatry, regardless of whether one calls the existence of different models in psychiatry psychiatric conceptual cacophony or euphony.

Finally, although he presents himself as an advocate of pluralism, Ghaemi, judging by the last pages of his book, turns out to be more the supporter of the new perspectivism in the sense that Michael A. Schwartz and Osbrone P. Wiggins (1988) gave to this term, than a pluralist. When he says that empirical evidence will tell us which kind of treatment is the most efficient for a particular disorder, he actually installs "positivist method of inquiry as the only acceptable one." As Gheami knows, empirical evidence cannot be obtained without the use of statistical analyses of clinical trials of groups of patients, without "highly specified techniques and procedures, careful definitions, standardization, treatment manuals, and the like." And these procedures and techniques are an integral part of the hypothetic-deductive approach, and more broadly of the medical model.

Pragmatic Approach

David H. Brendel is the author of the pragmatic approach in psychiatry. He has presented his ideas in several papers published in journals such as "Harvard Review of Psychiatry," "Journal of Clinical Ethics," "Journal of Medicine and Philosophy" and "Philosophy, Psychiatry and Psychology." The book *Healing Psychiatry. Bridging the Science/Humanism Divide* (2006) is his major work.

There are a few authors—for example, Arnold Goldberg (2002), George J. Agich (2002) and Peter Zachar (2002)—who have written along similar lines as Brendel.

On the basis of Brendel's educational background, one might say that he is the right person to articulate a concept that will heal psychiatry, meaning that he will resolve "the conceptual dichotomy between science and humanism so that patients in the twenty-first century can receive the best possible mental health care" (2006: 3). Brendel graduated in medicine and philosophy. He also completed a specialization in psychiatry. He works at Harvard Medical School, at McLean Hospital, Massachusetts General Hospital and the Boston Psychoanalytic Institute.

Brendel first states that it is opportune to criticize both the view of those who endorse a scientific approach and the view of those who favor a humanistic approach in psychiatry. When talking about the former he means the medical approach, and when discussing the latter he has in mind the psychological, mostly psychoanalytical approach. Brendel claims that in *Of Two Minds: Growing Disorder in American Psychiatry* (2000) Tanya M. Luhrmann has provided an accurate account of the deep divide in American psychiatry between those who espouse the scientific-empirical approach and those who are the proponents of a humanistic stance.

Brendel believes that he has found a remedy that will help cure psychiatry. *Pragmatism* is the name of the remedy. "It is by way of clinical pragmatism that the conceptual wounds in psychiatry and the emotional wounds in the lives of individuals can begin to heal" (2006: 6).

According to pragmatism, to remind the reader, explanations are valid if they are useful, if they provide benefit. The practical usefulness of a concept is the only reliable indicator of its truthfulness.

Brendel is of the opinion that philosophical pragmatism, which originated in the United States and has its proponents in William James, John Dewey, and Charles S. Pierce, provides principles and instruments which psychiatrists can use to bridge the divide between science and humanism, a divide that drags psychiatry backward.

Brendel is right when he writes that it is the attitude of psychiatrists towards the said divide and their ability to bridge it that will determine the quality of mental health care, research and education in the mental health field in the twenty-first century. It is not only a theoretical and practical matter but also an ethical issue because psychiatrists have a professional and ethical obligation to provide the best possible assistance to patients. And such assistance is presumed on bridging the divide between science and humanism. Hence those who ignore or pay lip service to the need to cross the divide behave unethically.

Brendel has recognized instruments in the four major principles of pragmatism that will lead psychiatry out of the crisis in which it has been for a long time. To be able to heal wounds psychiatrists have to nurture the following approaches: practical, pluralistic, participatory, and provisional. If they do that they will provide patients the best possible care.

I will analyze each of these principles (approaches) in turn. Their implementation, according to Brendel, shows how pragmatism can help psychiatry to address its foreboding disintegration.

Practical approach. Brendel writes: "Clinical psychiatrists ought to regard their theories not as ends in themselves but rather as tools for dealing with the practical challenges they confront each day in the clinic" (2006: 38). No matter how good a concept or theory sounds, only practical consequences matter. "Psychiatric explanations are coherent and plausible," Brendel adds, "insofar as they are effective in the course of clinical care and are subjected to continual questioning, testing, and reassessment" (2006: 38).

Pluralistic approach. There is considerable proof that biological, psychological and social-cultural factors co-determine the origin of mental disorders, their clinical presentation and outcome. Therefore, only an approach that is pluralistic, meaning an approach that comprises all the sides of mental disorders, is well-grounded. In other words, the principles of all three models (medical, psychological, social-cultural) should be applied. These models are complementary because each of them is focused on one dimension of the mentally disordered. The weak points of individual models should not be a reason to shun them. Each model should be acknowledged for the specific knowledge it provides, regardless of its downsides. And there is no psychiatric model that is not useful, i.e., helpful to some extent and in some regards.

"Clinical judgment, of course is very difficult to define, but its core elements would include evidence-based hypothesis formation, consideration of a wide range of diagnostic possibilities, careful observation of a broad spectrum of clinical phenomena, flexibility to revise a clinical formulation on the basis of new evidence, and open-mindedness to consultation with other colleagues in situations that are characterized by complexity, confusion, and uncertainty" (2006: 40).

The pluralistic approach should enable psychiatrists to find a conceptual synthesis of differing positions of individual models. What is important is to strike the optimal balance between scientific and humanistic views.

Participatory approach. The patient and possibly those who are close to them should partake in designing the therapeutic plan. The psychiatrist's opinion alone about what the therapeutic plan should be like does not suffice. The patient's view, as well as the view of those they live with, has to be taken into consideration. If the patient participated in defining the therapeutic plan, they are more likely to accept it and implement it. The same holds for people living with the patient. If they have a say in the articulation of the plan, they will more easily understand it, in particular its usefulness. Also they will more readily support the patient in the implementation of the plan, and will be more willing to monitor how strictly the patient follows therapeutic guidelines. Briefly said, a deliberative and collaborative approach is a genuine possibility for psychiatry.

Provisional approach. Pragmatism says that there are no ever-enduring truths, that concepts that proved unhelpful in the past might prove helpful in the future. Correspondingly, psychiatrists should not be fully committed to a particular view and believe that there is no other and never will be any other more useful view that will profit patients. New discoveries might easily make flawed a concept which we believe to be so congruent to reality that we take it for granted. A critical view of reality makes us humble and cognizant of how tentative beliefs arc. The conviction that a concept will withstand the test of time is by and large futile.

The reader of the preceding lines rightly wonders what pragmatism offers to psychiatry that is new, what is the point in applying the principles of pragmatism in psychiatry, how can pragmatism help psychiatry heal the wounds caused by the science/humanism divide. Before Brendel taught us this, we knew that good practice is the best theory. There was no need to tell us that no model can encompass the totality of mental illness. There is also nothing new in the assertion that a paternalistic attitude towards the mentally disordered is harmful and that the patients themselves and those living with them should be included in the therapeutic process and in particular in the so-called resocialization of the mentally ill. Finally, all those who have read the history of psychiatry or have been in psychiatry for several decades know quite well that nothing is durable in the world of psychiatric ideas about the origin and nature of mental disorders and the best possible treatment.

Brendel fell short of answering the key question, the importance of which he clearly pointed out: how would it be possible to resolve, or to use his phrase to heal the deep wounds that the confronting conceptual approaches have left on the face of psychiatry (Brendel, 2004), conceptual wounds that have resulted from dividing the human individual into an object of scientific scrutiny and a subject of personal experience.

In order to show that pragmatic psychiatry does not offer anything new, least of all a fix for the conceptual cacophony in psychiatry, I will present Brendel's recommendations about what a pragmatic psychiatrist should do when someone in need approaches them. First, they focus on achieving the possible treatment outcome, and do not wonder whether or not they are doing their job according to the principles of a particular model. Second, their approach is pluralistic; it includes the consideration of both scientific data and the patient's specific existential (psychological, interpersonal) position. Third, they ask the patient and whenever possible those who live with them or are close to them, to partake in deciding what kind of approach is satisfactory and useful, and if this is the patient's request, they integrate two or more models. Fourth, they acknowledge that any decision they have made, any plan they have formulated is only provisional in view of the long-term treatment. "This pragmatic model may entail a creative combination of psychotherapy and psychopharmacology, which is increasingly recognized by both psychotherapists and psychopharmacologists as more efficacious in many situations than either modality alone" (Brendel, 2004).

Brendel's effort to formulate pragmatic psychiatry is worthwhile. However, he does not explain how psychiatrists will deal with combining or harmonizing the principles and treatment techniques of different models in everyday practice. When I say "how psychiatrists will deal with" I mean how can psychiatrists be equally good at providing pharmacotherapeutic and psychotherapeutic services, how can they reconcile antagonistic positions of the medical and the psychological model, or in Brendel's terms, how can psychiatrists heal the wounds created by scientific/humanistic discord? The above-mentioned principles or approaches of pragmatic psychiatry do not teach psychiatrists how to achieve this noble goal.

There is no better way to show how hard it is to carry out the *devoirs* which, according to Brendel, a psychiatrist should perform in the process of diagnosing and treating patients, than to cite Brendel himself. "The pragmatic psychiatrist will make use of every applicable explanatory concept along the biopsychosocial continuum in order to collaborate with patients toward the goal of achieving integrative and beneficial treatment outcomes. This pursuit will heed and incorporate any scientific evidence that may apply to the clinical situation at hand, but will do so in a flexible, interactive way, and humanistic fashion. It can and ought to be done without falling into the trap of postmodernism's lack of theoretical and practical clarity" (2006: 48). It sounds good as a goal, a norm, a declaration. But the question arises as to will psychiatrists be able to make use of every applicable concept that emerges in biomedical or somatic psychiatry, in psychological psychiatry and social psychiatry? First of all, will they be able to follow all the innovations in the cited fields; second, will they be able to learn how to apply them; third, will they be able to reconcile different concepts and practices of the different and antagonistic models that are covered by the notion of biopsychosocial continuum?

In the introductory part of his book Brendel admits that "at this time, unfortunately, there is no well-defined and widely accepted third option that navigates between both sides of the science/humanism divide" (2006: 23). And it is not "forces in contemporary sciences (and in society in general)" that are to be blamed for the lack of a well-defined and widely accepted third option, as Brendel claims, but rather the fact that a mentally disturbed person lives in two worlds and there is no all-encompassing concept of both the mentally ill and the mentally sound, of mental disorder and mental health. Only such a concept, or concepts, can pave the way towards a psychiatric *supermodel* which will harmonize and above all unite opposing psychiatric models.

By its basic assumptions and the design of its practice, provided by Brendel, pragmatic psychiatry certainly is not such a sought-after third option, or supermodel. Pragmatic psychiatry is but one of many failed attempts to resolve the psychiatric conceptual cacophony or appease it at the very least.

Conclusion

There are many models in psychiatry. They are largely opposed and even mutually exclusive in terms of epistemology, conceptualization of the genesis of mental disorders and prescribing the most efficient type of treatment.

The existence of a great many models is not common in other medical disciplines. This is one of the specificities of psychiatry. In no medical discipline other than psychiatry is it appropriate to ask about a particular doctor's theoretical-practical orientation. On the other hand, prior to seeking psychiatric help, it is recommendable to get information about the model that potential care provider espouses.

There is no scientific or any other evidence that any model is superior to others in regard to how its proponents interpret the origin of mental disorders and treat those who suffer from them. That is one of the key reasons why all models are legitimate. The truth is that in various periods no more than one or two models have been considered as the most plausible. Nevertheless, the dominance of one or two models at a particular time, caused mostly by social circumstances and financial interests, has not made other models totally obsolete.

The result is conceptual cacophony as a stumbling block, or one of the stumbling blocks, in psychiatry. It is such a powerful disintegrating force within psychiatry that the future of psychiatry greatly depends on whether psychiatric conceptual heterogeneity will be resolved or at least reduced.

Moreover, conceptual discord tarnishes the public image of psychiatry and psychiatrists. Thus, Neil McLaren maintains that comparatively frequent changes of the dominant model in psychiatry prevent people from taking psychiatry seriously. "On the theoretical basis of psychiatry there is no agreement," writes McLaren. "Granted, the dominant approach to mental disorder today that is termed biological psychiatry ... tomorrow could see yet another of the vertiginous swings which have characterized psychiatry for the past one hundred years. These types of swings have led some perfectly sensible people to ask why they should take psychiatry seriously" (2007: X).

Conceptual cacophony has a negative impact on relations within the psychiatric community as well. Professional communication is in a fair number of cases is confined to practitioners of one and the same model. Those who are committed to the cause of a particular model are quite often not keen on learning what their colleagues on the other side of the fence think about a particular patient, which kind of problems they face, how far they have gone in detecting pathways leading to mental illness. There is no doubt that such a state of affairs within the psychiatric community hinders dialogue between the holders of different views. And it is dialogue rather than its absence that might assist psychiatrists in their efforts to bridge the science/humanist divide.

Even though mental disorder does not include the impairment of all mental functions, one might say that a mentally disturbed person is disturbed in all aspects of their existence. Therefore, an approach that respects the complexity of human beings has the greatest chance of proving helpful. By focusing only on one aspect of the mentally ill people individual psychiatric models have missed that chance.

Attempts to define a new approach that would correct the deficiencies of the individual models (the biopsychosocial model, pluralistic approach, pragmatic approach) have not provided a satisfactory response embraced by most psychiatrists to the psychiatric conceptual puzzle. Eclecticism is not a seemly option, either.

As far as the creation of conceptual unity is concerned, psychiatry is at a dead-end at this stage. The most worrisome thing is that the majority of psychiatrists are not aware of the extent of the damage caused by conceptual cacophony. They simply ignore both the conceptual cacophony and the damage it has done.

In "Introduction" to *Philosophical Issues in Psychiatry. Explanations, Phenomenology, and Nosology* Kenneth S. Kendler writes: "How can we develop a frame of reference in which we can anchor our multiple perspectives, lest our pluralism degenerate into a disorganized list of facts that could more confuse than enlighten?" (2008: 5).

My answer to this question would be that, at this stage, nothing suggests that psychiatrists are likely to develop such a frame of reference any time soon.

Notes

1. Aaron Lazare (1973) mentions four models: *the medical, the psychological, the behavioral* and *the social*. Paul R. MacHugh and Philip R. Slavney, in the book *The Perspectives of Psychiatry* (1983) agree with Lazare as far as the number of psychiatric models is concerned, but dub them differently: *the concept of disease, the concept of dimensions, the concept of behaviors, and the concept of life stories*. Miriam Siegler and Humphry Osmond, in their book *Models of Medicine, Models of Madness* (1974), take schizophrenia as a paradigm of mental disorder, and enumerate eight models of mental disorders: *the medical model, the moral model, the impaired model, the psychoanalytic model, the social model, the psychedelic model, the conspiratorial model, the family interaction model*. Thaddeus Weckowicz, in the book entitled *Models of Mental Illness. Systems and Theories of Abnormal Psychology* (1984), talks about two groups of psychiatric models. *Medical* and *psychological models* constitute the first group. Weckowicz holds that these models are scientific models. *Philosophical-moral models* constitute the second group. *The philosophical-moral models* are: *the philosophical-hermeneutical model, the phenomenological-existential model, the humanistic model* and *the moral-legal model*. Peter Tyrer and Derek Steinberg, in the book entitled *Models of Mental Disorder* (1987), cite four psychiatric models: *the disease model, the psychodynamic model, the behavioral model*, and *the social model*. Sanford L. Drob, in the paper "The dilemma of contemporary psychiatry" (1989) mentions the following approaches or orientations within psychiatry: *biological psychiatry, behavioral psychiatry, cognitive theories, family-systems approaches, psychodynamic approaches*, and *existential-interpersonal psychiatry*. Peter Zachar and Kenneth S. Kendler, in the text "Psychiatric disorders: a conceptual taxonomy" (2007) mention two psychiatric models: the medical model and alternative models of psychiatric disorders. There are four versions of the medical model: the organic disease model, the altered function model, the biopsychosocial model, and the harmful dysfunction model. And there are "several alternative models of psychiatric disorder that adopt positions on the dimensions of categorization not taken by the medical models": two different uses of nominalism, dimensional models, and the practical kinds of model.

2. Rachel Cooper suggests that it is possible to have multiple paradigms in mental health because there is an abundance of investigators in these areas. In her view, "when only a small number of scientists work in some discipline, the whole community has to work under one paradigm for progress to be made." Today, the sheer number of mental health professionals who conduct research means that multiple paradigms can be supported (2007: 89). I disagree. In the first place is there any relationship between the number of professionals in a discipline and the number of paradigms in it? Indeed, there is only one paradigm in many disciplines and sub-disciplines that have many more professionals than psychiatry has. As the number of mental health professionals increases every year, does this mean, following Cooper's line of reasoning, that the "reason that it is possible to have multiple paradigms in mental health" is getting weightier as well?

3. Michael A. Schwartz and Osborne P. Wiggins write: "What is crucial is the *openness* of the psychiatrist toward *various* interpretations: the facts pertaining to the patient may make sense within one perspective, but they may make better sense within another. And we wish to emphasize that by speaking of such 'openness' we do not mean a passive attitude of receptivity to whatever may disclose itself. We mean rather an active attitude of alertness and vigilance.... In many cases, of course, it may seem 'obvious' that one perspective rather than the others makes better sense of the patient's distress. But this 'obviousness' in order not to be carelessness, must

issue from the long experience of a psychiatrist who has acquired such a facility in applying the four perspectives that he or she can quickly recognize the data that fall within one rather than the others." (1988, emphasis in the original)

I agree, the openness of psychiatrists toward various interpretations is *crucial*. But it is just this kind of openness that is lacking in most psychiatrists' practice. Moreover, how many psychiatrists have acquired "a facility in applying the four different perspectives that he or she can quickly recognize the data that fall within one rather than the others?" It is also questionable whether the long experience of a psychiatrist makes him or her more or less alert to different perspectives. It is not so rare that psychiatrists who have practiced for many years become more entrenched into one model than psychiatric novices.

4. Assen Jablensky observes that "over-valued beliefs and nostrums are not uncommon in medicine, but perhaps nowhere do so many ideologies flourish as in psychiatry" (2010).

5. The pervasive contemporary pluralism is not specific to psychiatry. Psychology has been facing up to the same problem for decades. Frederick J. Wertz addressed this issue in the paper "Multiple methods in psychology: Epistemological grounding and the possibility of unity" (1990). Wertz writes: "Pluralism in psychology has a long history of being viewed as a core disciplinary problem in that fragmentation leads to incompatible knowledge claims and incompatible results..., leaving us without a clear, integrated picture of psychological life, hence disciplinary incoherence. The 'hodge podge of methods' (Yanchar, 1997: 152) leads us into an epistemic relativism in which we lack overarching rules for evaluating knowledge claims...."

    After stating that the methodological pluralism has become a disciplinary nightmare Wertz, on a half-optimistic, half-pessimistic note, maintains: "Even though that the solutions to these difficult disciplinary challenges are available, I do not expect a consensus to be forthcoming anytime soon."

6. Ahmed Okasha, formerly president of World Psychiatric Association, in the Foreword to *Oxford Textbook of Philosophy and Psychiatry* by K.W.M. (Bill) Fulford, Tim Thornton and George Graham, refers to Kendler (2001) who said that the psychiatrist traverses many times the mind-brain divide, and adds: "Therefore, as a discipline, psychiatry should be deeply interested in the mind-body problem, the answer to which, if there is one, cannot be sought without help from philosophy" (2006: XXIX).

7. Allen J. Frances recently remarked along the same lines: "The good news is that the remarkable revolutions in neuroscience, molecular biology, and genetics over the past three decades have given us great insights into the functioning of the normal brain. The bad news is that out understanding of psychopathology is fairly primitive and may remain so for some time. With apologies to Tolstoy's *Anna Karenina*, it appears that normal brains tend to be normal in more or less the same way, while the causes of psychopathology are likely to be wildly heterogeneously complex. Although there have been many tantalizing putative biological findings for particular disorders, all reflect no more than group mean differences and none has achieved anything close to the needed sensitivity and specificity to qualify as a diagnostic test. Thus, it is obvious that our field lacks the fundamental understanding of pathogenesis that will be required before we can take the next meaningful step forward towards a paradigm-shift etiological model of diagnosis" (2009a).

8. It is hard to explain why Rachel Cooper included psychoanalysis in "psy-sciences," that is, multi-paradigm sciences. Psychoanalysis is mono-paradigm science, if science at all. Cooper herself uses psychoanalysis as an example of mono-paradigm science in her book *Psychiatry and the Philosophy of Science* (2007: 95).

9. Now and then some authors are keen on negating the reductionist character of the medical model. That is the case with, for example, Premal Shah and Deborah Mountain. They define the medical model in the paper entitled "The medical model is dead—long live the medical model," that was published in the British Journal of Psychiatry. "The 'medical' model is a process whereby, informed by the best available evidence, doctors advise on, coordinate or deliver interventions for health improvement" (2007). When the medical model is defined as loosely and vaguely as Shah and Mountain did, any pros and cons about the medical model are senseless.

10. K.W.M. (Bill) Fulford and Anthony Colombo write about different approaches of various psychiatric team members as follows: "Doctors approach mental disorders on the model of physical diseases (in terms of symptoms, syndromes, and test results); social workers find medical diagnoses 'labels', unhelpful, focusing rather on the social context of mental distress; psychologists are interested in behaviour (bodily and cognitive) and their contingencies; psychotherapists understand mental distress and disorder in terms of partially hidden affect and conation; and family therapists work by reference to family systems" (2004).

11. Paul R. McHugh and Phillip R. Slavney defined the notion of perspective as "channel of knowledge which reveals certain aspects of patients while obscuring others" (1983: 3), and Michael A. Schwartz and Osborne P. Wiggins as "fundamentally different modes of conceptualization and reasoning" (1988).

12. Roy R. Grinker's definition of *eclecticism* in his paper "Struggle for eclecticism" (1964) clearly shows the vagueness of this notion. Grinker writes that he and the people who worked with him realized, in the 1950s, the limitation of the psychoanalytical approach. This prompted them to introduce in educational curricula, apart from psychodynamic theory, milieu therapy, group therapy, family dynamics, basic principles of biology, genetics including social psychiatry, as well. Such their ideas brought them into conflict with the dominant attitude in psychiatry at that time, "and also brought us," writes Grinker, "into a struggle for what I should call, for want of a better name, eclecticism. It is our attempt to preserve what is valuable, question what is doubtful, and reject what is useless, not only in the psychodynamic-psychoanalytic field but in all others" (1964). It sounds good, but it is imprecise.

13. S. Nassir Ghaemi shares this opinion of the biopsychosocial model. Ghaemi, in the "Introduction" to the second edition of the book *Psychiatric Movements. From Sects to Science* (2005) by Leston L. Havens, writes: "Psychiatry today is adrift. Both dogmatisms of psychoanalysis and biological psychiatry have shown their inadequacies over the last century. The biopsychosocial model is a poor compromise. It fails to give guidance to clinicians about what to do for specific conditions, in specific circumstances, for specific patients" (2005: XIII).

14. The distinction should be made between the two-person treatment model and combined therapy (pharmacotherapy plus psychotherapy). The difference is that in the case of the two-person treatment a psychopharmacologist provides pharmacological, and a psychotherapist provides psychotherapeutic services to one and the same patient. As for combined treatment, if it is not specified that it is the two-person model, then one and the same therapist provides both kinds of services.

There is a huge body of literature indicating that combined therapy is more efficient than monotherapy. See, among others, the following writings: Hogarthy, G.E., Anderson, C.M., Reiss, D.J. et al. (1991) "Family psychoeducation, social skills training, and maintenance chemotherapy in the aftercare treatment of schizophrenia, II: two-year effects of a controlled study on relapse and adjustment"; Keller, M.B., McCullough, J.P., Klein, D.N. et al. (2000) "A comparison of nefazodone, the cognitive behavioral-analysis system of psychotherapy, and their combination for the treatment of chronic depression"; Thase, M.A., Greenhouse, J.B., Frank, E. (1997) "Treatment of major depression with psychotherapy or psychotherapy-pharmacotherapy combinations."

5

Ending and Beginning

I have pointed out a significant share of controversies and dilemmas in contemporary psychiatry.

The controversies and dilemmas in psychiatry are determined by various factors. That is why there is no solution of the type one-size-fits-all. Psychiatrists are unable to influence some of them (e. g., the nature of a person with mental disorder; how mental disorders are expressed). A second group is more of a matter for philosophers than psychiatrists (e. g., articulation of the mind-body relationship). A third group will probably be resolved by the discovery of the organic basis of most mental disorders (e. g., diagnostics and the classifications of mental disorders). The contradictions belonging to the fourth group are more artificial than real. For example, some of them could be removed by psychiatrists' acknowledgment of one of the social roles they perform, the role of the agents of social control.

Only those who have little knowledge of psychiatry or too much faith in psychiatry can expect psychiatrists to resolve all controversies and dilemmas in psychiatry. As the reader has seen, psychiatry is fraught with controversies and dilemmas; probably more than any other medical discipline. They are trade-mark of psychiatry. With a bit of exaggeration one can say that if we take controversies and dilemmas out of psychiatry there will be not much psychiatry left.

To designate and analyze the quandaries in psychiatry does not mean to put psychiatry in question. It should rather be the mark of a reflective view of psychiatry.

Critics of psychiatry of whatever orientation challenge the basics of psychiatry, its foundation. They blow up—one might say, abuse—the imperfections of psychiatry so as to dismiss it.

On the other hand, there are psychiatrists—and their number is quite large— who turn a blind eye to the controversies and dilemmas in psychiatry. If they are aware of them they choose to ignore them. If they are not aware of them they are reluctant to hear people talking about them. In any case, rosy is the only color in which they see psychiatry.

This book is a defense of psychiatry against both critics of psychiatry and those who are short of a critical view of the job they do. It is a defense of psychiatry against *psychiatry iconoclasts* and *psychiatry iconoclasters* (or iconophiles).

If the book induces some to look for other controversies and dilemmas in psychiatry, or to try to resolve some of those which I found difficult to solve, or to look for a more appropriate answer to those whose solution I expounded, it has fulfilled its purpose.

References

Abroms, E. M. 1983. "Beyond eclecticism," *American Journal of Psychiatry* 140: 740-745.

Agich, G. A. 2002. "Implications of a pragmatic theory of disease for the DSMs," in J. Z. Sadler (ed.) *Descriptions and prescriptions: values, mental disorders, and the DSMs*. Baltimore: The Johns Hopkins University Press, pp. 96-113.

American Psychiatric Association. 1980. *Diagnostic and Statistical Manual of Mental Disorders*, third edition, DSM-III. Washington, DC: American Psychiatric Association.

American Psychiatric Association. 1994. *Diagnostic and Statistical Manual of Mental Disorders*, fourth edition, DSM-VI. Washington, DC: American Psychiatric Association.

American Psychiatric Association. 2000. *Diagnostic and Statistical Manual of Mental Disorders*, fourth edition, DSM-IV-TR. Washington, DC: American Psychiatric Association.

American Psychiatric Association. 2010. DSM-5 Development. http://www.dsm5.org/Pages/Default.aspx

Andreasen, N.C. 1995. "Validation of psychiatric diagnoses: New models and approaches," *American Journal of Psychiatry* 152: 161-162.

Angermeyer, M.C. 2000. "Schizophrenia and violence," *Schizophrenia Bulletin* 102 (suppl. 407): 63-67.

Angermeyer, M. C., and S. Dietrich. 2006. "Public beliefs about and attitudes towards people with mental illness: A review of population studies," *Acta Psychiatrica Scandinavica* 133: 163-179.

Aragona, M. 2009. "The concept of mental disorder and the DSM-V," *Dialogues in Philosophy, Mental and Neuro Sciences* 2: 1-14.

Arboleda-Florez, J. 2003. "Considerations on the stigma of mental illness," *Canadian Journal of Psychiatry* 48: 645-650.

Ausubel, D. 1961. "Personality disorder is a disease," *American Psychologist* 16: 69-74.

Bastide, R. 1965. *Sociologie des maladies mentales*. Paris: Flammarion.

Bauer, J.J., D.P. McAdams, and J.L. Palls. 2008. "Narrative identity and eudaimonic well-being," *Journal of Happiness Studies* 9: 81-104.

Beigel, A. 1995. "A proposed vision for psychiatry at the turn of the century," *Comprehensive Psychiatry* 36: 31-39.

Bentall, R. 2004. *Madness Explained. Psychosis and Human Nature*. New York: Penguin.

Bentall, R. 2009. *Doctoring the Mind. Why Psychiatric Treatments Fail*. London: Allen Lane.

Bertelsen, M., P. Jeppesen, L. Petersen *et al.* 2008. "Five-year follow-up of a randomized multicenter trial of intensive early intervention vs. standard treatment for patients with a first episode of psychotic illness," *Archives of General Psychiatry* 65: 762-771.

Biswas-Diener, R., and E. Diener. 2001. "Making the best of a bad situation. Satisfaction in the slums of Calcutta," *Social Indicators Research* 55: 392-352.

Biswas-Diener, R., T.B. Kashdan, and L.A. King 2009. "Two traditions of happiness research, not two distinct types of happiness," *Journal of Positive Psychology* 4: 208-211.

Bloch, S. 1997. "Psychiatry: an impossible profession?," *Australian and New Zealand Journal of Psychiatry* 31: 172-183.

Boehm, W.W. 1955. "The role of psychiatric social work in mental health," in A.M. Rose (ed.) *Mental Health and Mental Disorder*. New York: Norton.

Bolton, D. 2008. *What is Mental Illness? An Essay in Philosophy, Science, and Values.* Oxford: Oxford University Press.

Boorse, C. 1975. "On the distinction between disease and illness," *Philosophy and Public Affairs* 5: 49-68.

Boorse, C. 1976. "What a theory of mental health should be," *International Journal for the Theory of Social Behavior* 6: 61-84.

Bowers, L. 1998. *The Social Nature of Mental Illness*. London: Routledge.

Bracken, P., and P. Thomas. 2005. *Postpsychiatry*. Oxford: Oxford University Press.

Brendel, D.H. 2004. "Healing psychiatry: a pragmatic approach to bridging the science/humanism divide," *Harvard Review of Psychiatry* 12: 150-157.

Brendel, D.H. 2006. *Healing Psychiatry. Bridging the Science/Humanism Divide.* Cambridge, MA: MIT Press.

Brock, G., and Q.D. Atkinson. 2008. "What can examining the psychology of nationalism tell us about our prospects for aiming at the cosmopolitan vision?," *Ethic Theory and Moral Practice* 11: 165-179.

Brown, P. 1987. "Diagnostic conflict and contradiction in psychiatry," *Journal of Health and Social Behavior* 28: 37-50.

Brown, P. 1989. "Psychiatric dirty work revisited: Conflicts in servicing non-psychiatric agencies," *Journal of Contemporary Ethnography* 2: 182-201.

Brown, P., and B. Tierney. 2009. "Religion and subjective well-being among the elderly in China," *Journal of Socio-Economics* 38: 310-319.

Bullmore, E., Fletcher, P., and Jones, P.B. 2009. "Why psychiatry can't afford to be neurophobic," *British Journal of Psychiatry* 194: 293-5.

Bushfield, J. 1986. *Managing Madness. Changing Ideas and Practice.* London: Hutchinson.

Byrne, P. 2001. "Psychiatric stigma," *British Journal of Psychiatry* 178: 281-284.

Campbell, T. 1983. "Two distinct routes beyond kin selection to ultrasociality: Implications for the humanities and social sciences," in D. Bridgeman (ed.) *The Nature of Prosocial Development: Theories and Strategies*. New York: Academic Press, pp. 11-41.

Cannon, T. D., B. Cornblatt, and P. McGorry. 2007. "Editor's introduction: The empirical status of ultra-high risk (prodromal) research paradigm," *Schizophrenia Bulletin* 33: 661-664.

Caroll, J. 2007. "Most Americans are 'very satisfied' with their personal lives," *Gallup Daily News*, December 31.

Carpenter, W.T. 2009. "Anticipating DSM-V: Should psychosis risk become a diagnostic class?," *Schizophrenia Bulletin* 35: 841-843.

Carver, C.S., and M.F. Scheier. 1999. "Origins and functions of positive and negative affect: A control-process view," *Psychological Review* 97: 19-35.

Cavenar, J.O. Jr., and I. Walker. 1983. "Normality," in J.O. Cavenar, Jr. and H.K.H. Brodie (eds.) *Signs and Symptoms in Psychiatry*. Philadelphia: J.B. Lippincott, pp. 19-36.

Chang, M.M., and G. Bidder. 1985. "Noncomparability of research results that are related to psychiatric diagnosis," *Comprehensive Psychiatry* 26: 195-207.

Chedru, F., F. Feldman, and A. Ameri *et al.* 1996. "Visual and auditory hallucinations in a psychologically normal woman," *Lancet* 28 September, 348.

Chou, K., and K. Mak. 1998. "Attitudes to mental patients among Hong Kong Chinese: A trend study over 2 years," *International Journal of Social Psychiatry* 44: 215-224.

Clinton, H.R. 2000. "Mental disease is a disease," in T.L. Roleff, and L. Egendrof (eds.) *Mental Illness. Opposing Viewpoints*. San Diego, CA: Greenhaven Press.

Cloninger, R.C. 1999. "A new conceptual paradigm from genetics and psychobiology for the science of mental health," *Australian and New Zealand Journal of Psychiatry* 33: 174-186.

Cloninger, R.C. 2004. *Feeling Good: The Science of Well-Being*. New York: Oxford University Press.

Cloninger, R.C. 2006. "The science of well-being: An integrated approach to mental health and its disorders," *World Psychiatry* 5: 71-76.

Cohen, H. 1955. "The evolution of the concept of disease," *Proceedings of the Royal Society of Medicine* 48: 155-160.

Coleman, J.V. 1971. "Adaptive integration of psychiatric symptoms in ego regulation," *Archives of General Psychiatry* 24: 17-21.

Colombo, A., G. Bendelow, B. Fulford *et al.* 2003. "Evaluating the influence of implicit models of mental disorder on processes of shared decision making within community-based multi-disciplinary teams," *Social Science and Medicine* 56: 1557-1570.

Colvin, C.R., and J. Block. 1994a. "Do positive illusions foster mental health? An examination of the Taylor and Brown formulation," *Psychological Bulletin* 116: 3-20.

Colvin, C.R., and J. Block. 1994b. "Positive illusions and well-being revisited: Separating fiction from fact," *Psychological Bulletin* 116: 28.

Conrad, D.C. 1952. "Toward a more productive concept of mental health," *Mental Hygiene* 36: 456-466.

Cooper, J.E., R.E. Kendell, B. Gurland, *et al.* 1972. *Psychiatric Diagnosis in New York and London*. Maudsley Monograph No. 20. London: Oxford University Press.

Cooper, R. 2007. *Psychiatry and Philosophy of Science*. Stocksfield: Acumen.

Corrigan, P. W., and D.L. Penn. 1999. "Lessons from social psychology on discrediting psychiatric stigma," *American Psychologist* 54: 765-776.

Culver, C.M., and B. Gert. 1982. *Philosophy in Medicine. Conceptual and Ethical Issues in Medicine and Psychiatry*. Oxford: Oxford University Press.

Deci, E.L., and R.M. Ryan. 2008. "Hedonia, eudaimonia, and well-being: An introduction," *Journal of Happiness Studies* 9: 1-11.

De Koning, M.B., O.J.N. Bloemen, T.A.M.J. van Amlsvoort *et al.* 2009. "Early intervention in patients at ultra high risk of psychosis: benefits and risks," *Acta Psychiatrica Scandinavica* 119: 426-442.

Demjaha, A., K. Morgan, C. Morgan *et al.* 2009. "Combining dimensional and categorical representation of psychosis: The way forward for DSM-V and ICD-11," *Psychological Medicine* 39: 1943-1955.

Denys, D. 2007. "How new is the new philosophy of psychiatry?," *Philosophy, Ethics and Humanities in Medicine* 2:22.

De Rosa, L.M.C., and A. Fiorello. 2004. "Perception of patients' unpredictability and beliefs on the cause and consequences of schizophrenia," *Social Psychiatry and Psychiatric Epidemiology* 39: 410-416.

DeRubeis, R.J., G.J. Siegle, and S.D. Hollon, 2008. "Cognitive therapy versus medication for depression: treatment outcomes and neural mechanisms," *Nature Reviews Neuroscience* 9: 788-796.

Devereux, G. 1970. *Essais d'ethnopsychiatrie générale*. Paris: Gallimard.

Devereux, G. 1980. "Normal and abnormal," in G. Devereux (ed.) *Basic Problems of Ethnopsychiatry*. Chicago and London: The University of Chicago Press, pp. 3-71.

Devereux, G. 1980. "Ethnopsychiatry as a frame of reference in clinical research and practice," in G. Devereux (ed.) *Basic Problems of Ethnopsychiatry*. Chicago and London: The University of Chicago Press, pp. 72-90.

Dew, R.E. 2009. "Why psychiatry is the hardest specialty," *American Journal of Psychiatry* 166: 16-17.

Dewhurst, D.I., and P.B. Watson, 1996. "Unity and diversity in psychiatry: Some philosophical issues," *Australian and New Zealand Journal of Psychiatry* 30: 382-391.

Dhossche, D., R. Ferdinand, J. van der Ende *et al.* 2002. "Diagnostic outcome of self-reported hallucinations in a community sample of adolescents," *Psychological Medicine* 32: 619-627.

Diener, E. 1984. "Subjective well-being," *Psychological Bulletin* 95: 542-575.

Diener, E. 1995. "Subjective well-being in cross-cultural perspective," in H. Grad, A. Blanco, and J. Georgas (eds.) *Key issues in cross-cultural psychology*. Lisse: Swets and Zeitlinger, pp. 319-338.

Diener, E., and C. Diener. 1996. "Most people are happy," *Psychological Science* 7: 171-185.

Diener, E., E.M. Suh, and S. Oishi. 1997. "Recent findings on subjective well-being," *Indian Journal of Clinical Psychology* 25: 25-41.

Drob, S.L. 1989. "The dilemma of contemporary psychiatry," *American Journal of Psychotherapy* 43: 54-67.

Eaton, W.W., A. Romanoski, J.C Anthony *et al.* 1991. "Screening for psychosis in the general population with a self-report interview," *Journal of Nervous and Mental Disease* 179: 689-693.

Ehrenreich, B. 2009. *Smile or Die: How Positive Thinking Fooled America and World*. London: Granta.

Eisenberg, L. 1977. "Mindlessness and brainlessness in psychiatry," *British Journal of Psychiatry* 148: 497-508.

Ellison C.G. 1991. "Religious involvement and subjective well-being," *Journal of Health and Social Behavior* 32: 80-89.

Engel, G. 1977. "The need for a new medical model: a challenge for biomedicine," *Science* 196: 129-136.

Engel, G. 1980. "The clinical application of the biopsychosocial model," *American Journal of Psychiatry* 137: 535-544.

Eriksen, K., and V.E. Kress. 2005. *Beyond the DSM Story: Ethical Quandaries, Challenges, and Best Practices*. Thousand Oaks, CA: Sage.

Esterberg, M.L., and M.T. Compton. 2009. "The psychotic continuum and categorical versus dimensional diagnostic approaches," *Current Psychiatry Reports* 11: 179-184.

Fabrega, H., Jr. 1993. "A cultural analysis of human behavioral breakdowns: an approach to the ontology and epistemology of psychiatric phenomena," *Culture, Medicine, and Psychiatry* 17: 99-132.

Falk, G. 2001. *Stigma: How We Treat Outsiders*. New York: Prometheus Books.

Feelgood, S.R., and A.J. Rantzen. 1994. "Auditory and visual hallucinations in university students," *Personality and Individual Differences* 17: 293-296.

Felker, B., J.J. Yazel, and D. Short. 1996. "Mortality and medical co-morbidity among psychiatric patients: a review," *Psychiatric Services* 47: 1356-1363.

Finzen, A., and U. Hoffmann-Richter. 1999. "Mental illness as a metaphor," in J. Guimon, W. Fischer, and N. Sartorius (eds.) *The Image of Madness*. Basel: Karger, pp. 13-19.

Frances, A.J. 1991. "A to Z guide to DSM-IV conundrums," *Journal of Abnormal Psychology* 100: 407-412.

Frances, A.J. 1994. "Foreword," in J.Z. Sadler, O.P. Wiggins, and M.A. Schwartz (eds.) *Philosophical Perspectives on Psychiatric Diagnostic Classification*. Baltimore: The Johns Hopkins University Press, pp. VII-IX.

Frances, A.J. 2009a. "Whither DSM-V," *British Journal of Psychiatry* 195: 391-392.

Frances, A.J. 2009b. "Issues for DSM-V: The Limitations of field trials: A lesson from DSM-IV," *American Journal of Psychiatry* 166: 1322.

Frances, A.J. 2010. "DSM 5 'Psychosis Risk Syndrome'—far too risky," *Psychology Today* March 18, 2010.

Frances, A. J., T.A. Widiger, and M. Sabshin. 1991. "Psychiatric diagnosis and normality," in D. Offer and M. Sabshin (eds.) *The Diversity of Normal Behavior*. New York: Basic Books, pp. 3-38.

Fredrickson, B.L. 2008. "Promoting positive affect," in M. Eid and R.J. Larsen (eds.) *The Science of Subjective Well-Being*. New York: Guilford, pp. 449-468.

Freeman, D. 2006. "Delusions in the non-clinical population," *Current Psychiatry Reports* 8: 191-204.

Freeman, D. 2007. "Suspicious minds: The psychology of persecutory delusions," *Clinical Psychology Review* 27: 425-457.

Freeman, D., and J. Freeman. 2008. *Paranoia. The 21st Century Fear*. Oxford: Oxford University Press.

Freeman, D., P.A. Garety, P.A. Bebbington *et al.* 2005. "Psychological investigation of the structure of paranoia in non-clinical population," *British Journal of Psychiatry* 186: 427-435.

Freides, D. 1960. "Toward the elimination of the concept of normality," *Journal of Consulting Psychology* 24: 128-133.

Friis, S. 2010. "Early specialized treatment for first-episode psychosis: Does it make a difference," *British Journal of Psychiatry* 196: 339-340.

Fromm, E. 1954. "The psychology of normalcy," *Dissent* 1: 139-143.

Fromm, E. 1968. *The Sane Society*. London: Routledge and Kegan Paul.

Fulford, K.W.M. 1999. "Nine variations and a coda on the theme of an evolutionary definition of dysfunction," *Journal of Abnormal Psychology* 108: 412-420.

Fulford, K.W.M. 2001. "What is (mental) disease: An open letter to Christopher Boorse," *Journal of Medical Ethics* 27: 80-85.

Fulford, K.W.M., and A. Colombo. 2004. "Six models of mental disorders: a study combining linguistic-analytic and empirical methods," *Philosophy, Psychiatry and Psychology* 11: 129-144.

Fulford, K.W.M., T. Thornton, and G. Graham. 2006. *Oxford Textbook of Philosophy and Psychiatry*. Oxford: Oxford University Press.

Fuller, T. E. 1994. "Violent behavior by individuals with serious mental illness," *Hospital and Community Psychiatry* 45: 653-677.

Gabbard, G., and J. Kay. 2001. "The fate of integrated treatment: Whatever happened to the biopsychosocial psychiatrist," *American Journal of Psychiatry* 158: 1956-1963.

Gafoor, R., D. Nitsch, P. McCrone *et al.* 2010. "Effect of early intervention on 5-year outcome in non-affective psychosis," *British Journal of Psychiatry* 196: 372-376.

Ghaemi, N.S. 2003. *The Concepts of Psychiatry. A Pluralistic Approach to the Mind and Mental Illness.* Baltimore: The Johns Hopkins University Press.

Ghaemi, N.S. 2007. "Pluralism in psychiatry: Karl Jaspers on science," *Philosophy, Psychiatry, and Psychology* 14: 57-66.

Ghaemi, N.S. 2009. "The rise and fall of the biopsychosocial model," *British Journal of Psychiatry* 195: 3-4.

Gips, R.G.T. 2003. "Illnesses and likenesses," *Philosophy, Psychiatry, and Psychology* 10: 255-259.

Glenmullen, J. 2000. *Prozac Backlash.* New York: Simon and Schuster.

Gold, I., and L. J. Kirmayer. 2007. "Cultural psychiatry on Wakefield's procrustean bed," *World Psychiatry* 6: 165-166.

Goldberg, A. 2002. "American pragmatism and American psychoanalysis," *Psychoanalytic Quarterly* 71: 235-254.

Goldberg, D. 2000. "Plato versus Aristotle: Categorial and dimensional models for common mental disorders," *Comprehensive Psychiatry* 41 (suppl. 1): 8-13.

Goodwin, F.K., and K.R. Jamison. 1990. *Manic-Depressive Illness.* New York: Oxford University Press.

Gray, A. J. 2001. "Attitudes of the public to mental health: A church congregation," *Mental Health and Religious Culture* 4: 71-79.

Greenfeld, L. 2005. "Nationalism and the mind," *Nations and Nationalism* 11: 325-341.

Grinker, R. R. 1964. "A struggle for eclecticism," *American Journal of Psychiatry* 121: 451-457.

Grube, M. 2006. "Towards an empirically based validation of intuitive diagnostic: Rumcke's 'Praecox Feeling' across the schizophrenia spectrum: Preliminary results," *Psychopathology* 39: 209-417

Guimon, J. 1989. "The biases of psychiatric diagnoses," *British Journal of Psychiatry* 154 (suppl. 4), 33-37.

Guimon, J., W. Fischer, and N. Sartorius.1999. "Introduction," in J. Guimon, W. Fischer, and N. Sartorius (eds.) *The Image of Madness: The Public Facing Mental Illness and Psychiatric Treatment.* Basel: Karger, pp. VIII-XIV.

Hartmann, H. 1939. "Psycho-Analysis and the concept of health," *The International Journal of Psychoanalysis* 20: 308-321.

Havens, L.L. 1973. *Approaches to the Mind: Movements of the Psychiatric Schools from Sects towards Science.* Boston: Little and Brown.

Havens, L.L. 2005. *Psychiatric Movements: From Sects to Science.* New Brunswick: Transaction Publishers.

Heckers, S. 2009. "Who is at risk for a psychotic disorder?," *Schizophrenia Bulletin* 35: 847-850.

Held, B.S. 2004. "The negative side of positive psychology," *Journal of Humanistic Psychology* 44: 9-46.

Hempel, C.G. 1965. "Fundamentals of taxonomy," in C.G. Hempel (ed.) *Aspects of Scientific Explanation and Other Essays in the Philosophy of Science.* Glencoe,IL: Free Press, pp. 137-154.

Hempel, C.G., and P. Oppenheim. 1948. "Studies in the logic of explanation," *Philosophy of Science* 15: 135-175.

Henriques, G.R. 2002. "Harmful dysfunction analysis and the differentiation between mental disorder and disease," *Scientific Review of Mental Health Practice* 1: 157-173.

Heyward, P., and J. Bright. 1997. "Stigma and mental illness: A review and critique," *Journal of Mental Health* 6: 345-354.

Hinshaw, S.P. 2007. *The Mark of Shame: Stigma of Mental Illness and an Agenda for Change*. Oxford: Oxford University Press.

Hirst, P., and P. Woolley. 1982. *Social Relations and Human Attributes*. London: Tavistock Publications.

Hoffman, M. 1978. "Philosophical aspects of 'mental disease'," *Australian and New Zealand Journal of Psychiatry* 12: 29-33.

Hogarthy, G.E., C.M. Anderson, D.J. Reiss *et al*. 1991. "Family psycho-education, social skills training, and maintenance chemotherapy in the aftercare treatment of schizophrenia, II: two-year effects of a controlled study on relapse and adjustment," *Archives of General Psychiatry* 48: 340-347.

Hollingshead, A.B., and F.C. Redlich. 1958. *Class and Mental Illness*. New York: Wiley.

Horwitz, A.V. 2002a. *Creating Mental Illness*. Chicago: University of Chicago Press.

Horwitz, A.V. 2002b. "Outcomes in sociology of mental health and illness: where have we been and where are we going," *Journal of Health and Social Behavior* 43: 143-151.

Horwitz, A.V., and J.C. Wakefield. 2007. *The Loss of Sadness. How Psychiatry Transformed Normal Sorrow into Depressive Disorder*. New York: Oxford University Press.

IGDA Workgroup, WPA. 2003. IGDA.8: Idiographic (personalised) diagnostic formulation," *British Journal of Psychiatry* 182 (suppl. 45), s55-s57.

Jablensky, A. 2010. "Psychiatry in crisis"," *World Psychiatry* 9: 29.

Jablensky, A., and R.E. Kendel. 2002. "Criteria for assessing a classification in psychiatry," in M. Maj, W. Gaebel, and J. J. Lobez-Ibor (eds.) *Psychiatric Diagnosis and Classification*. New York: John Wiley, pp. 1-23.

Jahoda, M. 1958. *Current Concepts of Positive Mental Health*. New York: Basic Books.

Jamison, K.R. 2009. *Nothing Was the Same*. Carlton North: Scrible Publications.

Jaspers, K. 1997/1913. *General Psychopathology*. Baltimore: The Johns Hopkins University Press.

Joce, P. 2008. "Classification of mood disorders in DSM-V and DSM-VI," *Australian and New Zealand Journal of Psychiatry* 42: 851-862.

Johns, L.C., M. Canon, N. Singleton, *et al*. 2004. "Prevalence and correlates of self-reported psychotic symptoms in the British population," *British Journal of Psychiatry* 185: 298-310.

Jones, E. 1942. "The concept of a normal mind," *The International Journal of Psycho-Analysis* 23: 1-8.

Jorm, A.F. 2000. "Mental health literacy—Public knowledge and beliefs about mental disorders," *British Journal of Psychiatry* 177: 396-401.

Jorm, A.F. and E. Oh. 2009. "Desire for a social distance from people with mental disorders: a review," *Australian and New Zealand Journal of Psychiatry* 43: 183-200.

Judd, L.L., H.S. Akiskal, J.D. Maser *et al*. 1998. "A prospective 12-year study of subsyndromal and syndromal depressive symptoms in unipolar major depressive disorders," *Archives of General Psychiatry* 55: 694-700.

Kaelbling, R., and R.M. Patterson. 1966. *Eclectic Psychiatry*. Springfield, IL: Charles C. Thomas.

Kandel, E.R. 1998. "A new intellectual framework for psychiatry," *American Journal of Psychiatry* 155: 457-469.

Kandel, E.R. 1999. "Biology and the future of psychoanalysis," *American Journal of Psychoanalysis* 156: 505-524.
Kandel, E.R. 2005. *Psychiatry, Psychoanalysis and the New Biology of Mind.* Washington, DC: American Psychiatric Association.
Kashdan, T.B., R. Biswas-Diener, and L.A. King. "Reconsidering happiness: The costs of distinguishing between hedonics and eudaimonia," *Journal of Positive Psychology* 3: 219-233.
Katschnig, H. 2010. "Are psychiatrists an endangered species? Observations on internal and external challenges to the profession," *World Psychiatry* 9: 21-28.
Kecmanovic, Dusan. 1998. "Should the notion of pathological be reserved for individual psycho(patho)logical manifestations?," *Psychiatria Danubina* 10: 439-444.
Kecmanovic, D. 2006. "Physical diseases and mental disorders: should they be differentiated?," *Acta Medica Academica* 35: 94-106.
Kecmanovic, D. 2007. "Nationalism and mental health: A critique of Greenfeld's recent views of nationalism," *Nationalism and Ethnic Politics* 13: 273-295.
Kecmanovic, D. 2009a. "Is there such a thing as reactive mental disorders?," *Current Topics in Neurology, Psychiatry and Borderline Disciplines* 17: 1-7.
Kecmanovic, D. 2009b. "Medical causalisation and destigmatization," On-line *British Journal of Psychiatry* 17 April 2009.
Kecmanovic, D. 2010. "Is subjective well-being a measure or the measure of mental health," *Acta Medica Academica* 39: 95-108.
Kecmanovic, D., and D. Hadzi-Pavlovic. 2010. "Psychiatric journals as the mirror of the dominant psychiatric model," *The Psychiatrist* 34: 172-176.
Keller, M.B., J.P. McCullough, D.N. Klein *et al.* 2000. "A comparison of nefazodone, the cognitive-behavioral analysis system of psychotherapy, and their combination for the treatment of chronic depression," *New England Journal of Medicine* 342: 1462-1470.
Kendell, R.E. 1975a. *The Role of Diagnosis in Psychiatry.* Oxford: Blackwell Scientific Publications.
Kendell, R.E. 1975b. "The concept of disease and its implications for psychiatry," *British Journal of Psychiatry* 127: 305-315.
Kendell, R.E. 1988. "Diagnosis and classification," in R. E. Kendell and A.K. Zealey (eds.) *Companion to Psychiatric Studies.* Fourth Edition. Edinburgh: Churchill Livingstone, pp. 207-223.
Kendell, R.E. 1993. "The nature of psychiatric disorders," in R.E. Kendell and A.K. Zealey (eds.) *Companion to Psychiatric Studies.* Fifth Subedition. Edinburgh: Churchill Livingstone, pp. 1-7.
Kendell, R.E. 2001. "The distinction between mental and physical illness," *British Journal of Psychiatry* 178: 490-493.
Kendell, R.E. 2002. "Five criteria for an improved taxonomy of mental disorders," in J. E. Helzer and J. J. Hudziak (eds.) *Defining Psychopathology in the 21st Century.* Washington, DC: American Psychiatric Publishing, pp. 3-18.
Kendell, R.E. 2004. "Why stigma matters" (Foreword), in A.H. Crisp (ed.) *Every Family in the Land. Understanding Prejudice and Discrimination against People with Mental Illness.* London: The Royal Society of Medicine, pp. XXI-XXIII.
Kendell, R.E., and I.F. Brockington. 1980. "The identification of disease entities and the relationship between schizophrenia and affective psychoses," *British Journal of Psychiatry* 137: 324-331.
Kendell, R.E., J.E. Cooper, and A.J. Gourlay *et al.* 1971. "Diagnostic criteria of American and British psychiatrists," *Archives of General Psychiatry* 25: 123-131.
Kendell, R.E., and A. J. Gourlay. 1970. "The clinical distinction between psychotic and neurotic depression," *British Journal of Psychiatry* 117: 257-260.

Kendell R.E., and A. Jablensky. 2003. "Distinguishing between the validity and utility of psychiatric diagnoses," *American Journal of Psychiatry* 160: 4-12.

Kendler, K.S. 1980. "The nosologic validity of paranoia (simple delusional disorder). A review," *Archives of General Psychiatry* 37: 699-706.

Kendler, K.S. 2005. "Towards a philosophical structure of psychiatry," *American Journal of Psychiatry* 162: 433-440.

Kendler, K.S. 2008. "Introduction," in K. S. Kendler, J. Parnas (eds.) *Philosophical Issues in Psychiatry*. Baltimore: The Johns Hopkins University Press, pp. 1-18.

Kendler, K.S., and C.O. Gardner, Jr. 1998. "Boundaries of major depression: An evaluation of DSM-IV criteria," *American Journal of Psychiatry* 155: 172-177.

Kessler, R.C., P. Berglund, O. Demler *et al.* 2005. "Life-time prevalence and age-of-onset distributions of DSM-IV disorders in the National Comorbidity Survey replication," *Annales of General Psychiatry* 62: 593-602.

Kessler, R.C., C. Chin-Yu, O. Demler, *et al.* 2005. "Prevalence, severity, and comorbidity of 12-month DSM-IV disorders in the National Comorbidity Survey replication," *Archives of General Psychiatry* 62: 617-627.

Kessler, R.C., K.A. McGonagle, S. Zhao *et al.* 1994. "Lifetime and 12-month prevalence of DSM-III-R psychiatric disorders in the United States. Results from the National Comorbidity Survey," *Archives of General Psychiatry* 51: 8-19.

Kessler, R.C., K.R. Merikangas., P. Berglund *et al.* 2003. "Mild disorders should not be eliminated from the DSM-V," *Archives of General Psychiatry* 60: 1117-1122.

Keyes, C.L.M. 2002. "The mental health continuum: From languishing to flourishing in life," *Journal of Health and Social Behavior* 42: 207-222.

Keyes, C.L.M. 2005. "Mental illness and/or mental health? Investigating axioms of the complete state model of health," *Journal of Consulting and Clinical Psychology* 73: 539-548.

Keyes, C.L.M. 2006. "Subjective well-being in mental health and human development research worldwide: An introduction," *Social Indicators Research* 77: 1-10.

Killian, T.M., and L.T. Killian. 1990. "Sociological investigations of mental illness: A review," *Hospital and Community Psychiatry* 41: 902-911.

King, L. 1954. "What is disease?," *Philosophy of Science* 2: 193-202.

King, L.A. 2001. "The hard road to the good life: The happy, mature person," *Journal of Humanistic Psychology* 41: 51-72.

Kirk, S.A. 2005. "Introduction: critical perspectives," in S.A. Kirk (ed.) *Mental Disorders in the Social Environment. Critical Perspectives*. New York: Columbia University Press, pp. 1-17.

Kirk, S.A., and H. Kutchins. 1992. *The Selling of DSM: The Rhetoric of Science in Psychiatry*. New York: Aldine de Gruyter.

Klein, D.F. 1978. "A proposed definition of mental illness," in R. L. Spitzer and F.D. Klein (eds.) *Critical Issues in Psychiatric Diagnosis*. New York: Raven Press, pp. 41-71.

Klerman, G. and G. Schecher. 1981. "Ethical aspects of drug treatment," in S. Bloch, P. Chodoff (eds.) *Psychiatric Ethics*. Oxford: Oxford University Press, pp. 117-130.

Knight, J. 1995. "Psychiatry: eclecticism and empiricism," *Australasian Psychiatry* 3: 407-410.

Korman, M. 1961. "The concept of normality: A reply to Freides," *Journal of Consulting Psychology* 25: 267-269.

Kraepelin, E. 1917. *Lectures on Clinical Psychiatry*. Third edition. New York: William Wood and Company.

Kraepelin, E. 1971/1919. *Dementia Praecox and Paraphrenia*. Huntington, NY: Krieger, pp. 74-75.

Kubie, L. 1954. "The fundamental nature of the distinction between normality and neurosis," *Psychoanalytic Quarterly* 23: 163-204.

Kuhn, T. 1962. *The Structure of Scientific Revolutions*. Chicago: University of Chicago Press.

Kupfer, D. J., M. B. First, and D.A. Regier. 2002. "Introduction" in D.J. Kupfer, M.B. First, and D.A. Regier (eds.) *Research Agendas for DSM-V*. Washington, DC: American Psychiatric Association, pp. XV-XXIII.

Kutchins, H., and S. Kirk. 1997. *Making Us Crazy: The Psychiatric Bible and the Creation of Mental Disorders*. New York: Free Press.

Lacoff, A. 2005. *Pharmaceutical Reason: Knowledge and Value in Global Psychiatry*. New York: Cambridge University Press.

Lagnado, M. 2003. "Increasing the trust in scientific authorship," *British Journal of Psychiatry* 182: 3-4.

Laing, R.D. 1967. *The Politics of Experience and the Bird of Paradise*. Harmondsworth, UK: Penguin Books.

Lambley, P. 1971. "Scientific status of technical eclecticism: a critical note," *Psychological Reports* 28: 91-97.

Langenbach, M. 1993. "Conceptual analyses of psychiatric languages: reductionism and integration of different courses," *Current Opinion in Psychiatry* 6: 689-703.

Larsen, T.K., S. Friis, U. Haahr, *et al.* 2001. "Early detection and intervention in first-episode schizophrenia: a critical review," *Acta Psychiatrica Scandinavica* 103: 323-334.

Law, J., and J. Urry. 2004. "Enacting the social," *Economy and Society* 33: 290-310.

Lazare, A. 1973. "Hidden conceptual models in clinical psychiatry," *New England Journal of Medicine* 288: 345-351.

Leary, M.R.,and L.S. Schreidendorfer. 1998. "The stigmatization of HIV and AIDS: Rubbing salt in the wound," in V. Derlega, A. Barbee (eds.) *HIV Infection and Social Interaction*. Thousand Oaks, CA: Sage Publications, pp. 12-29.

Lemert, E. 1951. "Mental disorder"," in E. Lemert (ed.) *Social Pathology*. New York: McGraw-Hill, pp. 387-443.

Lemert, E. 1972. "Social structure, social control and deviation," in M.B. Clinard (ed.) *Anomie and Deviant Behavior*. New York: The Free Press, pp. 82-83.

Lewis, A. 1951. "Social aspects of psychiatry," *Edinburgh Medical Journal* 58: 214-247.

Lewis, A. 1953. "Health as a social concept," *British Journal of Sociology* 4: 109-124.

Lewis, A. 1967. *The State of Psychiatry: Essays and Addresses*. New York: Science Book.

Lilienfeld, S.O., S.J. Lyn, J. Ruscio *et al.* 2010. *50 Great Myths of Popular Psychology*. Chichester, UK: Wiley-Blackwell.

Lilienfield, S.O., and L. Marino. 1999. "Essentialism revisited: Evolutionary theory and the concept of mental disorder," *Journal of Abnormal Psychology* 108: 400-411.

Lilienfeld, S.O., R.L. Spitzer, and M.B. Miller. 2005. "A response to a nonresponse to criticisms of a nonstudy. One humorous and serious rejoinder to Slater," *Journal of Nervous and Mental Diseases* 193: 745-746.

Lincoln, T.M. 2007. "Relevant dimensions of delusions: Continuing the continuum versus category debate," *Schizophrenia Research* 93: 211-220.

Link, B., J. Ohelan, M. Bresnaham *et al.* 1999. "Public conceptions of mental illness: labels, causes, dangerousness and social distance," *American Journal of Public Health* 89: 1328-1333.

Littlewood, R. 1998. "Cultural variation in the stigma of mental illness," *Lancet* 352: 1056-1057, September 26.

Lolas, F. 2010. "Psychiatry: a specialized profession or a medical specialty," *World Psychiatry* 9: 34-35.

Luhrmann, T.M. 2000. *Of Two Minds: The Growing Disorder in American Psychiatry*. New York: Vintage.

Macklin, R. 1972. "Mental health and mental illness: some problems of definition and concept formation," *The Philosophy of Science* 39: 341-365.

MacLaren, N. 1992. "Is mental disease just brain disease?," *Australian and New Zealand Journal of Psychiatry* 26: 270-276.

MacLaren, N. 2007. *Humanizing Madness: Psychiatry and the Cognitive Sciences*. Ann Arbor, MI: Future Psychiatry Press.

Magliano, L., C. de Rosa, and A. Fiorello. 2004. "Perception of patients' unpredictability and beliefs on the cause and consequences of schizophrenia," *Social Psychiatry and Psychiatric Epidemiology* 39: 410-416.

Maj, M. 2005. "'Psychiatric comorbidity': an artefact of current diagnostic systems," *British Journal of Psychiatry* 186: 182-184.

Major, B., and C.P. Eccleston. 2005. "Stigma and social exclusion," in D. Abrams, M.A. Hogg, and J.M. Marques (eds.) *The Social Psychology and Inclusion and Exclusion*. New York: Psychology Press, pp. 63-88.

Malinovski, B. 2008/1944. *The Scientific Theory of Culture and other Essays*. London: Routledge.

Marcuse, H. 2007/1964. *One-Dimensional Man. Studies in the Ideology of Advanced Industrial Society*. London and New York: Routledge.

Margolis, J. 1976. "The concept of disease," *The Journal of Medicine and Philosophy* 1: 238-255.

Margree, V. 2002. "Normal and abnormal: Georges Anguilhem and the question of mental pathology," *Philosophy, Psychiatry and Psychology* 9: 299-312.

Marshall, M., S. Lewis, A. Lockwood *et al.* 2005. "Association between duration of untreated psychosis and outcome in cohorts of first-episode patients," *Archives of General Psychiatry* 62: 975-983.

Marshall, M., and J. Rathbone. 2010. "Early intervention for psychosis (Review)," *Cochrane Database of Systematic Reviews, The Cochrane Library*, Issue 3. http://www.thecochranelibrary.com Accessed 6 May 2010.

Martin, J.B. 2002. "The integration of neurology, psychiatry, and neuroscience in the 21st century," *American Journal of Psychiatry* 159: 695-704.

Maslow, A. H. 1950. "Self-actualizing people: A study of psychological health," Personality, Symposium No 1, pp. 11-34.

Maslow, A.H. 1968. *Toward a Psychology of Being*. Second edition. New York: Van Nostrand Reinhold Co.

Maslow, A.H., and B. Mittelman. 1951. "The meaning of 'healthy' ('normal') and of 'sick' ('abnormal')," in A.H. Maslow, and N. Mittelmann (eds.) *Principles of Abnormal Psychology: The Dynamics of Psychic Illness*. New York: Harper, pp. 12-21.

Mayers, D.G. 2000. "The funds, friends, and faith of happy people," *American Psychologist* 55: 56-67.

McGlashan, T.H. 2005. "Early detection an intervention in psychosis: an ethical paradigm shift," *British Journal of Psychiatry* 187 (suppl. 48): s113-s115.

McGorry, P., M. Nordentoft, and E. Simonssen. 2005. "Introduction to 'early psychosis: a bridge to the future'," *British Journal of Psychiatry* 187 (suppl. 48), s1-s3.

McGorry, P.D., I.B. Hickie, A.R. Yung. *et al.* 2006. "Clinical staging of psychiatric disorders: a heuristic framework for choosing earlier, safer and more effective interventions," *Australian and New Zealand Journal of Psychiatry* 40: 616-622.

McGorry, P., E. Killackey, and A. Yung. 2008. "Early intervention in psychosis: Concepts, evidence, and future directions," *World Psychiatry* 7: 148-156.

McHugh, P.R. 2005. "Striving for coherence. Psychiatry's efforts over classification," JAMA 293: 2526-2528.

McHugh, P.R. 2006. *The Mind has Mountains. Reflections on Society and Psychiatry.* Baltimore: The Johns Hopkins University Press.

McHugh, P.R. and P.S. Slavney. 1982. "Methods of reasoning in psychopathology: Conflict and resolution," *Comprehensive Psychiatry* 23: 197-215.

McHugh, P.R., and P.S. Slavney. 1983. *The Perspectives of Psychiatry.* Baltimore: The Johns Hopkins University Press.

Menninger, K.A. 1930. "What is healthy mind," in N.A. Crawford and K.A. Menninger (eds.) *The Healthy-Minded Child.* New York: Coward-McCann.

Merton, R.K. 1968. *The Social Theory and Social Structure.* New York: The Free Press.

Mezzich, J.E. 1989. "An empirical prototypical approach to the definition of psychiatric illness," *British Journal of Psychiatry* (suppl. 4), s42-s46.

Mezzich, J.E. 2002. "Comprehensive diagnosis: A conceptual basis for future diagnostic systems," *Psychopathology* 35: 162-165.

Mezzich, J.E. 2005. "Values and comprehensive diagnosis," *World Psychiatry* 4: 91-92.

Micale, M.S. 1996. "Paradigm and ideology in psychiatric history writing. The case of psychoanalysis," *Journal of Nervous and Mental Disease* 184: 146-152.

Millikan, R.G. 1989. "Biosemantics," *Journal of Philosophy* 86: 281-297.

Millon, T. 1991. "Classification in psychopathology: Rationale, alternatives, and standards," *Journal of Abnormal Psychology* 100: 245-261.

Mills, C.W. 1959. *Sociological Imagination.* London: Oxford University Press.

Moncrieff, J., and M.J. Crawford. 2001. "British psychiatry in the 20th century—observations from a psychiatric journal," *Social Science and Medicine* 53: 349-356.

Moore, M.S. 1980. "Legal conceptions of mental illness," in B.A. Brody, and H.T. Engelhardt Jr. (eds.) *Mental Illness: Law and Public Policy.* Dordrecht: D. Reidel, pp. 158-173.

Munk-Jorgensen, P. 1995. "Decreasing rates of incident schizophrenia cases in psychiatric services," *European Psychiatry* 10: 129-141.

Murphy, D. 2005. "The concept of mental illness—where the debate has reached and where it needs to go," *Journal of Theoretical and Philosophical Psychology* 25: 116-132.

Murphy, D. 2006. *Psychiatry in the Scientific Image.* Cambridge, MA: The MIT Press.

Murray, C.J.L., and A.D. Lopez. 1996. *The Global Burden of Disease. A Comprehensive Assessment of Mortality and Disability from Diseases, Injuries, and Risk Factors in 1990 and Projected to 2020.* Cambridge, MA: Harvard School of Public Health.

Neuberg, S. L., D.M. Smith, and T. Asher. 2000. "Why people stigmatize: Toward a biocultural framework," in T.F. Heatherton, R.E. Kleck, M.R. Hebl, and J.G. Hull (eds.) *The Social Psychology of Stigma.* New York: Guilford Press, pp. 31-61.

Offer, D. and M. Sabhin. 1966. *Normality. Theoretical and Clinical Concepts of Mental Health.* New York: Basic Books

Offer, D., and M. Sabshin. (eds.) 1991. *The Diversity of Mental Health. Further Contributions to Normatology.* New York: Basic Books.

Okasha, A. 2006. "Foreword (from clinical practice)"," in K.W.M. Fulford, T. Thornton, and G. Graham (eds.) *Oxford Textbook of Philosophy and Psychiatry.* Oxford: Oxford University Press, pp. XXIX-XXXI.

Olfson, M., W. E. Broodhead, M.M. Weissman, *et al.* 1996. "Subtreshold psychiatric symptoms in a primary care groups practice," *Archives of General Psychiatry* 53: 880-886.

Olfson, M., R. Lewis-Fernandez, M. M. Weissman *et al.* 2002. "Psychotic symptoms in urban general medical practice," *American Journal of Psychiatry* 159: 1412-1419.

Oyserman, D., H.M. Coon, and M. Kemmelmeier. 2002. "Rethinking individualism and collectivism: evaluation of theoretical assumptions and meta-analyses," *Psychological Bulletin* 128: 3-72.

Parker, G. 2008. "How should mood disorders be modeled?," *Australian and New Zealand Journal of Psychiatry* 42: 841-850.

Parker, G. 2009. "Antidepressants on trial: how valid is the evidence?," *British Journal of Psychiatry* 194: 1-3.

Parnas, J. 2005. "Clinical detection of schizophrenia-prone individuals," *British Journal of Psychiatry* 187 (suppl. 48): s111-s112.

Parnas, J., P. Bovet, and D. Zahavi. 2002. "Schizophrenic autism: clinical phenomenology and pathogenetic implications," *World Psychiatry* 1: 131-136.

Parnas, J., and D. Zahavi. 2002. "The role of phenomenology in psychiatric diagnosis and classification," in M. Maj, W. Gaebel, J.J. Lopez-Ibor et al. (eds.) *Psychiatric Diagnosis and Classification.* Chichester, UK: John Wiley, pp. 137-162.

Parsons, T. 1958. "Definitions of health and illness in the light of American values and social structure," in E.G. Jaco (ed.) *Patients, Physicians, and Illness. Sourcebook in behavioral science and medicine.* New York: Free Press, pp. 165-187.

Pasamanick, B. 1961. "A survey of mental disease in an urban population, IV, An approach to total prevalence rate," *Archives of General Psychiatry* 5: 151-155.

Pearlin, L.I., W.R Avison, and E.M. Fazio. 2008. "Sociology, psychiatry, and the production of knowledge about mental illness and its treatment," in W.R. Avison, J.D. McLeod, and B.A. Pescolido (eds.) *Mental Health, Social Mirror.* New York: Springer, pp. 33-53.

Perkins, D.O., H. Gu, K. Boteva, *et al.* 2005. "Relationship between duration of untreated psychosis and outcome in first-episode schizophrenia: a critical review and meta-analysis," *American Journal of Psychiatry* 162: 1785-1804.

Perring, Ch. Mental illness http://plato.stanford.edu/entries/mental-illness Accessed 9 March 2009.

Phillips, J. 2005. "Idiographic formulation, symptoms, narratives, context and meaning," *Psychopathology* 38: 180-184.

Phillips, M.R. 2009. "Is distress a symptoms of mental disorders, a marker of impairment, both or neither," *World Psychiatry* 8: 91-92.

Pickering, N. 2003. "The Likeness argument and the reality of mental illness," *Philosophy, Psychiatry and Psychology* 10: 243-254.

Pilgrim, D., and A.E. Rogers. 2005. "Psychiatrists as social engineers: A study of an anti-stigma campaign," *Social Science and Medicine* 61: 2546-2556.

Pincus, H.A. 1998. "Clinical significance and DSM-IV," *Archives of General Psychiatry* 55: 1145-1148.

Pincus, H.A., W.W. Davis, and L.E. McQueen. 1999. " 'Subtreshold' mental disorders," *British Journal of Psychiatry* 174: 288-296.

Polanyi, M. 1998. *Personal Knowledge. Towards a Post Critical Philosophy.* London: Routledge.

Posey, T.B., and M.E. Losch. 1983. "Auditory hallucinations of hearing voices in 375 normal subjects," *Imagination, Cognition and Personality* 2: 99-113.

Post, J.M. 1995. "The health of presidents and presidential candidates: Dilemmas and controversies," *Political Psychology* 16: 757-771.

Poulton, A., T.E. Caspi, M. Moffitt. *et al.* 2000. "Children's self-reported psychotic symptoms and adult schizophreniform disorder: a 15-year longitudinal study," *Archives of General Psychiatry* 57: 1053-1058.

Price, B.H., R.D. Adams, and J.T. Coyle 2000. "Neurology and psychiatry: Closing the great divide," *Neurology* 54: 8-14.

Redlich, F.C. 1976. "Editorial Reflections on the Concepts of Health and Disease," *The Journal of Medicine and Philosophy* 1: 269-280.

Regier, D.A., J.K. Myers, M. Kramer, *et al.* 1984. "The NIMH epidemiologic catchment area program: historical context, major objectives, and study population characteristics," *Archives of General Psychiatry* 41: 934-941.

Richters, J.E. and S.P. Hinshaw. 1999. "The abduction of disorder in psychiatry," *Journal of Abnormal Psychology* 108: 438-455.

Robins, L.N. 1994. "How recognizing 'comorbidities' in psychopathology may lead to an improved research nosology," *Clinical Psychology: Science and Practice* 1: 93-95.

Robins, E., and S.B Guze. 1970. "Establishment of diagnostic validity in psychiatric illness: Its application to schizophrenia," *American Journal of Psychiatry* 126: 107-111.

Robins, L.N., and D.A. Regier. 1991. *Psychiatric Disorders in America. The Epidemiological Catchment Area Study*. New York: Free Press.

Rosenhan, D.L. 1973. "On being sane in insane places," *Science* 179: 250-258.

Rossi, A., and E. Daneluzzo. 2002. "Schizotypical dimensions in normals and schizophrenic patients: a comparison with other clinical samples," *Schizophrenia Research* 54: 67-75.

Roth, M., and J. Kroll. 1986. *The Reality of Disease*. Cambridge: Cambridge University Press.

Rümcke, H.C. 1948. "Het Kernsymptoom der Schizophrenie en het Pracoxgevoel" (The nuclear symptoms of schizophrenia and the praecox feeling). First published in *Studies en Voordrachten over Psychiatrie*. Amsterdam: Scheltema and Holkema, pp. 53-58.

Ruscio, J. 2004. "Diagnoses and behaviors they denote: A critical examination of the labeling theory of mental illness," *Scientific Review of Mental Health Practice* 3: 5-22.

Ryan, R.M., and E.L. Deci. 2001. "On happiness and human potentials: A review of research on hedonic and eudaimonic well-being," *Annual Review of Psychology* 52: 141-166.

Ryff, C.D. 1989. "Happiness is everything, or is it? Explorations on the meaning of psychological well-being," *Journal of Personality and Social Psychology* 57: 1069-1081.

Ryff, C.D., and C.L.M. Keys. 1995. "The structure of psychological well-being revisited," *Journal of Personality and Social Psychology* 69: 719-727.

Ryff, C.D. and B.H. Singer. 1998. "The contours of positive human health," *Psychological Inquiry* 9: 1-28.

Ryff, C.D., and B.H. Singer. 2008."Know thyself and become what you are: a eudaimonic approach to psychological well-being," *Journal of Happiness Studies* 9: 13-39.

Sabshin, M. 1989. "Normality and the boundaries of psychopathology," *Journal of Personality Disorders* 3: 259-273.

Sabshin, M. 1990. "Turning points in twentieth century American psychiatry," *American Journal of Psychiatry* 147: 1267-1274.

Sachdev, P.S. 2007. "An agenda for neuropsychiatry as a 21st century discipline," *Acta Neuropsychiatrica* 19:2-5.

Sadler, J.Z. (ed.) 2002. *Description and Prescriptions: Values, Mental Disorders, and the DSMs*. Baltimore: The Johns Hopkins University Press.

Sadler, J.Z., and Y.F. Hugus. 1992. "Clinical problem solving and the biopsychosocial model," *American Journal of Psychiatry* 149: 1315-1323.

Sadock, B. J., and V.A. Sadock, V. A. 2005. *Kaplan's and Sadock's Comprehensive Textbook of Psychiatry*, 8th edition. Baltimore: Lippincott, Williams and Wilkins.

Sandanger, I., J.F. Nygard and T. Sorensen. 2002. "The concept of psychiatric illness—a core problem in psychiatric epidemiology," *Norsk Epidemiology* 12: 181-187.

Sartorius, N. 2002. *Fighting for Mental Health. A Personal View*. Cambridge: Cambridge University Press.

Sartorius, N. 2006. "Good news or bad? The processes of revision of the classification of mental disorders have started," *Psychiatria Danubina* 18: 2-3.

Sartorius, N., and H. Schulze. 2005. *Reducing the Stigma of Mental Illness: A Report from a Global Programme of the World Psychiatric Association*. Cambridge: Cambridge University Press.

Sass, L.A. 1996. *Madness and Modernism. Insanity in the Light of Modern Art, Literature, and Thought*. Cambridge, MA: Harvard University Press.

Scadding, G.J. 1967. "Diagnosis: the clinician and the computer," *Lancet* ii: 877-882.

Scheff, Th. J. 1963. "The role of the mentally ill and the dynamic of mental disorder: A research framework," *Sociometry* 26: 463-453.

Scheff, T. J. 1966. *Being Mentally Ill: A Sociological Theory*. Chicago: Aldine.

Scheff, T.J. 1968. "The role of the mentally ill and the dynamics of mental disorder: a research framework," in S. P. Spitzer and N. K. Denzin (eds.) *The Mental Patient: Studies in the Sociology of Deviance*. New York: McGraw-Hill, pp. 8-22.

Scheff, T.J. 1974. "The labeling theory of mental illness," *American Sociological Review* 39: 444-452.

Schreier, H.A. 1999. "Hallucinations and nonpsychotic children: more common than we think," *Journal of the American Academy of Child and Adolescent Psychiatry* 38: 623-625.

Schwartz, M.A., and O.P. Wiggins. 1985. "Science, humanism, and the nature of medical practice: a phenomenological view," *Perspectives in Biological Medicine* 28: 331-336.

Schwartz, M.A., and O.P. Wiggins. 1988. "Perspectivism and the methods of psychiatry," *Comprehensive Psychiatry* 29: 237-251.

Sedgwick, P. 1982. *PsychoPolitics*. Cambridge: Harper and Row.

Seligman, M.E.P. 1992. *Learned Optimism*. North Sydney: Random House Australia.

Seligman, M.E.P. 2002. "Positive psychology, positive prevention, and positive therapy," in C.R. Snyder and S. J. Lopez (eds.) *Handbook of Positive Psychology*. New York: Oxford University Press, pp. 3-9.

Seligman, M.E.P. 2002. *Authentic Happiness*. North Sydney: Random House Australia.

Shah, P. and D. Mountain. 2007. "The medical model is dead—long live the medical model," *British Journal of Psychiatry* 191: 375-377.

Sheldon, K.M. and L.A. King. 2001. "Why positive psychology is necessary?," *American Psychologist* 56: 216-217.

Shils, E., and H. Finch. 1949. *Max Weber on the Methodology of Social Sciences*. New York: Free Press.

Siegler, M., and H. Osmond. 1974. *Models of Madness, Models of Medicine*. New York: MacMillan.

Silove, D. 1990. "Biologism in psychiatry," *Australian and New Zealand Journal of Psychiatry* 24: 461-463.

Simsek, O.F. 2009. "Happiness revisited: Ontological well-being as a theory-based construct of subjective well-being," *Journal of Happiness Studies* 10: 505-522.

Singer, P. 1995. *Where Are We To Live. Ethnics in an Age of Self-Interest.* Amherst, NY: Prometheus Books.

Slater, L. 2004. *Opening Skinner's Box: Great Psychological Experiments of the Twentieth Century.* London: Bloomsbury.

Slater, L. 2005. "Reply to Spitzer and colleagues," *Journal of Nervous and Mental Disease* 193: 743-744.

Slavney, P.R., and P.R. McHugh. 1987. *Psychiatric Polarities. Methodology and the Practice.* Baltimore: The Johns Hopkins University Press.

Slife, B. 1987. "The perils of eclecticism as therapeutic orientation," *Theoretical and Philosophical Psychology* 7: 94-103.

Smith, A.D. 2001. *Nationalism.* Cambridge: Polity.

Sontag, S. 1991. *Illness as Metaphor. AIDS and Its Metaphors.* London: Penguin Books.

Spiegel, A. 2005. *The Dictionary of Disorder.* Newyorker, January 3.

Spitzer, M. 1988. "Psychiatry, philosophy and the problem of description," in M. Spitzer, F.A. Uehlein, and G. Oepen (eds.) *Psychopathology and Philosophy.* Berlin: Springer, pp. 3-18.

Spitzer, R. L. 1975. "On pseudoscience in science, logic in remission, and psychiatric diagnosis: A critique of Rosenhan's 'On being sane in insane places'," *Journal of Abnormal Psychology* 84: 442-452.

Spitzer, R.L. 1991. "An outsider-insider's views about revising the *DSMs*," *Journal of Abnormal Psychology* 100: 294-296.

Spitzer, R.L. 1999. "Harmful dysfunction and the DSM definitions of mental disorder," *Journal of Abnormal Psychology* 108: 430-432.

Spitzer, R.L., and J. Endicott, J. 1978. "Mental and medical disorder. Proposed definition and criteria," in R.L. Spitzer, F. Klein (eds.) *Critical Issues in Psychiatric Diagnosis.* New York: Raven Press, pp. 15-40.

Spitzer, R.L., S.P. Lilienfeld, and M.B. Miller. 2005. "Rosenhan revisited. The scientific credibility of Lauren Slater's pseudopatient diagnosis study," *Journal of Nervous and Mental Disease* 193: 734-738.

Spitzer, R.L., and J.C. Wakefield. 1999. "Diagnostic criterion for clinical significance: does it help solve the false positive problem," *American Journal of Psychiatry* 156: 1856-64.

Spitzer, R.L., and J.B. Williams. 1982. "The definition and diagnosis of mental disorder," in W.R. Grove (ed.) *Deviance and Mental Illness.* Beverly Hills, CA: Sage, pp. 15-31.

Stangor, C., and C.S. Crandall. 2000. "Threat and the social construction of stigma," in T.F. Heatherton, R.E. Kleck, M.R. Hebl *et al.*, (eds.) *The Social Psychology of Stigma* (eds.). New York: Guilford Press, pp. 62-87.

Stärker, A. 1921. "Psycho-analysis and psychiatry," *International Journal of Psychoanalysis* 2: 360-372.

Stein, D.J., K.A. Phillips, D. Bolton. *et al.*, 2010. "What is mental/psychiatric disorder? From DSM-IV to DSM-V," *Psychological Medicine*, Published online by Cambridge University Press, 20 January 2010.

Stransky, E. 1904. "Zur Auffassung gewisser Symptome der Dementia Praecox," Neurologishes Zentralblatt 23: 1137-1143.

Szasz, T.S. 1961. *The Myth of Mental Illness.* New York: Harper and Row.

Taylor, S.E., and J.D. Brown. 1988. "Illusion and well-being: a social psychological perspective on mental health," *Psychological Bulletin* 103: 193-210.

Taylor, S.E., and J.D. Brown. 1994. "Positive illusions and well-being revisited: separating fact from fiction," *Psychological Bulletin* 116: 21-27.

Telfer, E. 1990. *Happiness*. New York: St. Martin's Press.

Thase, M.A., J.B. Greenhouse, and E. Frank. 1997. "Treatment of major depression with psychotherapy or psychotherapy-pharmacotherapy combination," *Archives of General Psychiatry* 54: 1009-1015.

Thompson, A.H., H. Stuart, R.C. Bland. *et al.* 2002. "Attitudes about schizophrenia from the pilot side of the WPA worldwide campaign against the stigma of schizophrenia," *Social Psychiatry and Social Epidemiology* 37: 475-482.

Thornicroft, G. 2006. *Shunned: Discrimination against People with Mental Illness.* Oxford: Oxford University Press.

Thornton, T. 2007. *Essential Philosophy of Psychiatry.* Oxford: Oxford University Press.

Thornton, T. 2008. "Should comprehensive diagnosis include idiographic understanding," *Medicine, Health Care and Philosophy* 11: 293-302.

Tien, A.Y. 1991. "Distribution of hallucinations in the populations," *Social Psychiatry and Psychiatric Epidemiology* 26: 287-92.

Tucker, G.J. 1998. "Putting DSM-IV in perspective," *American Journal of Psychiatry* 155: 159-161.

Turner, M.A. 2003. "Psychiatry and the human sciences," *British Journal of Psychiatry* 182: 472-74.

Tyrer, P., and D. Steinberg. 1987. *Models of Mental Illness.* Chichester: John Wiley and Sons.

Valenstein, E.S. 1998. *Blaming the Brain. The Truth about Drugs and Mental illness.* New York: The Free Press.

Varelius, J. 2009. "Defining mental disorder in terms of our goals for demarcating mental disorder," *Philosophy, Psychiatry, and Psychology* 16: 35-52.

Veatch, R.M. 1973. "The medical model: its nature and problems," *The Hastings Center Studies* 1: 59-76.

Verdoux, H., S. Maurice-Tison, B. Gay *et al.* 1998. "A survey of delusional ideation in primary-care patients," *Psychological Medicine* 28: 127-134.

Verdoux, H., and J. van Os. 2002. "Psychotic symptoms in non-clinical populations and the continuum of psychosis," *Schizophrenia Research* 54: 59-65.

Verhaeghe, P. 2008. *On Being Normal and Other Disorders. A Manual for Clinical Psychodiagnostics.* London: Karnac.

Wakefield, J.C. 1992. "The concept of mental disorder. On the boundary between biological facts and social values," *American Psychologist* 47:373-88.

Wakefield, J.C. 1996. "DSM-IV: Are we making diagnostic progress," *Contemporary Psychologist* 41:646-52

Wakefield, J.C. 1999a. "Evolutionary versus prototype analyses of the concept of disorder," *Journal of Abnormal Psychology* 108: 374-99.

Wakefield, J. C. 1999b. "The measurement of mental disorder," in A. V. Horwitz, T. L. Scheid (eds.) *A Handbook for the Study of Mental Health. Social Contexts, Theories, and Systems.* Cambridge: Cambridge University Press, pp. 29-57.

Wakefield, J. C. 2006. "What makes a mental disorder mental?," *Philosophy, Psychiatry and Psychology* 13: 123-131.

Wakefield, J.C. 2005. "Disorders versus problems of living in DSM: rethinking social work's relationship to psychiatry," in S.A. Kirk (ed.) *Mental Disorders in the Social*

Environment. Critical Perspectives. New York: Columbia University Press, pp. 83-95.

Wakefield, J.C. 2007. "The concept of mental disorder: diagnostic implications of the harmful dysfunction analysis," *World Psychiatry* 6: 149-156.

Wakefield, J.C. and M. First. 2003. "Clarifying the distinction between disorder and nondisorder: Confronting the overdiagnosis ('false positive') problem in DSM-V," in K.A. Phillips, M. First, and H.A. Pincus (eds.) *Advancing DSM: Dilemmas in Psychiatric Diagnosis*. Washington, DC: American Psychiatric Association, pp. 23-56.

Wakefield, J. C., and R.L. Spitzer. 2002. "Lower estimates—but of what?," *Archives of General Psychiatry* 59: 129-130.

Warner, R. 2005. "Problems with early and very early intervention in psychosis," *British Journal in Psychiatry* 187 (suppl. 48): s104-s107.

Waterman, A.S., S.J. Schwartz, and R. Conti. 2006. "The implications of two conceptions of happiness (hedonic enjoyment and eudaimonia) for the understanding of intrinsic motivation," *Journal of Happiness Studies* 9: 41-79.

Watson, A.C., E. Otey, A.L. Westbrook *et al.* 2004. "Changing middle-scholars' attitudes about mental illness through education," *Schizophrenia Bulletin* 30: 563-572.

Weckowitz, T.R. 1984. *Models of Mental Illness. Systems and Theories of Abnormal Psychology*. Springfield, IL: Charles C. Thomas.

Weiner, E. 2009. "Happiness is low expectations," *International Herald Tribune* 22 July.

Wertz, F.J. 1990. "Multiple methods in psychology: epistemological grounding and the possibility of unity," *Journal of Theoretical and Philosophical Psychology* 19: 131-166.

WHO. 1948. *Official Record of the WHO*. No 10. Geneva: WHO, p. 10.

WHO. 1979. *Schizophrenia: An International Follow-up Study*. Chichester, UK: John Wiley and Sons.

WHO. 2001. *Mental Health: New Understanding, New Hope*. The world health report. Geneva: World Health Organization.

Wiggins, O. P., and M.A. Schwartz. 1994. "The limits of psychiatric knowledge and the problem of classification," in J. Sadler, O.P. Wiggins and M. Schwartz (eds.) *Philosophical Perspectives on Psychiatric Diagnostic Classification*. Baltimore: The Johns Hopkins University Press, pp. 89-103.

Wilson, C., R. Nairn, J. Coverdal *et al.* 1999. "Mental illness depictions in prime-time drama: identifying the discursive resources," *Australian and New Zealand Journal of Psychiatry* 33: 232-239.

Wing, J.K. 1978. *Reasoning about Madness*. Oxford: Oxford University Press.

Wittchen, H.U., C.B. Nelson, and G. Lachner. 1998 . "Prevalence of mental disorders and psychosocial impairment in adolescents and young adults," *Psychological Medicine* 28: 109-26.

Woolfolk, R.L. 2002. "The power of negative thinking: Truth, melancholia, and the tragic sense of life," *Journal of Theoretical and Philosophical Psychology* 19: 27.

Wootton, B. 1959. *Social Science and Social Pathology*. London: George Allen and Unwin.

Yang, L.H., A. Kleinman, B.G. Link *et al.* 2007. "Stigma: adding moral experience to stigma theory," *Social Science and Medicine* 64: 1524-1535.

Yung, A.R., B. Nelson, K. Baker *et al.* 2009. "Psychosis-like experiences in a community sample of adolescents: implications for the continuum model of psychosis and prediction of schizophrenia," *Australian and New Zealand Journal of Psychiatry* 43: 118-128.

Yung, A.R., and P. McGorry. 2007. "Prediction of psychosis: setting the stage," *British Journal of Psychiatry* 191 (suppl. 51): s1-s8.

Yung, A.R., H.P. Yuen, G. Berger *et al.* 2007. "Declining transition rate in ultra high risk (Prodromal) services: dilution or reduction of risk," *Schizophrenia Bulletin* 33: 673-681.

Zachar, P. 2002. "The practical kinds model as a pragmatist theory of classification," *Philosophy, Psychiatry and Psychology* 9: 219-227.

Zachar, P., and K. S. Kendler. 2007. "Psychiatric disorders: A conceptual taxonomy," *American Journal of Psychiatry* 164: 557-565

Zarin, D.A. and F. Earls. 1993. "Diagnostic decision making in psychiatry," *American Journal of Psychiatry* 150: 197-206.

Author Index

Subject Index